LONELINESS AND ITS OPPOSITE

LONELINESS AND ITS OPPOSITE

sex, disability, and the ethics of engagement

DON KULICK AND JENS RYDSTRÖM

DUKE UNIVERSITY PRESS :: DURHAM AND LONDON :: 2015

© 2015 Duke University Press
All rights reserved
Printed in the United States of
America on acid-free paper ∞
Designed by Amy Ruth Buchanan
Typeset in Minion by Westchester
Publishing Services

Library of Congress Cataloging-in-Publication
Data
Kulick, Don.
Loneliness and its opposite : sex, disability, and
the ethics of engagement / Don
Kulick and Jens Rydström.
pages cm
Includes bibliographical references and index.
ISBN 978-0-8223-5821-3 (hardcover : alk. paper)
ISBN 978-0-8223-5833-6 (pbk. : alk. paper)
ISBN 978-0-8223-7584-5 (e-book)
1. People with disabilities—Sexual
behavior—Denmark. 2. People with
disabilities—Sexual behavior—Sweden.
3. Sex—Anthropological aspects.
I. Rydström, Jens. II. Title.
HQ30.5.K85 2015
305.9'08—dc23
2014032511

Cover art: Judith Scott, *Untitled*, 1991, fiber
and found objects, 51 × 10 × 7 inches (left);
Untitled, 1991, fiber and found objects,
61 × 11 × 6 inches (right). Copyright
Creative Growth Art Center. Photos by
Leon Borensztein.

DEDICATED TO THOSE
WHO MAKE LOVE
AND
EROTIC RELATIONSHIPS
POSSIBLE.

:: We know much more about the public
    dimension of disability than about its
    private dimension; we are at the begin-
    ning of a period of sexual investigation
    for disabled people, where information
    is scarce and ethnography and sharing
    of practices need to be pursued.
    —Tobin Siebers, *Disability Theory*

:: When it comes to sexuality, every
    handicapped person knows exactly
    what they're not allowed to do. The
    problem is that most of them don't
    know what they *are* allowed to do.
    —Vivi Hollænder, Danish sexual advisor

:: Sometimes the most radical gesture of
    all can be to say, "I can't do it myself."
    —Christine Bylund, Swedish disability
    rights activist

CONTENTS

Acknowledgments, xi

1 :: The Subject of Sex, *1*

2 :: The Roots of Engagement, *39*

3 :: How to Impede and How to
Facilitate the Erotic Lives of
People with Disabilities, *78*

4 :: Shifting Boundaries, *119*

5 :: Paying for Sexual Services, *174*

6 :: Why the Difference? *217*

7 :: Disability and Sexuality—
Who Cares? *262*

*Appendix: Breakdown
of Interviews, 297*

Notes, 299

Bibliography, 325

Index, 345

ACKNOWLEDGMENTS

Composing the acknowledgments—the opening note of gratitude and debt—is the time when promises of anonymity become a lamentable bind for anyone writing a book. It is the moment when it finally hits home that ensuring that individuals can't be identified means not being able to thank them in print. That we can't name names is particularly painful in this case, because our greatest debt is to the many women and men with disabilities who spoke to us during this study, and who permitted Don access to intimate details about their lives when he lived with them in group homes.

Since we can't thank those people by name, we offer them this study, in the hope that they may recognize how much they have taught us about engagement and social justice, and also in the hope that their experiences, documented in a book like this, might play a galvanizing role in generating awareness of and support for the crucial work being done in Denmark, and also in inciting reform in Sweden and perhaps in other places in the world, too, where adults with disabilities, when it comes to sexuality, are still treated and disciplined as though they were children.

:: :: ::

Don: In addition, I especially thank Finn Kudsk, for helping me in numerous ways to manage in Denmark, and Jeannette Grubb Bramming, Vivi Hollænder, and Lone Qvist—three remarkable *sexualvejledere*—who opened up the world of sex and disability for me. Many others, who work in particular group homes or in the sex industry, must remain anonymous here, but please know that I am eternally grateful to all of you. The following individuals in Denmark and Sweden, whom I interviewed in their capacity as people who have discussed issues of sexuality and disability in the press or on television, can be acknowledged by name, with gratitude: Stefan Balogh, Gert-Inge Brander, Gunnel Brander, Pye Jakobsson, Glenn Hanzen, Britt Hermannsen, Annika Hildebrandt, Henriette Holmskov, Birgitta Hulter, Janne Liliendal, Lotta Löfgren-Mårtenson, Sosso Milegrim, Michelle Miller, Peder Mondrup, Frigg Birt Müller, Lars Nielsen, Tor Martin Møller, Johan Nordansjö, Margareta Nordeman, Sören Olsson, Jonas Pedersen, Asgerbo Persson, Annette Sandström, Simon Simonsen, Veronica Svensk, and Iren Åhlund.

Heartfelt thanks also to the following colleagues and friends, who facilitated the writing of this book either by reading and commenting on drafts of chapters or in a variety of other, deeply appreciated, ways: Hanne Brodersen, Ana Deumert, Morris Fred, Annie Heffernan, Lena Lennerhed, Lenore Manderson, Emily Martin, Helle Rydstrøm, Steven Sampson, Donna Schwan, Cory Silverberg, Christopher Stroud, Margaret Willson, and, as always, Jonas Tillberg.

I thank the John Simon Guggenheim Foundation for the fellowship that facilitated the writing of this book, the University of Chicago for granting the research leave that permitted me to write, and the Department of Comparative Human Development for providing an exceptionally supportive intellectual and collegial environment.

:: :: ::

Jens: I especially want to thank my Danish history colleagues Peter Edelberg and Klaus Petersen, who gave me deeper insights in Danish history and culture in general, and Karsten Løt, who contributed facts about Danish disability history. Lone Barsøe and Jørgen Lenger went out of their way to explain different aspects of Danish social and political life. Lisa Ledin from the Swedish Institute of Assistive Technology (SIAT) helped me find Inger Nordqvist's missing archives. Lale Svensson at the Swedish National Archives, Per-

Anders Pennlöv at the Archives of the Swedish Parliament, and Ole Henrik Sørensen at the Danish Royal Library were particularly helpful in other contexts, and I thank them.

The following individuals in Denmark and Sweden generously shared their memories from their activist and professional lives: Axel Brattberg, Vilhelm Ekensteen, Karl Grunewald, Sten Hegeler, Finn Hellman, Claes Hultling, P. O. Lundberg, Gunvør Munch, Bibi Nordström, and Ingrid Sjöstrand-Möllborg.

I want to thank Robert McRuer, Margrit Shildrick, and students of Linköping University for constructive comments about the project. I am indebted to my colleagues at the Gender Studies Department of Lund University for creating a friendly and intellectually stimulating environment. And I thank the following friends and colleagues for contributing to the project by reading drafts, providing information, or discussing the work as it progressed: Elisabet Apelmo, Giulia Garofalo, Christian Graugaard, Kristofer Hansson, Ulrika Holgersson, Lotta Löfgren-Mårtenson, Urban Lundberg, Diana Mulinari, Eva Österberg, Tiina Rosenberg, René Ruby, Matilda Svensson, and, most lovingly, Martin Loeb.

:: :: ::

We would both like to thank the following public figures, whom we interviewed either together or separately on different occasions: Lone Barsøe, Lone Hertz, Ole Lauth, Karsten Løt, and Anne Skov. Very special thanks also to Helene Ahrens, Nanna Munch Larsen, and Maria Sandberg for transcribing interviews and media material. We are enormously grateful to Ashley Shelby for her work editing this manuscript, and to Duke University Press's three external readers, two of whom, Tom Shakespeare and Fiona Williams, identified themselves to us. We thank Tom, Fiona, and the third anonymous reader for generous and constructive feedback and extremely helpful critique.

The research that has resulted in this book was financed by a grant from the Swedish Research Council (Vetenskapsrådet), which we gratefully acknowledge.

We conceived this project together and conducted research independently, in conversation with one another. We discussed the analysis during the writing of the book. Don wrote chapters 1, 3, 4, 5, and 7. Jens wrote chapters 2 and 6, which were revised and edited by Don. Throughout the process we added material and analysis to each other's chapters.

CHAPTER 1 :: the subject of sex

Axel Branting is a Swedish man in his late fifties who has worked in sex education, in various capacities, for many years. Partly because he has a minor disability himself, he has developed a special expertise on the subject of sexuality and disability, and he earns some of his income by counseling people who have a variety of physical and intellectual impairments.

A few years ago, a woman in her early thirties came to Branting for advice. The woman had been in an accident a decade earlier and was paralyzed from the neck down. She told Branting that she had a sexual problem: after having been unable to experience any erotic sensation since her accident, she'd recently discovered that whenever her male assistants lifted her out of her wheelchair to bathe her, she had an orgasm.

Branting was baffled. "So what's the problem?" he asked her.

The problem, the woman explained, was that her male assistants had noticed that she found being lifted arousing, and so they had begun avoiding lifting her. Whenever they could, they waited for female assistants to do the lifting—something the woman did not find erotically titillating at all.

It took Branting only a moment to guess why the male assistants had responded as they had. They were probably afraid. They were afraid that any hint of erotic frisson from the woman, even if it arose as a result of an innocent and necessary act, like lifting her out of her wheelchair to bathe her, might open them to accusations of sexual abuse. They must have talked among themselves and agreed to stop lifting her, Branting thought.

But they never discussed any of this with the woman, and she didn't know how to bring it up with them. She felt humiliated and depressed, and she lamented the loss of her only possibility of erotic sensation.

Branting was only visiting the area where he met the woman and had no chance of intervening by talking to the assistants. Yet he was distressed that the woman was being treated so callously. And so he offered her the only piece of counsel he could think of. Turning centuries of advice prescribed to sexually unfulfilled women on its head, Branting told her that next time one of the male assistants lifted her, "Close your eyes and pretend like you're *not* having an orgasm."

:: :: ::

A quadriplegic woman like the one who came to Axel Branting for help with her sex life challenges a number of assumptions and boundaries. Not only does the woman clearly have a sexuality (something which, in itself, may surprise many people), but her dependency on personal assistants to help her experience that sexuality raises vexing issues about where a boundary might be drawn between intimate assistance and erotic involvement.

The woman's anguish over the loss of her only opportunity for sexual pleasure also raises the question of what sex *is*, given that the activity that led to her achieving orgasm was nothing more than the simple experience of being lifted out of her wheelchair (Axel Branting guessed that her arousal probably had something to do with her blood pressure suddenly sinking as she was being lifted).

Situations like this are difficult. A main source of the difficulty is that they exist at all: they raise issues that many people feel are best left avoided. The sexual desires and lives of women and men with disabilities is a subject that makes many nondisabled people deeply uncomfortable. That discomfort often expresses itself in a curious combination of squeamishness and verbosity: nondisabled people don't like thinking about disabled people having sex, but are nevertheless surprisingly willing to express an opinion about whether or not women and men with disabilities have any sexual rights.

Individuals like the woman who came to see Branting are hard cases, but the most problematic ones of all involve adults with congenital disabilities, such as significant cerebral palsy or significant Down syndrome. Many non-disabled people may find it possible to express understanding of and sympathy for the sexual desires of, say, a good-looking, twenty-three-year-old hockey player who breaks his back and ends up a paraplegic in a wheelchair. But far fewer people have comparable levels of understanding and sympathy when the person with sexual desires is a fifty-four-year-old man with Down syndrome or a woman born with cerebral palsy so severe that she has no verbal language, drools occasionally, and has arms and legs that need to be strapped to a wheelchair to help control spasticity. That such a person has a sexuality that he or she might need help in understanding and realizing is a thought that disturbs many people, who would much rather not have to think about such things. These kinds of significantly disabled adults are the ones who need the most help in exploring their sexuality. They are the ones who present the biggest challenge to the way we think about things like equality, justice, and ethical engagement.

This book addresses that challenge by exploring the erotic lives of individuals with disabilities and by describing how those lives are either impeded or facilitated by people who work with and care for them. The material we present focuses on the most complex and difficult cases: of people with significant disabilities (such as severe forms of cerebral palsy or intellectual impairment) who either have no partners—and who, therefore, like the woman who came to Axel Branting for advice, are dependent on helpers and others to be able to experience sex—or who do have partners but whose partners also have mobility impairments that render them unable to engage in sexual activity without the assistance of a third party.

The people we will discuss have limited or no mobility in their limbs. Or they are individuals who have trouble understanding the boundary between public and private space—a difficulty compounded by the fact that many of them live in group homes where the boundary between public and private is anything but clear-cut. They are people who need assistance to perform basic activities like eating, bathing, going to the toilet—and masturbating or having sex with a partner. How is the sexuality of people like this expressed and recognized? How is it treated? How is it lived?

The context for this study is two different Scandinavian countries, Denmark and Sweden: two prototypical welfare societies that are usually portrayed in English-language literature as being both sexually progressive and at the forefront of rights for people with disabilities. As far as phenomena having to do with gender equality between women and men (such as equal pay, parental leave, and political representation), it is true that, by international standards, both Denmark and Sweden are impressively progressive. Both countries spend about 30 percent of their domestic budget on social services (as compared to 24 percent in the United Kingdom and 20 percent in the United States), and universal health care is largely free.[1] To people with significant disabilities, both countries provide state-sponsored pensions, housing in group homes, and personal assistance to those who choose to live in their own homes.

Denmark and Sweden also resemble each another when it comes to disability politics and disability activism. In both countries large national disability associations were established in the mid-1920s; in both countries, eugenics campaigns in the 1930s led to the coerced or forced sterilization of tens of thousands of people with various kinds of impairments; and in both countries, de-institutionalization in the 1980s made it possible for many people with disabilities to lead more independent lives.

Those structural and historical similarities make all the more perplexing the fact that one area where Denmark and Sweden diverge dramatically is, precisely, in ideologies and practices regarding the erotic lives of people with significant disabilities. Put as starkly as possible, the difference is this: in Sweden, the sexuality of people with disabilities is denied, repressed, and discouraged. In Demark, on the contrary, the sexuality of people with disabilities is acknowledged, discussed, and facilitated. Why does this difference exist? How is it experienced by people with disabilities and those who work with and care for them? What does it mean for more general understandings and practices of ethical engagement and social justice? Those are the questions we examine in this book.

The Significance of Sex

The sexual lives of adults with disabilities is not a new concern, but it is only very recently that it has begun to be discussed in any way other than incredulously, dismissively, or with punitive intent. A groundbreaking 1996 book titled *The Sexual Politics of Disability* spent two hundred pages presenting material from interviews and questionnaires in order to conclude that disabled people "*can* talk about sex. We can *have* sex—we *are* entitled to have sex and find love. We *do* face oppression, abuse and prejudice, but we can fight back and we can demand support and the space to heal" (emphasis in original).[2] That such startlingly self-evident truths needed to be asserted with such insistence as recently as twenty years ago testifies to the staggering resistance that confronts people with disabilities simply to be regarded as adults.

Deeply ingrained prejudices play a central role in that resistance. Many commentators have pointed out that the widespread belief that "disability = helplessness" encourages people to associate disabled adults with children and, hence, with sexual innocence and asexuality. Others have described alternative reasons that might explain the incomprehension and sometimes naked hostility that expressions of sexuality among disabled individuals can provoke in nondisabled people. Alison Lapper, a British artist born in 1965 with no arms and shortened legs, spent her childhood and youth in various institutions. At one point, when staff suspected she might be engaging in "activity below the waist" with a male friend, the couple were whisked away and interrogated separately by "a board consisting of the headmaster, the warden, the deputy warden and just about everybody else who had any rank." Lapper was forced to undergo a gynecological examination, and she and her male friend were forbidden to meet, talk, or even look at one another ever again. They were also both ordered to undergo separate sessions with a psychotherapist. The reason for this extreme (but, in the late 1970s, utterly common) reaction, Lapper thinks, is because

> the general view among the staff was that we shouldn't be thinking about sex at all. Having the kinds of impairments that we all exhibited meant in their eyes that it was our duty to turn our backs on the possibility of sex. It was a very prejudiced view that had two particular components. Firstly, they thought we were too repulsive physically for anyone able-bodied to possibly consider us sexually attractive. Secondly, there was something so fundamentally wrong about our shapes that it would not be right for us to contemplate any sexual activity even with each other, even if we felt the inclination. Ideally, we were to put that part of life aside.[3]

Well aware of experiences like the one Lapper describes, the disabled American author Anne Finger has remarked that "sexuality is often the source of our deepest oppression; it is also often the source of our deepest pain."[4] She goes on to critique disability rights activism for neglecting sexuality as a key element of struggle. Her critique hit a sore spot—it is widely cited in commentaries that point out that the disability rights movement has not exactly clamored for sexual rights: its activism has largely been concerned with the public domain—access, employment, discrimination. One disability rights activist and scholar summarized this approach pithily when he explained that "ending poverty and social exclusion comes higher on the list of needs than campaigning for a good fuck."[5]

Such an attitude is understandable, but the point made by critics like Finger is that neglect of sexuality has contributed to keeping the private sphere both under-theorized and under-politicized. This is unacceptable, not least because for many disabled people, especially those who live in group homes, or who need assistance to do things like bathe and dress, the line between public and private is blurred, and often it is neither acknowledged nor respected.

Ignoring sexuality, or believing that it should be a secondary focus of struggle, is also misguided because sexual agency is a decisive marker of adult status in society. The idea that people with disabilities somehow aren't interested in sex, or shouldn't be interested in it, both derives from and rein- forces the patronizing stereotype that disabled adults are like children. This is a prejudice, a furtive way of denying that disabled adults are adults—or even, in an important sense, that they are fully human beings. In his memoir about life in an iron lung, Mark O'Brien wrote that once, in a rehabilitation center, a doctor screened a movie about sexuality and disability for him and other people on his ward. Addressing the group after the film, the doctor said, "You may think you'll never have sex again, but remember . . . some people do become people again."[6]

Of course, the other prejudice that confronts people with disabilities is not that they are asexual, but, rather, that they are hypersexual. This old chestnut circulated around the globe with renewed vigor during the 2012 Paralympic Games in London via a report claiming that in only a few days, the Paralympic athletes had worked their way through 11,000 condoms and that organizers of the event had had to order more. A journalist writing for the British Channel 4 calculated that at the rate they were going, the just over 4,000 Paralympians would use almost 43,000 condoms by the time of the closing ceremony, "with an impressive condom per athlete ratio of 10.2 condoms each."[7]

This was a spicy item. It was featured on television and appeared in news- papers around the world as an amusing human interest story, a nudge-nudge, wink-wink reminder that crippled people shouldn't fool you—beneath their pity-inducing exteriors beat throbbing libidos just waiting to be unleashed. Unable to resist the opportunity to fondle a sagging cliché, the *Sunday Inde- pendent* newspaper even included a quote by an observer who volunteered that "I have noticed that people of small stature are often highly sexed and I have a theory that this is because they have, out of proportion to the rest of their bodies, large heads and genitals, thus probably have a higher proportion of testosterone whizzing around in their bodies."

Oversexed dwarves are the flip side of the asexual child coin. Both stereotypes denigrate adults with disabilities, and both function to imbue the topic of sex and disability with a sinister shadow of threat and danger: of sexuality out of control, of perversion, and of abuse.

All this is beginning to change. A major source of that change is people with disabilities, some of them feminist or queer, who understand that sexuality is a nexus of power, but many of them with no particular politics other than a desire to be treated like adults.

The large institutions that used to house people with disabilities were closed in most western European and North American countries in the 1970s and 1980s, and today large numbers of people with disabilities are living independently. Enabled by direct payment schemes, they hire personal assistants who are their employees, not their overseers. They have been empowered by disability rights activism to demand access, support, and respect. As part of their increased capability for independence, many are actively and unapologetically exploring their sexuality. They are finding partners, engaging in romantic relationships, and refusing to be told that a disability automatically disqualifies them from having an erotic life.

The days when people with disabilities could be made to feel "it was our duty to turn our backs on the possibility of sex" are over. Today, books of poetry and memoirs by disabled authors who discuss sex are not hard to find. A few random examples in English are Jillian Weise's volume *The Amputee's Guide to Sex* (2007), whose titular poem consists of three sections: "I. Removal of Prosthetic"; "II. Foreplay"; "III. Sex." *Cripple Poetics: A Love Story* (2008), a lusty book by Petra Kuppers and Neil Marcus, contains lines like, "How can I speak of cripple and not mention the wind / How can I speak of cripple and not mention the heart." Many of the poems in Mark O'Brien's volume *The Man in the Iron Lung* (1997) are about sex, and the chapter in his 2003 memoir titled "The Sex Surrogate" was recently made into *The Sessions*, a successful Hollywood feature film.

Examples of other memoirs by people with disabilities that discuss sex include Lucy Grealy's *Autobiography of a Face* (1994), Nancy Mairs's *Waist-High in the World* (1996), and Eli Clare's *Exile and Pride* (1999). Authors who contributed to the anthology *Queer Crips* (Guter and Killacky eds., 2004) have a great deal to say about sex, and sex and relationships make up a substantial part of anthropologist Gelya Frank's book *Venus on Wheels* (1999), a biography of Diane DeVries, a woman who has no limbs. Disabled comedian Greg Walloch's film *F**K the Disabled* (Kabilio dir., 2001) is explicitly about sex, as is playwright Krista Smith's series of monologues titled *True Story Project: Sex*, performed in New York in autumn 2006.

Another group of people who have been crucial in bringing about change with regard to sexuality and disability have been social workers, educators, and counselors who work with people with disabilities, as well as medical personnel who work with rehabilitation. One of the stories we will tell in some detail in the next chapter is the history of the adoption, in Denmark, of a document whose English title is *Guidelines about Sexuality—Regardless of Handicap*. That document, which was first issued in 1989 by the national Ministry of Social Affairs, provides concrete guidelines for how social workers and helpers might assist people with disabilities to discover their sexuality and have a sex life. Individuals with disabilities were consulted when the document was being written by civil servants working at the Ministry of Social Affairs, but the people who fought for the development of guidelines, and who did battle with conservative doctors and politicians who claimed that to even mention sex to disabled people was a form of sexual abuse, were social workers and educators who worked with adults with intellectual impairments. Those social workers defied superiors who wanted the topic dropped and insisted on pursuing it, even in the face of threats of prosecution for abuse.

Another important source of change has been the representation of people with disabilities in popular culture. Past decades produced at least one memorable depiction of sex and disability—the tender scene in Hal Ashby's *Coming Home* (1978), in which a buff paraplegic Vietnam veteran played by Jon Voight (nowadays better known as Angelina Jolie's father) has extended and relatively explicit sex with a young Jane Fonda.

A more significant pop culture breakthrough in terms of disability and sexuality, however, was the 2005 film *Murderball*, a documentary about paraplegic men who play wheelchair rugby. That film, which won numerous awards and was nominated for an Academy Award, brashly contravened a number of stereotypes. The disabled athletes featured in *Murderball* are not sweet cripples. Many of them are bellicose, boastful, hard-drinking jock chauvinists who have less than enlightened views about women and who talk a great deal about—and claim to have a great deal of—sex. Different viewers have different responses to the film: some find it refreshing; some find it depressingly patriarchal and heteronormative. Its significance is precisely that it provokes divisions of that sort among the people who watch it. One of the film's most explicit take-home messages is that people with disabilities are not necessarily chaste saints.

A number of other films in recent years have also highlighted sex and disability in ways that challenge stereotypes, partly by simply demonstrating that men and women with disabilities are not asexual. The 2005 documentary *39 Pounds of Love* begins with a moving portrayal of an unhappy infatuation that the film's protagonist—a thirty-six-year-old man who has spinal muscular atrophy—has with the young woman who works as his personal assistant. The BBC2 feature film *Every Time You Look at Me* (2004) is about a romance between a thalidomide-affected man and a woman with restricted growth. The year 2012 was a watershed for films portraying sexually active disabled people. The French film *Rust and Bone* contains sex scenes between a double amputee and her nondisabled partner. *The Intouchables*, another French film, features a scene in which the main character, a quadriplegic billionaire, tells his personal assistant that he finds having his ears massaged arousing. A later scene shows a prostitute doing just that. *Hyde Park on Hudson* shows a disabled Franklin Roosevelt pursuing a new mistress. And *The Sessions*, the Hollywood movie we mentioned earlier, includes recurring scenes of nudity and sex between the disabled protagonist and the female "sex surrogate" he hires to help him lose his virginity.

Academic scholarship has begun to take notice of sex and disability, but outside of medical contexts concerned with rehabilitation (where there are many publications with titles like *Is Fred Dead? A Manual on Sexuality for Men with Spinal Cord Injuries*), advice to professionals and parents (books like *Doing What Comes Naturally: Dispelling Myths and Fallacies about Sexuality and People with Developmental Disabilities*), or advice manuals (the best and most extensive of which is *The Ultimate Guide to Sex and Disability*), only a handful of book-length studies specifically address the topic.[8] The book mentioned earlier, *The Sexual Politics of Disability*, mapped out sexuality and disability as a field of concern to social scientists, and almost twenty years after its publication remains the most comprehensive study of the topic. Using data from questionnaires and from interviews with forty-two women and men of varying sexualities and physical disabilities, authors Tom Shakespeare, a sociologist and well-known disability studies scholar; Kath Gillespie-Sells, a community organizer; and Dominic Davies, a counselor, detailed the challenges and barriers that confront disabled women and men who want to explore and develop their erotic lives. The book discusses relationships, self-image, internalized oppression, parenting, and many other topics. The amount of ground it covers necessarily means that many issues are treated cursorily—"each of the chapters," the authors remark at the end, "could make several books, each subsection could be expanded into an article."[9]

Another interview-based monograph from Britain, published at about the same time as *The Sexual Politics of Disability*, is social work researcher Michelle McCarthy's book *Sexuality and Women with Learning Disabilities* (1999). McCarthy interviewed seventeen women about their knowledge of things like the clitoris and orgasm, and she asked her respondents to give her details about the types of sexual activity they engaged in. *Sexuality and Women with Learning Disabilities* is concerned primarily with sexual abuse. This focus seems to be partly because of McCarthy's particular interests and the manner in which she recruited her respondents (all of the women she interviewed had been referred to her by a group that provided sex education for adults with intellectual impairments) and partly because McCarthy says that the women she interviewed did not have very positive views of sexuality. Most of them had been victims of sexual abuse. She discusses reasons why this might be the case, and she ends her book with policy recommendations that might help improve sexual awareness among professionals and reduce sexual abuse among women with intellectual disabilities.

The only other scholarly books that discuss sex and disability outside the contexts of rehabilitation or advice are two recent anthologies that both have the same title: *Sex and Disability*. One, published in 2010 in the United Kingdom, is a collection of eleven conference papers that range in breadth from a discussion of the experiences of disabled men who go to Manchester's gay bars, to the difficulties that people with learning difficulties face when they express an interest in sex and relationships. The second anthology, published in 2012 in the United States, contains seventeen articles written by North American scholars on topics ranging from amputee devotees (men who are ardently attracted to amputees) to an analysis of *Murderball*.[10] Reflecting a general difference between British disability studies (which tend to be sociological and social policy–oriented) and U.S. disabilities studies scholarship (which is dominated by a more cultural studies perspective), the U.K.-published *Sex and Disability* volume focuses on interviews and policy, and the American anthology, whose contributors are mostly professors of literature, focuses on representation—on how sexuality and disability is depicted in memoirs, film, performance pieces, literature, and in culture and politics in general. Both books show how much there is to say about the topic of sex and disability. They demonstrate the vastness of the landscape that presents itself for exploration the moment one begins to seriously consider sex and disability in terms of culture, theory, meaning, and policy.

How This Study Emerged

The research we present in the chapters that follow is something of a hybrid between these two kinds of studies—British commitment to social relationships and social life, and North American interest in representation and cultural studies. The study emerged out of previous work that both of us have done in queer theory. We have both worked for many years in Sweden, and in the early 1990s we were among the first scholars in that country to work with queer theory, teach it, and explain it to curious journalists. Together with several other faculty members and students at Stockholm University, we started the country's first queer studies reading group, and this led, among other things, to the country's first large-scale research project that explored "heteronormativity" as a discourse and practice.[11]

Unlike in most other places, where queer theory has remained confined to literature and gender studies departments, in Sweden, queer theory struck a nerve among journalists, activists, and even some politicians: for example, on several occasions—in a development that could barely even be fantasized about in countries like the United States or the United Kingdom—Mona Sahlin, then minister for the environment and later leader of the Social Democratic Party (the largest political party in the country), called for "more queer in politics." The concept was quickly absorbed into mainstream commentary and analysis, and today words like *queer* (in English—the word never received a Swedish equivalent) and *heteronormativitet* (heteronormativity) are used habitually and fluently in daily newspapers, social commentaries, and political rhetoric.[12]

The popularity of "queer" helped to bring some of the issues that queer theory highlighted into wider public awareness and debate, especially issues concerning gender, such as transgender rights and the idea that drag queens are not inherently misogynist. But the mainstream popularity of the concept also resulted in its domestication. Any radical or transformative potential that queer theory may have had was eclipsed as academics, the mass media, and politicians consistently highlighted the least threatening aspects of the concept, such as gender-bending, drag, and the right of young gays and lesbians to be who they are. Sexual practices—particularly those that are controversial or uncomfortable for many people, such as gay male promiscuity, prostitution, and pornography (basically all the practices that Gayle Rubin famously included in her "Outer Circle" of sex acts[13])—fell from view, as people who identified with, or as, queer discussed hip new identities, like asexuality and polyamory, and celebrated the ingenuous queerness of ABBA. In Swedish there is an expression, "to hug to death" (*krama ihjäl*), and this is arguably what happened to queer theory there. It became so cute and harmless that it was hugged to death.[14]

In this context, Don attended a public lecture in about 2008 by Axel Branting, the counselor who told the story with which we began this chapter. Branting's story provoked an epiphany. Before Branting's talk, Don, like perhaps most people, had never given much thought to the sexual desires of people with significant disabilities. To the extent that he had ever thought about the topic at all, he imagined that a disability as severe as neck-down paralysis somehow disqualified a person from sexuality. It eliminated erotic feelings; it extinguished sexual desire.

But hearing Branting talk about the anguish of the anonymous paralyzed woman in the wheelchair, who reached orgasm when she was lifted and who was then denied that life-affirming pleasure by men who feared they would be accused of sexual assault, made Don realize that there was a whole population of people whose erotic lives were actively being suppressed by the same individuals the welfare state employed to care for them. It also made him realize that the sexuality of a woman such as the one who had come to Branting for counseling was far queerer and far more disturbing to some kind of sexual-political hierarchy than almost anything imagined by the Swedish journalists and queer theorists who spent their time discussing gender fluidity in the postmodern theater, or the Eurovision song contest.

Jens had a similar experience, independent of Don. In his youth, Jens had worked for a while as a driver for the Stockholm County disability transportation system. The people with disabilities he met at work never talked about sex, so Jens had never given the topic much thought. But then Jens became friends with Finn Hellman, a blind disability rights activist who was also an active member of the queer studies reading group at Stockholm University. Finn often said, only half in jest, that he felt he was the only queer in the blind community and the only blind person in the queer community. His insistence on discussing sexuality in relation to disability and vice versa was an eye-opener to Jens, and during many long, coffee-laden conversations in a small café in Stockholm, Finn and Jens wrestled with the idea that queer theory, as it was developing in the 1990s, might be useful also for thinking about disability.

In 2002 Finn attended a conference on disability and sexuality in California and returned to Sweden invigorated. He wrote an article about the conference for the leftist *Stockholm's Independent Newspaper* (*Stockholms Fria Tidning*) rejoicing at having finally figured out that "queer theory is an unbeatable way to understand disability and vice versa—whether to analyze bodies or shame, invisibility, power, norms, or anything else."[15]

At this juncture a mutual friend suggested starting a reading group on crip theory, the new amalgamation of queer studies and disability studies that had recently been formulated in the United States and was just beginning to be discussed in Europe. And so, in a parallel to what had happened at Stockholm University with queer theory in the early 1990s, a decade later a new reading group was born. At Finn's suggestion, the group was dubbed Lyttseminariet, from *lytt*, an old Swedish word for *crippled*. The Lytt-seminar attracted academics and a few activists who were searching for something fresh within disability studies and who were unhappy that disability rights organizations—which are committed to social change, not theoretical rumination—were not particularly supportive of intellectual debate.

The Lytt-seminar resulted in several publications, including the only book to date in Swedish on disability and intersectionality and a special issue of the journal *lambda nordica* on crip theory, the latter edited by Jens.[16] Those academic interventions, however, made little impact, and there is still very little discussion or debate in Sweden on sexuality and disability, except—as we will show—when the subject is sexual exploitation and sexual abuse. When the topic is sexual danger, Swedes working in a variety of professions can be articulate and prolix. On the topic of sexual pleasure, they have virtually nothing to say at all.

It was an effort to comprehend this vast imbalance, and a curiosity to understand how people with significant impairments actually experience and manage their erotic lives, that compelled Jens and Don to embark on this collaborative research project together.

Crip Theory?

Given the common background and interests in queer theory that we have just described, it might legitimately be expected that crip theory might provide a framework for the analysis of the material we present in this book. After all, crip theory, as the American disability studies scholar Robert McRuer has elaborated it, is a self-consciously direct offshoot of queer theory. Queer theory problematizes society from the perspective of marginalized sexualities, and it "queers" culture by looking at what happens to its claims and its institutions when the silences it encourages are examined and the categories and identities it takes for granted are interrogated.

In a series of identical analytical moves, but with a focus on disability rather than (or, in fact, in addition to) sexuality, McRuer's crip theory calls on scholars to explore the ways in which people with disabilities "crip" culture. They do this, he says, by drawing attention to "compulsory able-bodiedness," a term McRuer coined as a calque on Adrienne Rich's famous essay on "compulsory heterosexuality."[17] Disabled people crip culture by demonstrating how the compulsory able-bodiedness that stigmatizes them is a nimbus of power that defines and regiments identities, relationships, social structures, and cultural hierarchies of value.

Crip theory has helped refresh disability studies as a field of research. It has played a welcome and invigorating role in making a field that many people associate primarily with either medicine or activism seem vital, theoretically innovative, and even sexy. But even as one acknowledges that, one can also be skeptical about its usefulness as an analytic perspective. As social scientists, we are critical of the tendency in studies that invoke crip theory to focus so intently on disability as a cultural sign. Much of McRuer's *Crip Theory*, for example, as he summarizes himself, is an examination of "highly charged institutional and institutionalized sites where cultural signs of queerness and disability appear, and where in many ways, they are made to disappear to shore up dominant forms of domesticity and rehabilitation, respectively."[18] This interest in semiosis is an artifact of crip theory's origin in literary and cultural studies theory, and there is no doubt that it can produce valuable insights. At one point, for example, McRuer suggests intriguingly that "severely disabled" bodies can help us better understand and critique "the limited forms of embodiment and desire proffered by the system that would constrain us."[19] This is a potentially fertile idea, not least because it seems to invite researchers to really pay attention to disabled individuals who frequently get left out of discussions or theories about disability because they have intellectual limitations or because they are dependent on guardians and other caregivers to interpret their vocalizations or movements.

However, rather than actually engage with the life of anybody who is severely disabled, as soon as McRuer makes his suggestion about "severely disabled" he exemplifies the possibility of the critique he has in mind by enumerating groups of disabled activists who have launched protests: "The

Rolling Quads, whose resistance sparked the independent living movement in Berkeley, California; Deaf students shutting down Gallaudet University in the Deaf President Now action; . . . ACT UP storming the National Institutes of Health or the Food and Drug Administration"; and Audre Lorde's imaginary "army of one-breasted women descending on the [U.S.] Capitol."[20]

A list like this, apart from raising the question of what McRuer actually means by the phrase "severely disabled" (certainly it is an open question how many of the members of any of the groups he mentions would describe themselves as "severely disabled"), also immediately directs attention *away from* those who are most significantly disabled (many or perhaps most of whom aren't going to storm or shut down anything) toward, instead, precisely the kinds of politically aware, combative, independent, and articulate disabled subjects who have always been at the center of both disability activism and academic disability studies.

This implacable drift away from the least articulate people to the most articulate is, we think, a difficulty with crip theory, and also with similar perspectives that arguably align with it—for example, Margrit Shildrick's "postconventional" analysis of disability, which examines what she calls "anomalous embodiment," but mostly as a way of discussing the sociocultural imaginary. Or Tobin Siebers's "disability theory," which is a defense of identity politics and, hence, of overt and explicit forms of organization and alliance.[21]

The empirical material that most often gets examined in research that focuses on culture and representation is, precisely, material that represents: either mainstream cultural products like newspaper stories, novels, television shows, photographs or movies, or work by individuals with disabilities who are articulate—who write memoirs, create performances, make films, organize protests, or compete in sports like murderball. This is all unquestionably important: that those cultural products, those individuals' perspectives, and those protests are crucial to document, analyze, and understand goes without saying.

But less clear, to us anyway, is how cultural studies–based perspectives like crip theory contribute anything new to approaching or understanding the actual lives (as opposed to the cultural role and meaning) of people with disabilities who do none of those things—people who have little or no verbal language, who do not engage in cultural critique or political activism, who live in institutions or group homes, who require a great deal of assistance to manage basic activities like eating or communicating and getting by in their day-to-day lives. These people produce no cultural artifacts, they stage no protests, they make few or no demands, they write no poems, they throw no balls. They are passive, in a sense that we will have more to say about later but that here can mean simply that they require the intervention of more capable, caring others to be able to realize their basic human capabilities and potential. These are the people who interest us most in this book.

Of course we could use an exploration of the lives of people with significant impairments to argue that their existence and struggles crip things like understandings of normality, relationships, and space. It would not be difficult to argue, for example, that personhood is disaggregated ("cripped," "reterritorialized") in the relationships that significantly impaired individuals establish with their helpers. If I need other people's assistance to eat, dress, make lunch, scratch my itchy nose, convey meaning through my monosyllabic vocalizations, and engage in sexual relations with my equally disabled partner, then the locus of my personhood is dispersed—it resides not in my body, but across a network of relations that need to get coordinated in order to allow me to be able to flourish as an individual. The kind of relationships that some disabled people develop with their helpers, therefore, can teach us that the Western conception of personhood as situated in a single body is, in fact, inadequate.

The idea that intellectual and physical impairments reopen old certainties and pose challenges to commonplace perceptions is a pervasive message in crip theory as well as in a great deal of North American disability studies scholarship more generally. Much of that scholarship is animated by the conviction that people with disabilities can teach us something. They can teach us about bodies, about ability, about normality, about how to manage a staring encounter, about public and private space, about "the emergence of new forms of embodied selfhood that take account equally of the intersectionality of the socio-political context, the meaning of intimacy and the erotic, and the psychic significance of the cultural imaginary"—they can teach us about a whole range of issues about which we clearly ought to learn.[22]

Our view is: maybe they can. In the chapters that follow we will point out how a focus on the erotic lives of people with disabilities unavoidably complicates understandings of and practices pertaining to things like boundaries, sociality, and care. But we have found that we are uncomfortable with scholarly insistence that people with disabilities teach us something. We don't see why they should. And we worry that the pervasive focus in disability studies on teachability and on how people with disabilities "unsettle" this or "disrupt" that might deflect or defer a focus on the kinds of serious injustices that many of them face in their day-to-day lives.

Sexual Facilitation and Social Justice

Rather than suggest that the erotic lives of people with disabilities can teach us something novel about ourselves, our society, or about sex, therefore, the argument we pursue in this book focuses on ethical engagement and responsibility.

The empirical material we discuss presents a stark contrast. Two countries with similar cultural histories and social welfare policies have developed two very different ways of engaging with the sexuality of individuals with significant impairments. On the one hand, we have Demark, where the sexuality of people with disabilities, generally speaking, is acknowledged and assisted. On the other hand, we have Sweden, where the sexual lives of people with disabilities is denied and impeded. These very different forms of engagement tell us something about different understandings of what sexuality signifies and about what kinds of assistance people with disabilities are believed to be entitled to expect. They also tell us something about the vicissitudes of the public/private divide and the symbolic connotations of ability and disability.

But more important than what those differences *tell us* culturally or ideologically, in our view, is what they *do* socially and relationally. The differences have a profound impact on the lives of women and men with disabilities. They directly influence the possibilities that those women and men have to develop, explore, and thrive as fellow human beings with dignity.

Everything turns on the kind of engagement that nondisabled people who work with and assist disabled people are willing to extend. Swedes, we will see, engage most often through disavowal. They decline to engage, which is itself, of course, a particular kind of engagement. Swedish professionals routinely deny that significantly disabled people have sexual desires: people with disabilities desire affection, Swedes tell one another, not sex. Sex, in the context of disability, is an activity associated with danger. As we mentioned earlier, sex is readily discussed in terms of abuse. But as a source of enjoyment it is largely ignored. If erotic pleasure unavoidably must be acknowledged—for example, if an individual for whom one works as a personal assistant requests help turning the pages of a porn magazine or if a young man in a group home keeps trying to masturbate in the communal living room—then this will likely be regarded as a problem that needs to be contained and solved. The solution, which is sometimes arrived at with the help of elaborate pedagogical material like instructional films, is to make sure that the disabled person understands that sexuality is a resolutely private matter. It is an activity that must take place behind locked doors, alone or with a partner who requires no help from an assistant, and leave little or no trace upon its completion.

Danes engage with these issues very differently. Although Danish professionals, too, are concerned about sexual abuse, and produce materials that help prevent or stop it, they also devote a large amount of time and effort to discussing and promoting sexual pleasure. Social workers who want to learn how to help people with disabilities have a sexual life can enroll in an eighteen-month specialized program that trains them to be what are called "sexual advisors" (seksualvejledere). The set of national Guidelines about Sexuality—Regardless of Handicap mentioned earlier discusses how sexual advisors and other helpers can assist people with disabilities perform activities like masturbate, have sex with a partner, or purchase sexual services from a sex worker.

This explicit, articulate attention to sexual pleasure is not well known internationally—or, rather, it is known only through rumor and superficial or misleading accounts. Thanks to what they have read in their newspapers and have seen reported on television, most Swedes, for example, think that the sexual advisor certification program teaches Danish women how to sexually service handicapped men. And a myth that circulates widely, even in respectable English-language academic texts, is that the Danish state provides disabled men with a subsidy for the purchase of sexual services—allocating the money, one is perhaps supposed to presume, from a special "whore budget" that the national parliament magnanimously approves each fiscal year.[23]

In fact, there is no whore subsidy in Denmark. Nor do sexual advisors have sexual relations with the individuals with disabilities they assist. But the fact that urban legends like these exist suggests a vague awareness internationally that something is different in the state of Denmark. What exactly is different is a subject we will spend a great deal of time exemplifying in detail in the chapters that follow, partly by way of contrast with neighboring Sweden. And what difference that difference makes is a topic we will discuss as a matter of social justice.

Framing the question of sexuality and disability as a matter of social justice allows us to partly sidestep the dead-end question of rights. "Rights" are not completely irrelevant to sexuality and disability, as is evidenced not least by international protocols like the United Nation's Standard Rules on the

Equalization of Opportunities for Persons with Disabilities, which states that "persons with disabilities must not be denied the opportunity to experience their sexuality, have sexual relationships and experience parenthood."

But a considerable problem with the use of the word *rights* in the context of sexuality and disability is that it seems to encourage a reduction of the whole complicated issue to a tabloid truism. "Is sex a right?" the question is often phrased, in a way that makes the answer obvious: No. Because if sex is a right, what—or, more to the point, whom—is it a right to?

If sexuality, for people with disabilities, were simply a matter of access—like gaining admission to buildings, or services, or the labor market—then a question like "Is sex a right?" would generate minimal controversy. These days, it would be difficult to find many people who actively oppose making public space, social services, and jobs accessible to people with disabilities—even if, as anybody with a disability can readily testify, in practice, funds, knowledge, and the practical will to realize the goal of accessibility are often sorely lacking. But laws and regulations that promote access exist in many countries, and they can be used, and are used, to advance progressive change.

Sex is another matter. To the extent that sex can be phrased in terms of access, we are back to the question: access to what (or, again, to whom)? One scholar who has advocated thinking about sexuality and disability in terms of access is anthropologist Russell Shuttleworth. Shuttleworth wants "sexual access" to mean "the effect that sociopolitical processes and structures and symbolic meanings have on disabled people's sense of desirability, sexual expression and well-being, sexual experiences, and embodied sexual feelings, as well as the resistance they often deploy against sexual restrictions."[24] This abstract definition belies more mundane concerns. Shuttleworth worked with men who have cerebral palsy, and they told him that they felt that their sexuality was blocked by other people's prejudices, by their own insecurities (which, Shuttleworth points out, are nurtured by other people's prejudices and by the cultural value placed on flawless bodies), and by social settings that make it difficult for them to meet partners. So, for them, sexual access means admittance to social arenas where they might make erotic connections and the dispersion in society of more expansive ideologies about what constitutes attractiveness.

We agree with Shuttleworth that the ability to enter and participate in a variety of social spaces is an important aspect of sexual access for people with disabilities. A more enlightened culture of beauty would certainly help, too. But the more one thinks about it, the more one might wonder: what about any of that is specific to disability? Lots of people, many of whom have no physical or intellectual impairments to speak of at all, are hindered in their search for erotic fulfillment and love by other people's prejudices, their own insecurities, and by their lack of access (because they are the wrong race, age, class, etc.) to social arenas where they conceivably might meet an erotic partner. That those obstacles affect people with significant disabilities more than they affect people without disabilities is unquestionable. But what traction is gained on issues pertaining specifically to disability when the question of disability and sexuality is phrased in general terms of wanting people to be able to get out more, and wishing that cultural ideals of desirability weren't so restricted?

Our experience working in Sweden has shown us that discussing disability and sexuality in terms like those can easily result not in engagement with disabled people's sexuality, but in quite the opposite: the trivialization and dismissal of their concerns. "What are they complaining about?" is a not-uncommon riposte to anyone who raises the issue of sexuality in Sweden. "Lots of people don't have sex. What kind of special treatment do they want?" In responses like that, sexual access is understood to mean "special sexual favors" or "special sexual rights." And in that sense, it also rankles many people with disabilities, who object to what they see as the patronizing implication that they are so undesirable, or incapable, that they require charitable interventions in order to be able to have a sexual life.

In fact, many people with significant disabilities do require special interventions to be able to have a sexual life. But those interventions are of a very different nature from simply making it easier for them to get out more and hoping that others will find them fetching. The interventions we discuss in this book are not about demanding the right or the access to sex so much as they are about facilitating disabled individuals' capability to engage in a range of social and emotional relations with other people. These are interventions that show us that the critical question when thinking about sexuality and disability is not "Is sex a right?" or "Sexual access to what (or whom)?" It is "What can we do to help people develop their capability for forming attachments to other people, including attachments that involve sexual pleasure and love?"

Phrased like that, the question doesn't elicit a yes/no answer; it isn't something a tabloid newspaper can ask its readers to vote on. It isn't even necessarily about people with disabilities. It is a general question, one that pertains to everybody, and that addresses everybody. But posed in the context of people with disabilities, it invites a considered engagement with the lives of individuals who need particular kinds of assistance to be able to live a life of dignity.

In formulating our approach to the issue of sexuality and disability in terms of the facilitation of human capabilities, we draw on an understanding of social justice known as the "capabilities approach." Developed in economics by the Indian economist Amartya Sen and in philosophy by the American philosopher Martha Nussbaum, the capabilities approach to social justice argues that justice is a matter of fostering the circumstances that allow individuals to realize a life with human dignity. The approach defines justice in terms of how well a society provides affirmative measures that allow each individual to develop his or her capabilities to flourish and to engage with others to the fullest extent of his or her capacities. A society that provides an individual with the capability to do things that she or he has reason to value is a just society; a society that impedes that freedom by denying people the opportunity to try to do things or to be something they value is a society lacking in justice.[25]

In her recent work, Nussbaum has engaged extensively with the question of how theories of justice relate to people with disabilities, particularly individuals with significant intellectual disabilities. She argues that most theories of justice ignore people with disabilities, and even the approach she regards as the most comprehensive and powerful one we have (John Rawls's theory of justice as fairness) sidelines people with disabilities and treats them as subjects of charity or compassion rather than as subjects of primary justice. By examining what needs to happen to conceptions and practices of social justice if we respect people with disabilities as equal citizens and participants in human dignity, Nussbaum elaborates an approach to justice that extends reciprocity to people with significant disabilities and that helps us understand how disregarding them as persons worthy of regard is not just bad social policy or an indication of noninclusive politics—it constitutes a fundamental breach of social justice.

Understanding engagement with the sexual lives of people with disabilities as a question of basic social justice is the main point of this book. By examining two divergent ways of engaging with the sexuality of significantly disabled women and men we hope to make it clear why Danish policies and practices are more just than their Swedish equivalents—and, by extension, why they are more just than policies and practices everywhere else that engage with the sexuality of disabled people by ignoring and impeding it. We also hope to show how the capabilities approach can provide insight into the realm of sexual facilitation and assistance. Nussbaum's own work on disability and justice has little to say specifically on the topic of sexuality. Like most others who advocate for the greater inclusion of disabled people in social and political life, she is mostly concerned with the public sphere (education, participation in civic life, and access to public space and the labor market). But partly because her version of the capabilities approach originally arose out of her feminist involvement with women in India, she recognizes that the private sphere is both a significant vector of oppression and a necessary site of redress and progressive change. Nussbaum regards sexuality as a fundamental human entitlement, and she is explicit in asserting that a central feature of a life with dignity is being able to form attachments to other people and having opportunities to develop one's sexuality and seek sexual satisfaction.

We are going to use Nussbaum's arguments about capabilities and social justice to suggest a way forward in discussions about the sexual rights of people with disabilities. We do this in the book's concluding chapter. To get there, we start our exploration of these issues by documenting how it has come to be that Denmark and Sweden have developed such different ways of engaging with the sexuality of people with disabilities. Beginning with a discussion of two watershed conferences—one in Sweden in 1966, the other in Denmark in 1967—the next chapter traces the historical roots of disability activism and caring practices in the two countries and shows how they came to diverge on the issue of sexuality and disability. In both countries, what is known as the "normalization principle" guided reforms and legislation from the 1950s onward. But whereas Danes, over the years, came to debate a wide range of ethical, legal, and political problems concerning sexual education and sexual assistance, Swedes, having recognized sexuality and disability as a "problem," went on to largely ignore it, especially in relation to congenital disabilities.

Disability rights groups, too, differed in the way they discussed sexuality. In the 1970s, radical Marxist disability groups emerged in both Denmark and Sweden. They criticized the established disability movements for soliciting and relying on charity and also for what the young activists saw as their meek politics. Leftist activists insisted that disability was not an individual problem: it is a social and political position determined by society—a capitalist, crippling society. The Danish Marxist disability organization Handikamp (a play on the words *handicap* and *kamp*, literally meaning "handi-struggle" or "handi-battle") had a great deal to say about sexuality and liberation in its materialist analysis of society—including the coining of snappy, sex-positive slogans like "It's Sexy to Be Slack" (*Det er smukt at være slapt*). Handikamp's Swedish sister group, Anti-Handicap, was different. Although it, too, offered a socialist critique of capitalism, sexuality was absent from its discussions.

This historical background leads to chapter 3, which begins an exploration of the situation in both countries today. Here, we document the precise nature of the differences between Denmark and Sweden by detailing how the actions of people who work with and care for people with disabilities are guided by very different attitudes about engagement. In Sweden, two related mottoes or mantras are frequently invoked when social workers and personal assistants talk about sexuality and disability. The first is "Don't wake the sleeping bear"; that is, don't do anything (such as provide information or help) that might arouse a sexuality that seems dormant or absent. The second is "If I haven't done anything, at least I haven't done anything wrong." Those two expressions summarize and sustain a culture in which disabled people's sexuality is ignored and hindered.

We contrast this attitude, and the policies and practices that emerge from it, with the situation in Denmark. There, the *Guidelines about Sexuality— Regardless of Handicap* document explains how people who work with and care for adults with disabilities can help them discover and explore their sexuality and how they can assist them to perform activities like masturbation or engaging in sex with others. We discuss what that kind of assistance actually means in practice.

Once the general framework that structures different manners of engagement with disabled adults' sexuality in each of the two countries has been made clear, the next chapter continues our documentation of what it means in practice to either impede or help facilitate sexual lives. We discovered that a common way of talking about this is in terms of boundaries that get crossed and potentially violated. So chapter 4 discusses the kinds of boundaries that people with disabilities and the individuals who work with and care for them consider are challenged by sexuality. The boundaries we examine are the ones between public/private, work/intimacy, love/sex, affection/abuse, and sex/reproduction. How are boundaries between public and private established in places like group homes, which are both the homes of the residents who live there and the work places of the staff who are employed there? How far can a helper go before help *with* sex becomes engaging *in* sex? What is a mother to do when she realizes that her adolescent son can't understand why the love and physical assistance she has always provided can't extend also to helping him satisfy his sexual urges? What is the boundary between a disabled adult's right to explore sexuality—even to the point of having bad sex and unhappy relationships—and the responsibility of caring others to protect that adult from abuse? How do policies and practices that help facilitate sex take into consideration the possibility of pregnancy?

The chapter that follows that discussion is an extended examination of another kind of boundary, this one between sex and money. Chapter 5 discusses the vexed issue of disability and prostitution. Most people with disabilities—just like most people who don't have a disability—never purchase sexual services. But despite its relatively scarce occurrence in real life, prostitution almost inevitably arises as a topic of debate whenever sex and disability is discussed, perhaps at least in part because many nondisabled people seem to have a hard time imagining that disabled people, especially significantly disabled people, could ever hope to have sex, unless it is with somebody who has been paid to provide it. Discussions about prostitution are the most common contexts in which nondisabled people feel licensed to ventilate their opinions about whether people with disabilities have a right to sex, so the topic is perhaps popular also for that reason.

But what actually happens when a person with significant disabilities goes to a sex worker? How does an individual with limited ability to communicate and who lives in a group home even find out about sex workers or find one? What do sex workers think of disabled clients? How do they interact with them? Chapter 5 details what happens when people with significant disabilities purchase sexual services from sex professionals. We discuss both women and men who buy sex, and women and men who sell it.

By the end of chapter 5 we will have provided ample documentation of the significant differences that exist between Denmark and Sweden with regard to sexuality and disability. In chapter 6, we address the reasons for these differences. Why are two Scandinavian countries that are so similar in so many ways so different when it comes to this specific issue? Three factors seem especially important in accounting for the difference: historical and cultural differences that structure the relationship between the individual and the state; the different nature and reach of feminist discourse in the two countries during the past forty years; and the role that individual actors have played in either promoting or downplaying the role of facilitation in the sexual lives of adults with disabilities. By examining each of those factors, we show how the divergences we document are tied to broader cultural, political, and practical forces that extend far beyond specific concerns related to disability and sexuality.

The final chapter focuses on the question of why the sexual lives of people with disabilities pose an issue of ethical engagement and social justice. We review philosophical writing by scholars like Iris Marion Young, Jacques Derrida, and Emmanuel Levinas on vulnerability and responsibility, and we discuss that material in relation to work in disability studies that highlights the significance of intellectual and physical "impairment" as opposed to socially created "disability." As part of this discussion, we offer an explicit moral evaluation of the data we have discussed throughout the book. In order to be able to make that evaluation, we present an account of justice that provides a set of principles that can help us assess the policies and actions we have described. That account is the capabilities approach to social justice that we sketched above. We explain this approach in more detail, beginning with its roots in social contract models of justice (particularly that of political philosopher John Rawls) and going on to explain how the perspective has been elaborated by Martha Nussbaum. This leads to a final series of reflections about responsibility, and a review of some of the practical protocols for facilitating sexuality that we hope will provide a revitalizing basis for more general discussions about sex, disability, and the ethics of engagement.

The Empirical Material

The material on which we base our observations and analysis comes from three main sources: formal interviews, archival data, and ethnographic observation.

Interviews

We interviewed ninety-eight people, some several times, in conversations that lasted between twenty minutes and four-and-a-half hours. The interviews were conducted among a wide range of people, including individuals with a variety of disabilities, parents, authorities on sexuality, people who work in group homes or as personal assistants, and sex workers who accept clients with disabilities. A full breakdown of the interviews appears in the appendix.

To put our ninety-eight interviews into perspective, it may be useful to know how the material compares to previous studies on this topic. We have already noted that *The Sexual Politics of Disability* was based on questionnaires and interviews with forty-two women and men with various physical disabilities and that Michelle McCarthy's book on the sexual lives of women with intellectual disabilities was based on interviews with seventeen women.

Another study we have already mentioned is Russell Shuttleworth's, which was based on interviews he conducted in the mid- to late 1990s with fourteen men with cerebral palsy who lived independently in the San Francisco Bay Area and with seventeen "relevant others," such as parents, girlfriends, and personal assistants.[26] Psychologist Michel Desjardins interviewed fifteen parents (twelve mothers, three fathers) of intellectually disabled young people living in Montreal to discuss sexuality and sterilization.[27] Sociologist Sarah Earle interviewed ten people for a study on sexual facilitation and physical disability, and sociologist Teela Sanders, in researching an article on disabled men who pay for sex, spoke to six men who identified as having an impairment, and an unspecified number of sex workers who had some disabled people as clients.[28]

In Scandinavia, there is an early interview study done in 1977 by the Swedish social welfare researcher Inger Nordqvist. Nordqvist interviewed seventeen men and thirteen women who had either a mobility or visual impairment about sexual education, sexuality, and relationships. An important study that we refer to throughout this book is the Swedish social work researcher Lotta Löfgren-Mårtenson's monograph, *May I? ("Får Jag Lov?")*, on dances arranged for young people with intellectual disabilities. Löfgren-Mårtenson conducted fieldwork at fourteen dance evenings, and she interviewed thirty-seven people—thirteen young people with intellectual disabilities, thirteen staff members who worked in group homes and other centers serving the young people, and eleven parents (seven mothers, four fathers).

Another Swedish social work researcher, Julia Bahner, interviewed fifteen people for her PhD thesis on personal assistants and sexuality.[29] Swedish social work researcher Ove Mallander conducted participant observation in several group homes for adults with intellectual disabilities and interviewed six residents of the group homes and seven staff members. He has a short section on sexuality in his study.[30] Norwegian anthropologist Marit Sundet conducted ethnographic fieldwork in two group homes for people with disabilities, and her PhD thesis contains a chapter on sexuality. She followed five people for more than two years, and she conducted formal interviews with an unspecified number of staff members and others who had contact with the five people on whom she focused.[31]

This brief summary should make two things apparent: first, the relatively meager amount of social science research on the topic of sexuality and disability is based on fairly small samples. Second, the research that exists usually focuses on a particular group of people. For example, the authors of *The Sexual Politics of Disability* and Michelle McCarthy were interested in the perspectives of people with disabilities, so those are the only people they interviewed. Desjardins, interested in parents, interviewed only parents. Work based on a wider range of interviews, like Löfgren-Mårtenson's, Sundet's, and Shuttleworth's, restricts itself to a consideration of one kind of disability—in the first two cases, intellectual impairments; in the third, physical impairments.

Our concern in this study is different. We wanted not only to gather information about disabled people's experience of sexuality but also to understand the situation of people with disabilities in context: historical context, sociopolitical context, practical context. In order to do that, we concluded that we needed to talk not solely to the people most directly affected by attitudes, policies, and practices relating to sex and disability—that is to say, individuals with disabilities. We also needed to talk to significant others who contribute to the environments in which people with disabilities live and act (or are prevented from acting).

For those reasons, we cast a wide net and sought out and spoke with a wide array of individuals—people with disabilities, as well as many others who assert strong influence on those individuals' sexual lives, such as parents, sexual advisors, sex workers who accept disabled clients, and so on. We believe that this range has given us a solid sense of both dimensions of sex and disability about which we can offer generalizations, as well as those aspects of experience that vary among different people and between different contexts.

We also wanted to address the experiences and lives of both adults with physical impairments and adults with intellectual impairments. This perspective is rather unusual in the literature on disability. Some discussions of disability take this more integrative approach, especially when the subject is an individual who has both physical and intellectual impairments. Walker, the boy who is the subject of the 2011 memoir *The Boy in the Moon*, who has a rare disorder that has resulted in severe cognitive, developmental, and physical disabilities, is one example. The philosopher Eva Kittay's daughter Sesha, who has both cerebral palsy and intellectual impairments, and who has been discussed in several publications, is another. However, these are the exceptions. The more common approach to disability in scholarly studies or in memoirs is to focus on *either* physical disability *or* intellectual disability.[32] The majority of the scholarly work that has theoretically reinvigorated research in disability studies in the United States, for example—work by such scholars as Lennard Davis, Simi Linton, Robert McRuer, Tobin Siebers,

Rosemarie Garland-Thomson, and Susan Wendell—is on physical disability. In the United Kingdom, leading scholars, such as Michael Oliver, Tom Shakespeare, and Margrit Shildrick, also focus primarily on physical disability. *The Sexual Politics of Disability*, for example, is almost exclusively about adults with physical impairments.

Other work focuses mostly or exclusively on intellectual impairment. Michael Berubé's writing about his son Jamie is a well-known example, as is Martha Nussbaum's work on ethics and disability, which is mostly about intellectual impairment (or individuals like Sesha, who have multiple impairments).[33]

In Scandinavia, writing on disability and the welfare state tends to discuss all kinds of disability when it examines statistics and the consequences of legal reforms, such as the 1994 Swedish Law on Support and Services to Certain Disabled People (LSS) or the 2009 Danish Citizen-Controlled Personal Assistance Act (BPA).[34] But scholars who conduct interviews with or do fieldwork among people with disabilities write about intellectual disability (examples are the studies by Löfgren-Mårtenson, Mallander, and Sundet mentioned earlier) or they focus on people with physical impairments—and, until very recently, always in the context of rehabilitation.[35]

We have deliberately included both intellectual and physical disability in this study, partly for the simple reason that many individuals have both kinds of impairments, but mostly because we are concerned in this book with people who require the assistance of others to be able to have an erotic life. Whether a person's impairment is intellectual or physical is less important to us than is the fact that they need help to be able to flourish and live fulfilling lives. The nature of the assistance they receive may well be different, depending on whether the recipient's impairment involves trouble understanding things like why certain behaviors are not allowed in public, or if the impairment involves the absence of or the inability to control movement in legs and arms. But what links both kinds of cases, despite their differences, is that other people need to engage with and intervene on behalf of the person with the impairment. Examining what is similar and what is different with this kind of engagement in relation to different kinds of impairments allows us to explore the engagement's form, content, and potential. It also allows us to tell the stories of a wide range of people whose lives rarely get noticed when talk turns to intimacy and sexuality.

We interviewed several people with acquired disabilities and two men who are blind. But people whose only impairment is blindness tend to be much more independent and better integrated into society than are the more significantly disabled individuals we discuss, who need a great deal of assistance in many spheres of life, including sexuality. And people with acquired disabilities such as spinal cord injuries are in a completely different situation than individuals with congenital impairments like Down syndrome or cerebral palsy. Generally speaking, if you have acquired a disability, and especially if you are young and already have a partner, then it is relatively easy to find information and support to help you rehabilitate your sexual life. In Scandinavia and elsewhere, numerous brochures and films discuss sexuality after a spinal cord injury. Movies like some of the ones we've mentioned (*Coming Home, Murderball, The Intouchables*) represent spinal cord injury as being compatible with sex, and even sexy. In Scandinavia, a well-known private clinic called Spinalis offers rehabilitation services and counseling, including counseling about sexuality. But the rehabilitation Spinalis offers is premised on the idea that if you require assistance to have sex, then you will either already have a sexual partner who will willingly provide that assistance, or else you will be able to find such a partner. The focus on rehabilitation and on already having or being able to attract a romantic relationship bypasses the central problem that concerns us in this book, which is how people engage with the sexuality of disabled individuals who either do not have romantic partners or who have them but cannot manage an erotic life with them without assistance because the partners also require help to do things like move and position themselves.

We have purposely excluded several groups of individuals with disabilities from this study. Although it will be clear that many of the issues we discuss throughout this book are relevant to elderly people who live in assisted living facilities or who rely on personal assistants, we did not do research among elderly adults. We also did not include individuals with psychiatric impairments, or people with a hearing impairment. While people with psychiatric impairments like schizophrenia or mood disorders have historically been subjected to the same kind of institutionalization and medical interventions as people with intellectual impairments, the social worlds of people with congenital intellectual and physical impairments and those with psychiatric impairments tend nowadays to be quite separate, as is the expertise and practice of the professionals who work with them.

As for deafness, many people with hearing impairments object to the idea that they might be disabled. Furthermore, deaf people in Scandinavia, like deaf people in many other places in the world, have developed a robust and in many ways segregated community that is configured in ways that make their lives very different from the lives of people with physical and intellectual impairments who live in group homes or require personal assistants to be able to flourish. To include people with hearing impairments in this study would not only risk offending them, it would also raise specific issues that we believe ought to be studied much more carefully and extensively than we would have been able to do.

Historical Material

The archival material that we have relied on consists of both published and unpublished sources, supplemented with interviews with key agents in both countries. The archival situation is better in Sweden than in Denmark because many large disability organizations, such as the National Association of the Handicapped (De Handikappades Riksförbund, DHR), have deposited their older archives in larger institutions. Organizations in Denmark do not have the same tradition of delivering their material to state archives. Consequently, the Danish National Archives does not contain the same comprehensive collections of disability-related material as its Swedish counterpart. This means that our understanding of Danish disability history has relied mainly on printed material, such as the membership journals of a number of disability organizations, and parliamentary protocols. The Swedish material is more ample, and there we have also been able to study correspondence, minutes of meetings, course programs, and other types of unpublished material.

Jens has also systematically studied series of publications from the 1920s up to the present of a total of twenty-three organizations, twelve of which are concerned with physical disability and eleven of which are concerned with intellectual disability. The organizations concerned with intellectual disability included parental organizations (five) and professional organizations (six). Of all twenty-three organizations, fifteen were Swedish and eight were Danish. This has given us a solid understanding of the development of debates and discourses in both countries.

Ethnographic Fieldwork

A critical feature of our understanding of this subject was the fieldwork that Don conducted in three Danish group homes. A group home in Denmark is a communal house or a series of communal houses all located next to one another, often in an area set apart from other buildings or houses in the vicinity. Each house consists of five to ten rooms built around a common living and dining room, and a common kitchen. Each resident has his or her own room. The quality of the rooms, and of the houses more generally, varies widely and depends on when the houses were constructed. Those built when the large institutions for disabled people began to be phased out in the late 1970s are rather threadbare today. In one of the group homes where Don worked, for example, toilets and showers were shared, with two bathrooms per house shared by six residents. Group homes built in the 1990s and later have higher standards. Rooms are larger (about 60 square meters, or 645 square feet, as opposed to rooms as small as 10 square meters, or 107 square feet, in the older group homes), en suite bathrooms are standard, and big windows let in whatever light manages to sift through the heavy Danish sky.

Group homes are staffed around the clock by social workers who have specialized training to work with people with disabilities and by helpers who have less formal training but who often have worked in the group home for years or even decades. During the day, administrators work in offices, and in the larger group homes, maintenance workers keep the yards in order and re-pair wheelchairs or broken pipes. Breakfast and lunch are made by either the residents themselves, social workers, or the kitchen staff, which sometimes consists of a single cook. Residents take turns planning weekly dinner menus, and dinners are usually eaten together, though in the group homes for people with intellectual disabilities, residents are free to take their food and eat it in their own rooms or anywhere else they want. This is harder to do for people with mobility impairments who need assistance to eat, and they usually eat dinner together at the same time.

The main reason we wanted to include fieldwork in this research was to see how important sexuality actually is in the day-to-day lives of people with disabilities. Interviewing people about their erotic experiences or talking to people like the Danish sexual advisors, whose profession consists of help-ing people with disabilities develop their sexuality, it is easy to get the sense that sexuality is a profoundly important and ever-present dimension of life for people with disabilities. We wanted to temper that contrived impression with observations of the everyday lives of people with severe impairments in order to see whether sex seemed as important in daily life as it did when we highlighted it in interviews.

The fieldwork consisted of one month in a group home for young adults in their twenties with intellectual disabilities and two weeks in a group home for older adults (most between the ages of thirty-five and forty-nine) with ce-rebral palsy. One of those group homes is located in a suburb of Copenhagen;

the other is located a five-hour train ride away, in the northern province of Jutland.

Don lived in the group homes and was there twenty-four hours a day. In the case of the group home for women and men with cerebral palsy, he lived in one of the resident's rooms—a young man kindly agreed to let Don stay in his room while he was away in Spain on holiday. In the group home for people with intellectual disabilities, Don slept in a room in the house that was used for staff meetings among the sexual advisors and for some personal counseling sessions. He had free access to the other six houses where the residents lived, and he wandered between them, chatting with staff and visiting residents in their rooms, in the yards as they caught some sun and smoked or drank coffee, and in the common living rooms, where they watched television or played video games. He ate dinner with the residents in the various houses in the evenings and socialized afterward, joining people in their rooms to listen to music by such favorites as the dance band Kandis, watch a movie like *Kung Fu Panda*, or indulge in marathon video sessions of the beloved Danish police show *Anna Pihl*.

Fieldwork was also conducted in a third group home for young people in their twenties with cerebral palsy. This group home is located about an hour outside of Copenhagen. Don was invited to visit this group home by the sexual advisor who works there. He presented his research plans to the residents, and after he left they voted to invite him to come and live in the group home for a month in order to work with them. This invitation was overruled by a county administrator who was opposed—for reasons that were never publicly divulged—to having an anthropologist on the premises. The residents protested this decision, pointing out that the group home where they lived was, precisely, their home and that they should be able to invite whomever they want to come and stay with them. As a result of those protests, Don was granted permission to spend three full days at the group home as long as he did not sleep there. So he arrived shortly before 7 AM and left at about 10 PM for three consecutive days, hanging out, talking to people, and conducting interviews.

Fieldwork in group homes was carried out only in Denmark. The reason for this is that we wanted to document instances where the sexuality of people with disabilities is acknowledged and assisted. Anyone who knows anything about the subject of sexuality and disability—or who even thinks about it for a moment or two—can probably easily bring to mind stories or rumors that illustrate how disabled people's sexuality is disregarded and denied. Memoirs like Alison Lapper's, and historical studies about past treatment of disabled people, amply document repression and refusal. News stories on the topic tend consistently to highlight sexual abuse, not sexual fulfillment. It could surprise no one to learn that an overwhelming majority of group homes for people with disabilities, all over the world, do what they can to impede sex and repress it.

What is less common and much less well known are group homes for people with disabilities that have welcoming attitudes and affirmative policies regarding sex. This is what we wanted to study. We wanted to see what happens when policies and practices facilitate sexual lives, not prevent them. We wanted to focus on what in policy and management contexts is referred to as "best practices." And this is why participant observation ended up only taking place in Denmark. Don had originally planned to also conduct fieldwork in one or several Swedish group homes, and in the course of the year we spent interviewing people, we asked experts, practitioners, people with disabilities, parents—we asked every single person we spoke to in Sweden—for an example, anywhere in the country, of a group home that had affirmative policies toward sex. The response we heard from every person we asked was the same: there isn't one.

Perhaps there is a group home, somewhere in Sweden, that has affirmative practices that facilitate the sexual lives of people with disabilities. But if such a place exists, it is a well-guarded secret, unknown to or undisclosed by any of the professionals who work with and write about sex and disability and unknown also to any of the Swedes with disabilities to whom we spoke. We made a decision not to spend time living in a group home only to conclude that sexuality is not acknowledged. Anthropologist Marit Sundet's ethnographic study mentioned earlier has already illustrated that; her study focused on a group home in Norway for people with intellectual disabilities where the sexuality of residents was regarded as a problem that needed to be managed and contained. Sundet's study was not about sexuality, but it contains a chapter on sexuality, and her observations are acute. Her work demonstrates the kinds of insights that can be gained by paying attention to how talk about sex, and practices related to it, are structured so as to deny sexuality's importance or even its existence. We draw on Sundet's observations in chapter 3 because from everything we have understood, what she documents for Norway is also representative of the way the sexual lives of people with disabilities is engaged with throughout Sweden today.

Of course, the fact that we did not conduct fieldwork in Sweden ourselves leaves open the possibility that the practices related to sexuality in Swedish group homes are sometimes more complicated than the literature indicates and our interviews revealed. We leave that topic for future study, which we hope this book will motivate other researchers to undertake.

A Note on Language, and Political (In)Correctness

The Danish and Swedish alphabets have three letters that represent vowels that do not exist in English. Two of the letters are written differently in both languages, but the sounds are similar.

Danish	Swedish	Pronunciation
æ	ä	similar to English "ai" in "said"
ø	ö	similar to English sound "uh"
å	å	similar to English "o" in "hope"

As for the language we use in this book to denote disability, we follow the lead of disability studies scholars such as Simi Linton, Romel Mackelprang and Richard Salsgiver, and Susan Wendell, and we alternate between what is known as "person-first" language ("person with a disability") and "disability-first" language ("disabled person").[36] We use the word *impairment* in the standard way, to refer to physical or intellectual limitations that to varying degrees restrict an individual's ability to engage with the world unless accommodations are made or assistance is given. *Disability* is used to refer to the condition that results when those accommodations or assistance are not available. In practice, the difference between *impairment* and *disability* is difficult and sometimes impossible to maintain because impairments often correlate with disability—so a person with cerebral palsy who cannot control her limbs and has no verbal language, for example, is both (physically) impaired *and* (socially) disabled. For this reason, we often use *impairment* and *disability* interchangeably.

Translation of the Scandinavian material into English presents an interesting dilemma. English-language readers will recognize the way language is used to discuss disability in Sweden because there talk about disability is one of the most hawkishly policed spheres of language. The slightest lapse— saying "handicap" (*handikapp*), for example, instead of "disability" (*funktionshinder*), or "functionally impeded" (*funktionshindrad*) instead of the much more cumbersome but politically correct "person-first" principle, "person with functional reductions" (*person med funktionsnedsättning*)—will often elicit a sharp disapproving correction from anyone who knows better, con-

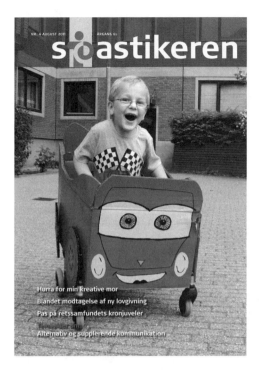

1.1 *The Spastic* (*Spastikeren*),
bi-monthly publication of
the Danish Association of
Spastics (Spastikerforeningen),
August 2011.

veyed in a tone suggesting that if you don't know the right words, you have
no business speaking at all.

Denmark is strikingly different on this front—there, there is little or no
political correctness when it comes to the language used to talk about disability. Even people who work most closely with and care most passionately
about people with significant disabilities habitually use words like *spastic*
(*spastiker*) when referring to people with cerebral palsy—and, indeed, people
with cerebral palsy call themselves spastics. The name of their advocacy organization is the Association of Spastics (Spastikerforeningen), and their bi-
monthly magazine is called *The Spastic* (*Spastikeren*).

Another telling example that succinctly sums up Denmark's unique relationship to politically correct language regarding disability is what happened
to the Danish Association for People with Restricted Growth (Landsforening
for Væktshæmmede). In June 2007, by a vote of its members, the association
officially changed its name *to* the Association of Dwarves (Dværgeforeningen). Their members' magazine is *Short and Sweet* (*Kort og Godt*).

And at one of the group homes where Don lived while conducting fieldwork, he sat outside one morning having a cup of coffee with a female social

worker in her sixties who had worked in that group home for twenty years. This woman was devoted to her job and clearly was much loved by the young men and women who lived in the group home. In between puffs of her cigarette, she turned to Don to tell him a story about a young woman who lived there. "Og så har vi den lille mongol," she said: "We have the little mongoloid." As soon she said "den lille mongol," the woman stopped and apologized, perhaps because she noticed that Don had nearly choked on his coffee.

"Oh, *undskyld*," she said. "Sorry; I know I shouldn't say 'little.' She's an adult."

:: :: ::

In thinking about how to translate language like this, we were confronted with a challenge: do we "clean up" the Danish words in English so that English speakers will not feel repelled by what they may perceive as Danish speakers' boorishness and insensitivity? Or do we translate the words literally, knowing that many English speakers will react with outrage? When a Dane says "handikapp," should we write "disability" in English, or do we write "handicap"? When a woman like the one just mentioned says "mongol," should we soften her words by writing "person with Down syndrome," or should we translate what she says literally, as "mongoloid"?

We have decided to translate the Danish terms in a way that preserves their unexpected and even scandalous connotations. To translate them otherwise would imply that the widespread concern throughout the United States and the United Kingdom (and Sweden) to speak about disability in politically correct ways is shared by Danes.

It is not.

We agree with the title of the well-known handbook on politically correct ways of talking about disability, that *Language Is More Than Just a Trivial Concern!*[37] How we talk about disability and about people with disabilities has real consequences both for the identities and feelings of individuals with disabilities and also for nondisabled people's sense of connection with and engagement toward people with disabilities. But even as we acknowledge this, it is also possible to observe that language is often hypostacized in discussions about disability. So much attention is paid to the right *language* that the right *policies* or the right *forms for ethical engagement* can get displaced or forgotten, as more scrutiny is sometimes devoted to how people talk than what they actually say. Talk in these situations can become a substitute for action; or, more accurately, talk can become the site where speakers can congratulate themselves for taking action. So when a Swede who works with people with disabilities, for example, polices the language of other speakers and swiftly corrects a word that he or she perceives to be out-of-date or offensive, that person can congratulate himself or herself that he or she has acted in a progressive, empathetic manner. By correcting another person's politically incorrect language, an individual can feel as though he or she has made a concrete contribution to the betterment of people with disabilities in society. Where language is perceived to be the site of progressive action, action is taken in language. Actions taken in other spheres can become less urgent and less necessary.[38]

In this context, Denmark emerges as an interesting and counterintuitive example. Language about disability there is politically incorrect to a massive degree. And although nondisabled Danes who use a word like *spastiker* may not feel that they are being politically incorrect, the theory of language behind political correctness is not relativistic. Not knowing that a word or phrase is politically incorrect is not an excuse—or it is an excuse that only works once. People committed to political correctness in language, such as the author of *Language Is More Than Just a Trivial Concern!* or Swedes who work with people with disabilities, would not, we suspect, be terribly receptive to the argument that, in Denmark, it is perfectly fine to call a person with Down syndrome a mongol. On the contrary, they would seek to educate Danes about why it is *not* perfectly fine at all. It is offensive, they would argue, it is demeaning, and it is wrong.

What we will present in this book, though, is the example of a country where wildly politically incorrect language about disability coexists with policies and practices that are both politically radical (for what they mean for the rights of people with disabilities as citizens) and ethically progressive (for what they imply about how disabled and nondisabled people might imagine and engage with one another). This contrasts starkly with Denmark's neighbor, Sweden. There, *language* about disability is constantly monitored and uncompromisingly judged. But policies and practices relating to the sexual lives of people with disabilities are politically retrogressive and ethically arrested. Significantly disabled individuals' access to sex is actively blocked—by the very same people who would be the first to correct you if you said "handicap" instead of "disability."

We want to highlight rather than downplay that contrast (which would be lost if we translated the Danish *mongol* into something like "person with Down syndrome") precisely in order to illuminate the misrecognized space that can exist between language and action. Danish political incorrectness does something theoretically interesting: it invites us to problematize the space that exists between language and action, and it pushes us to acknowledge that speech acts, for all their performative power, are not the same as, and cannot substitute for, concrete ethical practices of awareness, engagement, and justice.

CHAPTER 2 :: the roots of engagement

The once luxurious Hotel Apollonia in Sweden's capital city, Stockholm, is nowadays a rather drab building. In the 1960s, though, it was new, elegant, and modernly sleek, and its large conference room was used for important gatherings. It was in that room, in November 1966, that a state-supported organization called the Parents' Association for Mentally Retarded Children (Föräldraföreningen för Utvecklingsstörda Barn, FUB) organized a public debate. The theme of the debate was as modern as the hotel in which it took place: "The Mentally Retarded and the Sexual Question." The meeting featured an august panel assembled to provide expertise and opinion. Behind the podium sat representatives from the National Medical Board, educators who worked in institutions in which people with intellectual disabilities lived, members of the parents' association, and a legal expert.

Karl Grunewald, head of a department at the National Medical Board called Bureau for Handicap Issues (Byrån för Handikappfrågor), opened the two-hour discussion with a burst of optimism: "Ten years from now," he announced, "we will look back and say, 'Yes, of course, that was the year we brought up the sexual question for the first time.'"

The speakers who followed Grunewald were similarly optimistic. Agreeing that the time had come to begin concentrating on the "deeper concerns" of intellectually impaired women and men, the group discussed issues like sex education (Sweden was internationally renowned for its daring in this area—all nondisabled students had been receiving sex education since 1955), whether gender segregation in institutions was justified, whether staff working in institutions had the right to intervene to break up romances, and what parents should do when their intellectually impaired children start talking about love and sex. The legal expert commented on the irony of a situation where it was relatively difficult for a nondisabled person to be convicted of sexually exploiting a disabled person but where "it often doesn't take much before rather innocent behavior by a mentally retarded person creates pandemonium." Another speaker declared, "For too long, we have been hiding our heads in the sand." It was high time to address the question of sexuality.[1]

That time had also arrived in Denmark, Sweden's southern neighbor. Less than a year after the Apollonia meeting in Stockholm, a similar, but much larger and much longer, meeting was held in Nyborg, a sleepy town on the Danish seaboard. In February 1967 a subsection of the National Board of Social Services, called State Services for the Feebleminded (Åndssvageforsorgen), had decided that the theme of its annual meeting would be sexuality. The person who had made that decision was Niels Erik Bank-Mikkelsen, a towering figure who was to go on to become one of the most influential people in the world in the field of intellectual disability. A pensive gentleman always inpeccably dressed in bow tie and jacket, pipe in hand or tucked comfortably into the corner of his mouth, Bank-Mikkelsen was head of State Services for the Feebleminded. In this position, he had clout. He had developed, and for many years had been advocating for, what was known as the "normalization principle," which meant that the lives of people with disabilities should become as normal—that is, as similar to the lives of nondisabled people—as possible. And part of a normal life, Bank-Mikkelsen insisted, radically, was sexuality.

At the Nyborg meeting, Bank-Mikkelsen addressed sexuality by calling attention to and criticizing the eugenic ideas that continued to saturate thinking about the lives and the rights of people with intellectual disabilities. A law called the Feebleminded Act (Åndssvageloven), for example, still allowed doctors to sterilize people with intellectual disabilities without their consent. Bank-Mikkelsen knew that this law was about to be changed (which it was, in 1968), but he remained concerned that voluntary sterilization would continue to be offered with particular zeal to young people and adults with disabilities. He also condemned Danish marriage law. People with intellectual disabilities were required to undergo tests and get special permission to marry. Such a requirement was not reasonable, Bank-Mikkelsen observed. "Demanding things from the feebleminded that we would never dream of demanding from the rest of the population," he said, was unacceptable.[2]

In the discussions that followed Bank-Mikkelsen's speech, medical professionals, staff who worked in institutions, and parents all presented different views on sexual behaviors, relationships, parenthood, and a range of other issues. Most speakers agreed that the issue of sexuality needed to be dealt with, even though the ethical and practical problems that arose when one began to do so were considerable.

At the end of the two-day conference, Bank-Mikkelsen summed up the discussion and urged practical action. The issues the participants had raised, he said, could not wait another ten or twenty years before they were resolved. He personally guaranteed that professionals who worked with intellectually disabled men and women could count on the support of his department. Their backs were covered, he assured them. Now go out and devise practical solutions to the problems that had been discussed.

Foreshadowing a difference that would come to characterize the distinctive roads that Denmark and Sweden proceeded to follow with regard to disability and sexuality, the Stockholm meeting ended on a different note. Rather than highlighting practical solutions and urging professionals to get busy engaging with the problems they had identified, Karl Grunewald concluded the Apollonia meeting by downplaying the importance of sexuality. He told the audience that it was wrong to see sexuality as a kind of "quantum drive." Instead, it should be viewed as an "expression of the need for love, contact, attachment, trust, and care." Those needs were not as pronounced (*utpräglade*) in children who lived in institutions, he said; nor were they important for all intellectually impaired people. To parents, Grunewald offered the following advice: "If you can, give young people the opportunity to come to you with their problems. But don't burden them with your own understandings, don't theorize, and don't poke around in things they haven't asked for your help with."[3]

:: :: ::

It is no coincidence that these two meetings, both of which focused on the sexual lives of people with intellectual disabilities, and both of which were opened by nationally recognized authorities, took place around the same time in two neighboring Scandinavian countries. The meetings took place independently of each another, with no overlap in planning, speakers, or program. But they were both the outcome of a particular cultural zeitgeist around sexuality and also of a growing recognition, shared by many people around the world, that women and men with disabilities deserved to be treated like fellow citizens and not like social pariahs or children. That people with intellectual disabilities had sexual feelings had long been recognized. But it had been recognized only as a problem that had to be dealt with or stopped— through punishment, restraint, libido-inhibiting medication, lobotomies, sex-segregated living facilities, and through sneakier methods, such as overfeeding. Jørgen Buttenschøn, a pioneering Danish sexual reformer, once wrote that he had worked in an institution for people with disabilities "where one of the methods to make female residents less attractive, and perhaps also make them less interested in that part of their lives, was to give them compensation in the form of sweet things, cakes, candy, fatty food, etc. In other words, classic sublimation through compensatory eating."[4]

What began to change in the 1960s—as the forced sterilization of "the feeble minded" began to be seriously questioned and as the large institutions where many disabled people lived began to fall under critical scrutiny—and was reflected in the meetings in Stockholm and in Nyborg, was a growing recognition that people with disabilities had a right to have their sexuality acknowledged and respected. The 1960s was, of course, also the time of the so-called sexual revolution, in Scandinavia as elsewhere, which meant that it was a time when many of the old taboos around sexuality and relationships began to be challenged. In this context, it was perhaps inevitable that the erotic lives of individuals with disabilities, sooner or later, would emerge as a topic of concern and discussion.

What was less predictable was the outcome of those discussions.

Sweden and Denmark: A Brief Presentation

Sweden and Denmark are Scandinavian welfare states that resemble one another in many ways—so much so, in fact, that many non-Scandinavians have trouble telling them apart. Sweden is the bigger country, with currently just over nine million people spread across a vast area that arches up beyond the Arctic Circle and is roughly the size of the American state of California. Sweden is also the internationally better known of the two nations, largely because of its successful export of pop music (ABBA), melancholy movies (Ingmar Bergman), children's books and crime literature (*Pippi Longstocking* and *The Girl with the Dragon Tattoo*), tennis champions (Björn Borg), cheap furniture (IKEA), and expensive cars (Volvo and the now defunct SAAB).

Denmark, by contrast, is tiny—with just over five million citizens, it is about the same size as the U.S. state of Tennessee, or the Netherlands, but with only a third of the latter's population. (Denmark also governs the faraway, sparsely populated Faroe Islands and Greenland.) Denmark is known internationally primarily for its design and architecture (the Sydney Opera House, for example, was designed by a Dane, Jørn Utzon), for the twinkling storyteller Hans Christian Andersen and the troubled philosopher Søren Kirkegaard, for Lego building blocks, and, these days, for its production of bleak television series with verbless titles (*The Killing, The Castle, The Bridge*).

The languages spoken in Sweden and Denmark are grammatically very similar, and they share much of their lexicon, but pronunciation is divergent, so they are not really mutually comprehensible: literature is translated, television shows and movies are subtitled, and most speakers under thirty-five who try to converse in Danish with a Swede or vice versa tend to give up after a few minutes and switch to that increasingly flourishing Scandinavian language, English. Over the past seven centuries, Sweden and Denmark have been at war and at peace with each another many times. Royalty from the two countries have intermarried, and at different times parts of Denmark have belonged to Sweden, and parts of Sweden have belonged to Denmark. The Treaty of Roskilde of 1658, through which Denmark lost all of its rich eastern provinces to Sweden, established the boundaries between the two countries that exist today.

Both Sweden and Denmark have been at peace with each other, and with everybody else, for many years. Sweden's last war was fought in 1814, against Norway, which it defeated. And the last time Denmark mobilized as a nation was in 1864, in a disastrous war with Prussia and Austria that led to the country having to cede one-third of its land and almost half of its population.[5] Sweden and Denmark declared neutrality in both world wars, but during World War II, the German army occupied Denmark for five years, between 1940 and 1945. Denmark, but not Sweden, is a member of NATO, and both countries are members of the European Union, although, like the United Kingdom, both have opted to remain outside the Economic and Monetary Union so are not part of the Eurozone. They retain their national currencies (Swedish krona, Danish krone).

Sweden and Denmark are both prototypical welfare states. They were both relatively poor agrarian nations that industrialized late: after 1850 in Sweden and only after 1870 in Denmark. The agricultural sector remained strong for a very long time in both countries—in Denmark, it was only in the 1950s that the workforce in manufacturing overtook that of agriculture. In both countries, workers' movements emerged in the 1870s, but unlike many other European countries, communist parties remained insignificant. This left more moderate Social Democratic parties with the political initiative. In the 1930s, in both Denmark and Sweden, Social Democrats were voted into government. With support from agrarian parties, they implemented wide-ranging welfare reforms that were similar to—but much more far-reaching than— U.S. president Franklin Roosevelt's New Deal. Social Democratic parties in Denmark and Sweden created policies that would come to give Scandinavian welfare states their specific profiles: a large public sector with high taxes that guarantee their citizens generous pensions, unemployment benefits, and parental leave, as well as free health care, schooling, and higher education.

Although Denmark and Sweden are similar in many ways, there are important structural differences between them as welfare states. One important difference is that, in Denmark, the Social Democratic Party was almost never the sole governing party—it has most often governed in coalition with or with the support of the Radical Liberal Party (Radikale Venstre). And since World War II, Social Democratic governments have regularly lost elections and been replaced with center-right coalitions. In Sweden, on the other hand, the Social Democrats, once they were voted into power in 1932, reigned without interruption for the next forty-four years, until 1976 (and on and off for another fourteen years after that).

This different pattern of Social Democratic dominance has left its mark on the welfare policies of both countries: liberal and conservative parties have influenced the formation of welfare policies more strongly in Denmark. There, welfare schemes came to favor more small-scale solutions, such as allowing trade unions to organize pension schemes and health insurance. In Sweden, these were all centralized in national authorities.[6]

In terms of disability policies and politics, Sweden and Denmark share many developments. As mentioned earlier, national disability associations were established in both countries in the mid-1920s. These organizations lobbied for reforms and soon managed to influence government policies. Partly as a result of their efforts, both Denmark and Sweden developed social insurance schemes that came to substantially improve living conditions for people with disabilities—even though, at the same time, both countries also began implementing eugenics-based policies that ultimately led to the coerced or forced sterilization of tens of thousands of people with various kinds of impairments (we will discuss some of the legacies of those policies in chapter 4).[7]

Individuals with physical disabilities were guaranteed disability pensions in Denmark in 1933 and in Sweden in 1935.[8] Laws securing similar kinds of entitlements for individuals with intellectual impairments were passed twenty years later.[9] In Denmark, the Feebleminded Act of 1959 (Åndssvageloven) made the education of blind, deaf, and intellectually impaired young people the responsibility of the state, not private initiatives. A similar law was implemented in Sweden almost ten years later. The 1967 care law guaranteed all intellectually disabled people education, housing, and training for "activities of daily living" (ADL), that is, eating, communicating, or managing a household, depending on the type of impairment.[10]

The 1970s and 1980s were decades of major social reforms. The Danish Assistance Act (Bistandsloven), passed in 1974 and implemented two years later, was a sweeping law that decentralized social welfare and made it a municipal matter. It established the regulation of benefits for a wide range of people, such as elderly people and children, single mothers, and people with disabilities. Counseling, cash allowances (kontanthjælp), child care, practical assistance in one's home, assistive devices, rehabilitation—all of this became the responsibility of the municipality in which one lived. Similar reforms were carried out in Sweden in the 1980s.[11]

This was also the period when independent living became a possibility. Article 48 of the Danish Assistance Act of 1974 said that a person who lived at home and received out-patient care had the right to have the necessary "extra costs" (merudgifter) covered by the state. In 1976, when the act began to be implemented, a young disabled man (whose name has never been disclosed because of confidentiality restrictions) invoked article 48 and managed to get his local Bureau of Social Affairs (Socialforvaltning) to approve his request to move from the institution where he lived and receive the services he needed at home. This pioneering young man's case set a precedent, and word of his move spread quickly. This happened in Denmark's second-largest city, Århus (pronounced Orhoos), and within eighteen months more than forty people with disabilities in Århus had followed the example of the young man and moved out of institutions and into their own apartments. They received the same amount of money that a place in an institution would cost the city, and they were accountable to the local authorities for the use of the money.

This form of direct payment became known as the Århus arrangement (Århusordningen). It soon spread to other municipalities as well, but it became most established in Århus, and this feature of the city's political landscape earned it the reputation among people with disabilities as Denmark's most disability-friendly town—Århus, in other words, was the Berkeley of Denmark. In the years to follow, more and more people with disabilities moved to Århus, disability rights activism grew strong there, and disabled people became prominent voices in both local and national politics.[12]

The Århus arrangement was codified in 1986 by an amendment to the Assistance Act of 1974. However, it was up to each municipality to interpret the law, and the new law excluded individuals who were either considered incapable of managing the arrangements for their own assistance, or had an "insufficient level of activity" to require assistance.[13] These limitations remained in force until 2009, when the law was amended.

The new arrangement, called Citizen-Controlled Personal Assistance (Borgerstyret Personlig Assistance), or BPA after its Danish abbreviation, abolished the provision about having to attain a specific "level of activity." It retained the proviso requiring recipients to be able to manage their own assistance, but it was much more expansive about what this actually might mean, specifying that the recipient of assistance can "reach an agreement with a relative, a nonprofit association or a private enterprise" to manage the assistance for them.[14] An individual can receive reimbursement for up to 168 hours of assistance per week, which corresponds to around-the-clock help. The amount per hour is negotiated in each individual case and varies between 225 and 300 Danish kroner (about US$40–55) depending on the salary of the assistants (which in turn depends on their education, age, and work experience).[15]

In Sweden, welfare assistance to people with disabilities was much more centralized than it was in Denmark. When the Swedes finally did reform their system, however, change happened not gradually, as in Denmark, but all at once. In 1995, after years of preparations and a number of government commission reports, the Care Law of 1985 was replaced by a wide-ranging new law called the Law on Support and Service to Certain Disabled People (Lag om stöd och service till vissa funktionshindrade), or LSS after its Swedish abbreviation. The LSS law establishes that anyone who requires more than twenty hours of assistance per week can have that cost reimbursed from the central government. The municipality where one lives is responsible for reimbursing the costs of fewer than twenty hours of help.[16] Decisions about who is eligible to receive this assistance are made by the Swedish Social Insurance Agency (Försäkringskassan). Local offices of this centralized agency also decide how many personal assistants a person is entitled to have.[17]

As far as income is concerned, the maximum disability pension for individuals who have never been in the labor market is currently set at about US$1,270 a month (8,900 kronor) in Sweden and between about US$2,100 and US$3,100 (11,832–17,348 kroner) in Denmark, before tax. In Sweden, the actual amount of an individual's pension is decided by the Social Insurance Agency. In Denmark it is determined by individual municipalities, when they evaluate the degree of disability and the needs of an individual.[18] The pension levels between the two countries are not exactly comparable, since there are a number of other allowances that persons with a disability can apply for, such as compensation for necessary extra costs caused by their impairment (*helbredstilæg* in Danish, *handikappersättning* in Swedish), which is exempt from taxation, as well as housing allowances that are available to all citizens with low incomes.

Denmark and Sweden are representative of what sociologists and political scientists call a "Nordic model of disability protection." This model, which also includes Finland and Norway, is characterized by a high percentage of expenditures (nearly 4 percent of the gross domestic product, on average) on people with impairments, a consequently relatively high level of income parity between people with disabilities and the rest of the population, and a comparatively high percentage of people with disabilities in some form of remunerated employment. There are differences between the Nordic countries— for example, Denmark has a higher percentage of people with impairments living in institutions or service housing, such as group homes, than does Sweden, which grants more subsidies for personal assistants.[19] But compared to other countries in Europe, the Nordic model is fairly coherent.

The Normalization Principle

The political and theoretical framework that made much of this Nordic model possible is known as the normalization principle. The normalization principle is an approach to disability that emerged in Scandinavian countries. It bears some similarity to (but predates by about twenty years) the internationally better-known "social model of disability" developed in the United Kingdom by advocates like Michael Oliver and Colin Barnes in the

1970s. The British "social model" was given that name because it challenged an older "medical model" that saw disability as an individual, medical problem. The social model shifted the focus of attention and activism away from individuals with disabilities toward the society in which those individuals live. Disability was no longer to be seen as an individual problem to be remedied or overcome: disability was a social status, produced by society, a society that activists argued needed to change to become more inclusive and accommodating.

Already in the 1950s social workers and reformers in both Denmark and Sweden had adopted a similar approach when they began to challenge the idea that disability was best understood in medical terms. Niels Erik Bank-Mikkelsen, who formulated the term "normalization principle," used his considerable influence to have it codified in the Danish Feebleminded Act of 1959. As noted earlier, that act was radical in its declaration that social services should work to "create a life for the feebleminded as close to normal as possible."[20]

The normalization principle sprang from the practical work that Bank-Mikkelsen had done in cooperation with disability organizations, especially the Danish parental organization, National Association for the Well-Being of the Feebleminded (Landsforeningen Evnesvages Vel, LEV), which urged Bank-Mikkelsen to investigate the possibilities for legal reform. His collaboration with LEV led him to conclude that there was no justifiable reason to treat intellectually impaired women and men as anything other than "normal" people.[21]

In 1967, during a trip to the United States, Bank-Mikkelsen toured California's Sonoma State Hospital, a massive institution that housed thirty-four hundred children and adults with psychological and intellectual disabilities. What he saw there appalled him. In an interview with the *San Francisco Chronicle* he said it was the worst thing he had ever seen: "There were naked people there, naked people in crowds. I'm used to seeing damaged children and adults, but never in the midst of such neglect." He described how he saw fifty women crowded together on a cement floor, ten of them naked, the stench overpowering. In another part of the hospital he saw ninety men in one room that opened on to a toilet that also opened on to the room where the men ate. "We do not even treat cattle like that in Denmark," he said. "This is the responsibility of the politicians. They should ask themselves if they would want to live there or would want their children to live there."[22]

Bank-Mikkelsen maintained that disability was a resolutely political issue. The task was not to change intellectually disabled individuals and teach them to adapt to a "normal" life, which would be impossible to define anyway.[23] The task, he argued tirelessly, was to change society and create the conditions under which people with intellectual disabilities could live lives with dignity.

The normalization principle guided most Danish work for the intellectu-. ally impaired for decades, even if there was considerable resistance from members of the medical profession, who correctly perceived the normalization principle's rejection of the medical model as a threat to their position. However, as the head of State Services for the Feebleminded, Bank-Mikkelsen had enough power—and stubbornness—to push through normalization reforms with the support of progressive individuals who worked with and advocated for people with intellectual disabilities.[24] These reforms meant that, one by one, the old, large institutions were shut down and smaller group homes were created. Many people with disabilities moved out of the institutions and into their own apartments, and the rest stayed in smaller residential units where they had more influence over their daily lives and where the staff had more time for each resident.[25]

In Sweden in the 1960s and 1970s the normalization principle had its most important advocate in Bengt Nirje, a former Red Cross volunteer who had experience working with refugees and people with cerebral palsy. In 1961, Nirje was employed as ombudsman for the Parents' Association for Mentally Retarded Children (FUB, the organization that, in 1968, arranged the Apollonia meeting). During a study visit to Denmark in 1963, Nirje met Bank-Mikkelsen, who showed him how the normalization principle was formulated in documents that led to the Danish Feebleminded Act of 1959. The conversation with Bank-Mikkelsen was revelatory, and Nirje went on to develop the normalization principle and become one of its most renowned proponents and innovators. In 1968, Nirje proposed eight precepts of the principle. A normal life, he proposed, consists of

1. a normal daily rhythm,
2. a normal weekly rhythm,
3. a normal annual rhythm,
4. a normal life cycle,
5. a normal right to self-determination,
6. normal sexual patterns of one's culture,
7. normal economic patterns in one's country,
8. normal environmental demands in one's society.[26]

Sexuality was one of the eight characteristics of a normal life, and Nirje was highly critical of what he called the "unhappy and unnatural segregation" of women and men in institutions that housed people with intellectual impairments. Nirje distinguished between sensuality, sexuality, and love and wrote that all three are necessary for a good life. However, he studiously avoided discussion of concrete issues that might arise if one took him seriously and actually engaged with the erotic lives of individuals with intellectual disabilities.[27] Nirje's reluctance to discuss this is one of the most significant differences between how the normalization principle developed in Denmark and in Sweden. Questions concerning sexuality were better integrated in the Danish debates and provoked more productive conflicts than in Sweden. There, conscious endeavors to address the issue in ways that were uncontroversial resulted in much less challenging conversations and much more anemic proposals.

Sweden: The Middle Way

The advent of the sexual revolution in Sweden in the early 1960s resulted in very little discussion about sex and disability. The few individuals who did mention the topic—for example, in the *Swedish Cripple Journal* (*Svensk Vanföre-tidskrift*), published monthly by the National Association of Cripples (De Vanföras Riksförbund)—were timorous: they talked about how people with disabilities should have the right to a "normal emotional life," which was a decorous euphemism for "have sex."[28]

A more radical position was advocated by a Swedish medical student named Lars Ullerstam, who, in 1964, published one of the hot potato books of the sexual liberation era, *De erotiska minoriteterna*. Translated into English as *The Erotic Minorities: A Swedish View*—and into eight additional languages besides—Ullerstam's book is a catalogue of sexual perversions. There are entire chapters on incest, exhibitionism, algolagnia (Ullerstam's preferred term for sadomasochism), scoptophilia (voyeurism), pedophilia, homosexuality, and several other so-called erotic minorities. Ullerstam presented this parade in order to argue that the time for puritanical condemnation is past and that instead of ostracizing and criminalizing sexual deviance, society should acknowledge sexual variation and accommodate it.

People with disabilities get special mention in *The Erotic Minorities* when Ullerstam presents his proposals for reform. One of his suggestions is the establishment of state-run brothels staffed by what he calls "erotic Samaritans."

These Samaritans would be "cheerful, generous, talented, and ethically advanced persons" of both sexes who would be "held in great esteem" and who would work in the brothels, he thought, because they "would feel attracted to this humanitarian profession."[29] Although erotic Samaritans would serve many different kinds of people (such as adolescent boys, who Ullerstam felt should get reduced rates because they usually have no incomes), "the most important function of the brothel," he insisted, "would be to alleviate the misery of those who for various reasons cannot provide for themselves sexually, such as the handicapped and the perverted."[30]

Ullerstam's book garnered mixed reviews in Sweden. Historian Lena Lennerhed has written that the reception depended on "how literally" readers took him. Those who took all Ullerstam's proposals completely seriously dismissed the book as ridiculous. But, Lennerhed says, "more common was the view that even though Ullerstam certainly was not right in everything that he proposed, his agenda was important: to plead for tolerance. To not make already unhappy people even unhappier, and to be able to accept them as different—those were thoughts that many who participated in the debate found compelling."[31] Disability activist organizations and the disability press passed over *The Erotic Minorities* in silence. Perhaps they resented being pitied and lumped together with exhibitionists and necrophiliacs.

What did happen in Sweden was that Karl Grunewald, in the wake of the Apollonia meeting in Stockholm, and completely independently of anything having to do with Lars Ullerstam, commissioned an expert group, headed by a doctor, to prepare an information booklet aimed at staff members, parents, and any other individuals who might be concerned about disability and "the sexual question."

Three years later, in 1970, this group released a forty-page booklet titled *Issues in Relationships and Sexuality among the Mentally Retarded* (*Samlevnads och sexualfrågor hos psykiskt utvecklingsstörda*).[32] The booklet is a strikingly sensitive and nonpatronizing treatment of sexuality and intellectual disability. It stresses the desirability of the normalization principle and observes that in a time when, increasingly, the goal is to integrate intellectually disabled individuals into society through paid employment, nonsegregated living spaces, and participation in public spaces and social life, "is it so strange that he [the intellectually disabled individual] can fall in love, have a partner or, failing that, satisfy himself by masturbating? Today it is impossible to disregard the mentally retarded person's right to benefit and obtain satisfaction even from the sexual side of his existence."[33]

It is not clear who actually ever read or used this booklet, and it was completely forgotten in later writing on this topic (for example, neither sexologist Margareta Nordeman nor social work researcher Lotta Löfgren-Mårtenson, both of whom later wrote books on sexuality and intellectual disability, mentions it).

Nevertheless, the booklet is significant because it typifies the approach to sexuality and disability that turned out to be the Swedish way of handling the issue. A main feature of the approach is that it avoids the difficult issues of facilitation and practical help that came to occupy the Danes. The Swedish way of engaging with sexuality and disability never goes beyond recommending that staff, parents, and others should talk more. And in a move that is characteristic of Swedish writing and advocacy on this topic, the authors of the 1970 booklet make an explicit point of being noncontroversial. In the preface, they explain that it is hard to offer any general guidelines on sexuality, "because there is no sexual behavior or sexual morality that is generally accepted by everybody."[34] Therefore, they write that they have "purposely chosen a middle way, which we think will be acceptable to most people."

That "middle way" (which was exactly the phrase used by the American journalist Marquis Childs to characterize Swedish culture, in a best-selling 1936 book with that title) consists solely of providing information about sexuality and education.[35] *Issues in Relationships and Sexuality among the Mentally Retarded* informs readers that the sexual behavior of mentally retarded adults displays just as much variation as among "normal" adults. The difference is that disabled adults are under much more surveillance, and so any deviations from normal behavior stand out more. The booklet tells readers that masturbation is not harmful and that one should not react negatively to seeing it—one should respect privacy and help a young person or adult understand that masturbation should take place in private. It discusses how one should talk about these issues among staff members and provide sex education without embarrassment, with the goal of treating mentally retarded adults as adults, not children.[36]

But what the booklet nowhere considers is the question of facilitation and practical assistance. It recognizes that people with intellectual disabilities vary in many ways: the authors establish early on that "the group consists also of significantly retarded persons who because of complicated handicaps need help in the most basic situations."[37] But that this kind of variation might have consequences for sexuality, and might sometimes entail the need for sexual assistance that goes beyond the relaying of information—that dimension of sexuality is nowhere even hinted at.

This kind of evasion concerning the issue of practical help, and the insistence that the sexual problems of people with disabilities can all be solved if only people would talk more, is a core, structuring feature of the Swedish discourse on sex and disability that has continued to the present day.

The cautious attitude expressed in the *Issues in Relationships and Sexuality* booklet is characteristic of all of the work on sexuality and disability that took place in Sweden in the 1960s to the 1980s, even if this period actually was an era of initiatives and reform. In 1969, for example, the Swedish Central Committee for Rehabilitation (Svenska Centralkommittén för Rehabilitering, SVCR) organized the first Nordic Symposium on Relations and the Mobility Impaired (Rörelsehindrades Samlevnadsfrågor) in Stockholm. The symposium was attended by sixteen participants, who discussed topics ranging from physiological aspects of sexual intercourse to attitudes toward sexuality among parents and the staff of residential institutions. The main conclusion was that there was a need for more research and information.[38]

The person who had organized that symposium was a Swedish social worker named Inger Nordqvist. Nordqvist, who had a disability herself (rheumatoid arthritis), began working at SVCR in the late 1960s. She is the sole person in the country ever to have a paid position (by the government, a three-quarter time job) devoted to sexuality and disability, and until her retirement in 1998 she was the linchpin to everything that occurred in Sweden in this area.

As its name signals, the Swedish Central Committee for Rehabilitation focused on physical disabilities and on rehabilitation. Consequently, Nordqvist concentrated on physical disabilities. In 1970 she created a panel of experts consisting of a clinical sexologist, a psychologist, a social worker, and the vice-chairman of the Swedish Association of the Blind (De Blindas Förening). She named this panel the Handicap and Relationships Task Force (Gruppen för Handikapp och Samlevnadsfrågor, referred to as HS-gruppen, or the HS Task Force) and defined its purpose with an eleven-point charter. The aims of the HS Task Force were to

1. collect facts,
2. spread information,
3. organize hearings for rehabilitation staff,
4. organize seminars for sex educators,
5. create study packages and courses,
6. develop teaching materials for sexual education and counseling,

7. develop teaching methods in social sciences,
8. monitor teaching facilities on different levels,
9. stimulate the development of technical aids,
10. initiate research,
11. monitor international conferences.[39]

This was an ambitious agenda, but note that it was one where the question of sexual assistance was avoided. The closest the group came to broaching help with sex was the commitment in point 9 to "stimulate the development of technical aids." The main purpose of the HS Task Force was to collect facts and provide information. It was not a lobbying group, and even though one of its members was active in politics and later went on to become the deputy minister for social affairs in a Social Democratic government (this was the vice-chairman of the Swedish Association of the Blind, Bengt Lindqvist), there was no provision in the group's charter for trying to influence politicians or government policies.

Inger Nordqvist was diligent. She organized conferences and seminars, she wrote and edited several booklets and conference proceedings, she contributed a foreword to a Swedish translation of a book by a British physician titled *Entitled to Love*, and she helped set up a sexual counseling clinic for people with disabilities, north of Stockholm at Uppsala University Hospital.[40]

None of this work had any lasting effect whatsoever. The sexual counseling clinic received few clients—Nordqvist thought it was because doctors were reluctant to recommend it to their patients, and because people with disabilities were too insecure to dare to seek it out.[41] The conferences and seminars Nordqvist organized, and some of the literature she produced, undoubtedly raised awareness about sexuality and disability in some circles, but they resulted in no real advances. Inger Nordqvist died in 2003 at age sixty-eight. She remained isolated throughout her career, and despite (or perhaps because of) her unique position, she remained alone, lonely, and quite possibly ostracized.[42] In an interview in the *Swedish Handicap Journal* (*Svensk Handikapptidskrift*) in 1978 she lamented that there seemed to be so little willingness to address the issues she worked for. "Very few people understand what I aim for and what is important," she said. "Few people understand what I mean, and fewer still speak the same language. I confront the same kind of difficulties even from some established handicapped people, who don't have any loyalty to those who are worse off, as well as from different handicap organizations."[43]

The sad end result of Inger Nordqvist's nearly thirty years of work on disability and sexuality consists of a number of booklets and conference proceedings; a typewritten, stenciled two-volume report on sex aids it is doubtful anyone ever read; and forty boxes of correspondence and minutes from HS Task Force meetings that gathered dust for many years on bookshelves at her workplace and that were about to be unceremoniously dumped in an archive, when we discovered their existence.[44]

Nordqvist's position was not replaced when she retired, and to judge from everything that has been written in Sweden on the topic of sex and disability since the 1990s, her legacy is all but forgotten.

Denmark: Conflict and Change

In stark contrast to the "middle-way" politics that followed the Apollonia meeting in Sweden in 1966, the Nyborg conference in Denmark the following year became the starting point for vigorous activity and debate. Inspired by the conference, teachers and social workers employed at a vocational school for intellectually impaired young adults in Copenhagen, called the Mose Allé school, wrote an open letter to their professional journal, the *S.Å. Teacher* (*S.Å.-Pædagogen*, a journal for teachers employed by the S.Å., that is, Statens Åndssvageomsorg, or State Services for the Feebleminded).[45]

In the letter, the staff of Mose Allé school recounted that after returning from the Nyborg conference, they sat down together and made an inventory of the sexual needs that they perceived to exist among the young men and women who attended the school. Among other things, their discussion touched upon residents who seemingly did not know how to masturbate but who clearly signaled that they wanted to. There was general agreement among the staff that this group of students should be taught how to masturbate.

"But who is to teach them?" the staff asked in their letter. Some staff members thought they could cope with such a task, while others were unwilling. The letter suggested that assistance with learning to masturbate should perhaps be done by the staff only if parents would not do it. The letter also made the point that no real engagement with the sexuality of intellectually disabled people could occur unless "the question about covering the staff's back" was definitely resolved.[46]

The Mose Allé school staff's letter to *S.Å. Teacher* provoked a heated response from no less than Gunnar Wad, chief physician and the director of

Hammer Bakker institution, the largest institution in the country for people with intellectual disabilities, with nearly eight hundred "patients." In the next issue of the journal, Wad launched a vitriolic attack. He had one response to Mose Allé school staff's so-called work in this area, he wrote, and that response was an open threat: "If I get reliable information that any civil servant within the area where I am responsible or co-responsible for patients placed under the authority of the State Services for the Feebleminded . . . has followed the instructions given in the article in question—in other words, sexually abused our patients—I will, immediately and without any advance notice, see it as my fundamental duty to report them to the police."[47]

Having directed the Hammer Bakker institution since 1938, Gunnar Wad had high status and extensive contacts. He was a powerful man, and his promise to personally see to it that anyone who helped a disabled person learn to masturbate would be prosecuted for sexual abuse had a chilling effect. Its lasting historical importance was that it confronted progressive reformers with the question of the possible legal ramifications of engaging with the sexuality of people with significant disabilities. Wad's threats made it clear that the boundaries between what was allowed and what was prohibited needed to be clearly defined. Only after this was done would it be possible to develop a framework within which the sexual lives of people with disabilities could be engaged with on a practical level.

Wad's threats did not go uncontested. In the very next issue of the journal, Niels Erik Bank-Mikkelsen published a response. Bank-Mikkelsen first thanked the staff at Mose Allé school for their constructive input. He then pointed out that as someone who was not a trained pedagogue, he could not have any real opinion about the social or pedagogical merits of their proposal to assist significantly disabled individuals to learn how to masturbate. But since he was trained as a lawyer, he *did* have the capacity to evaluate Danish law. And in his professional opinion, Wad was wrong. The provisions of the penal code were not applicable on actions performed in connection with treatment or medical care. The penal code dealt with crime, Bank-Mikkelsen said. Helping people who needed assistance to perform activities they could not manage themselves was not a criminal act.[48]

Later that year Bank-Mikkelsen published a follow-up article in the journal *Mental Hygiene* (*Mental Hygiejne*). There he laid out for the first time what came to be the fundamental principles guiding sexual facilitation in Denmark. Bank-Mikkelsen prefaced those principles by reaffirming that the philosophy behind the activities of the State Services for the Feeble-minded in our country is that our clients have the same rights as other citizens. In addition to this, they have the right, because of their handicap, to get the necessary treatment in order to remedy their handicap or to be able to enjoy a better life with their handicap.

An outcome of this is that they have the right to a sexual life like other people. Furthermore, if their handicap so necessitates it, they have the right to receive help to administer their sexual life so that it can be adapted to the prevailing social norms at any given time.[49]

Bank-Mikkelsen wrote that sensible people working in some institutions for the feebleminded already provided sexual assistance to the residents who needed it, even if reactionary moralists—the wave at Gunnar Wad would not have escaped anyone familiar with this discussion—slowed down the development.[50] The principles for sexual facilitation that he went on to outline were later dubbed "Bank-Mikkelsen's Six Commandments." Professionals who work with people with intellectual disabilities, he wrote, have the following duties:

- to provide sexual education that respects the fact that the people receiving it have intellectual disabilities,
- to instruct about sexual practices,
- to provide access to family counseling and to help regarding marriage,
- to inform about contraception, including recommendations of voluntary sterilization, where appropriate,
- to arrange the living conditions in institutions so that it will be practically possible to have a sexual life,
- to inform about the rights of the clients in this area, in order to create a better understanding for these aspects of human rights in the general population, and among parents, relatives, and staff.[51]

After enumerating these duties, Bank-Mikkelsen repeated the assurance he had given at the Nyborg conference that staff who attempted to devise policies and practices that engaged with the sexuality of disabled adults had the full force of his support. "With the risk of being reported to the police for complicity in sexual crimes," he wrote, taunting Gunnar Wad, "I have ordered our staff members to continue working with these problems."[52]

Disability Activism and Sexuality

Questions about sexuality and disability were, of course, not only the province of teachers, social workers, and state employees like Inger Nordqvist or Niels Erik Bank-Mikkelsen. In the late 1960s and 1970s, leftist disability rights groups emerged in both Sweden and Denmark. Like many of their counterparts in countries like the United States and Britain, these new groups were sharply critical of both capitalist society and the established disability organizations, which, they maintained, had become complicit with an oppressive system.

In Scandinavia, one background for this critique was that established disability organizations like the Swedish National Association for the Handicapped (De Handikappades Riksförbund, DHR) and its Danish counterpart, the National Association of Cripples (Landsforeningen af Vanføre), had grown comfortable and wealthy during the 1950s and 1960s. Through charity campaigns and public funding, their economic situation improved, and they could afford to hire more staff, rent larger offices, and engage in costly projects, such as building accessible holiday facilities for their members. Although many politically engaged young people with disabilities benefitted from this kind of expansion, they came to see the dependence on charity as demeaning. Instead of relying on benevolence, young activists argued, people with disabilities should make demands based on their rights as citizens.

In 1968, a group of young Swedish radicals committed to reform established a group they named Anti-Handikapp. Like the radical British disability movement that was emerging at the same time, the new Swedish group lobbied for the introduction of a distinction between "disability" and "impairment." The activists argued that the term *handikapp* (handicap) should designate social and physical obstacles in society. A neologism they proposed, *funktionshinder* (functional impediment), was to be the word for a physical or intellectual impairment.[53] Hence, to be progressive and to advocate for the inclusion of disabled people in society was to be Anti-Handikapp.

The Anti-Handikapp group published a newsletter called the *A.H. Bulletin* (*A.H.-Bulletinen*), which quickly became an important forum for progressive discussions about disability politics. A recurring argument pursued by activists who contributed to it was that the main cause of the segregation of and discrimination against people with disabilities was capitalism. "Capitalism is the original, the fundamental handicap," they wrote. Since people are valued according to their market value as manpower, individuals with physical or intellectual impairments are accorded a very low value in contemporary society.[54] Moreover, in a profit-hungry economy, increasing numbers of workers were maimed by the high demands of productivity. More than four hundred people were killed each year in workplace settings, the activists wrote, and more than one hundred and thirty thousand were mutilated at their workplace. For workers generally, the tempo was constantly increasing so that everyone became worn down ever more quickly.

In this analysis, the way to overcome oppression was class struggle, just as it was for the larger Marxist movements from which the Anti-Handikapp activists drew their inspiration. And just as questions pertaining to sexuality were never very high on the agenda for any of those Marxist movements— frivolous details like sex, it was generally assumed, would sort themselves out in a politically correct manner after the revolution had triumphed—so was sexuality almost completely absent from the pages of *A.H. Bulletin*. In the entire ten years of its existence, there was *a single article* about sexuality: a two-page review of a book by a disabled Swedish journalist named Gunnel Enby. Enby's book, *We Must Be Allowed to Love* (*Vi måste få älska*), is a seventy-page memoir by a woman who had contracted polio as a child and spent most of her childhood and adolescence in an institution.[55] It is a plainly written and, therefore, all the more disquieting account of the absolute prohibition on sexuality in such institutions—which in reality were hospitals in which young people like Enby lived in single gurney beds, sharing rooms with senile and dying geriatric patients.

Enby describes the numerous degradations that she and other young people like her were subjected to: how one young woman managed to purchase a massage aid by mail-order, but because it buzzed when turned on, a nurse passing by in the corridor heard the woman using it and promptly confiscated it; how a semen stain on a sheet resulted in a couple in their midtwenties being forbidden to see each other ever again ("the girl . . . was deemed to be overerotic"). "The worst part is not having anywhere to go with one's friend," Enby wrote. "So humiliating to sneak into the morgue and the back corridors like dying elephants. So embarrassing to ask one's friends to keep guard outside the door—it's not like we were inside shooting up heroin."[56] Enby's solution to the problems she highlighted was simple. "All that's needed is one's own room, a key and the right to be alone with one's visitors," she wrote.

The reviewer of Enby's book in *A.H. Bulletin* agreed that "the handicapped should be given information about how they can, with the help of contraception and technical aids, achieve sexual satisfaction." The most important point, however, according to the reviewer, was that society must change. Shifting the focus, even in a discussion of a book about sexuality, away from sexuality back to class struggle, the reviewer declared: "We need a social system in which every individual is valued equally, and where people are the most important thing, not profit."[57]

In Denmark, the socialist alternative to the established disability movement originated from within an already well-established disability organization. The Youth Circle (Ungdomskredsen) of the National Association of Cripples was a lively forum for political discussion, and in 1976 it began publishing its own journal, *Handi-Kamp*, which means "handi-struggle" or "handi-battle." Like its Swedish counterpart, *Handi-Kamp* advocated a view of society grounded in historical materialism: capitalism was what produced cripples, activists explained, by injuring workers in its hunger for profit and by reducing everyone to nonhuman status as a means of production. Like the Swedes writing in *A.H. Bulletin*, the Danish activists who wrote in *Handi-Kamp* urged people with disabilities to resist capitalism.[58]

Unlike their Swedish counterparts, however, the Danes discussed sex frequently and with gusto. In contrast to the single article mentioning sex that appeared in the Swedish *A.H. Bulletin*, between 1979 and 1989 the Danish *Handi-Kamp* published a whopping *ten special issues* about sexuality.[59] In the first, the editor situated the sexual question firmly in an economic structure by pointing out that "a person's rights—also to sexual fulfillment—is determined in our society to a large extent by her or his profitable value."[60] But the discussion that ensued there and in the issues to follow was far from doctrinaire. Sexual variety, rather than conformity, was highlighted, both women's and men's sexualities were explored, and while certain forms of capitalist practices, such as commercial pornography, were critiqued, it was frequently pointed out that part of the problem for people with disabilities was that they were actively hindered from participating (because of prejudices and barriers that prevented access) in the kinds of erotic exchanges that nondisabled people took for granted. The special issues featured interviews, articles, and debates on topics like sexual counseling, masturbation, how different individuals handle the intimate ministrations of helpers, pornography, personal ads, performance anxiety, female erotica, masochism, and problems that confronted anyone living in institutions who wanted to have a sex life.

In May 1980 the Youth Circle associated with *Handi-Kamp* organized a weekend of sex and love and invited two men from the Danish Gay Liberation Front (Bøssernes Befrielses Front) to speak. A report on this event published in *Handi-Kamp*, by activist Lone Barsøe, begins by saying: "Maybe someone will wonder right away what the thoughts and problems of gay men [bøsserne] have to do with the handicapped and sex. Apart from the fact that there presumably are some handicapped people who are not sexually attracted to the opposite sex, we assert that the oppression that gay men are subject to has several parallels to what we experience as handicapped."[61]

Unlike Sweden, where gay rights and disability rights occupied separate universes, in Denmark, influential activists like Barsøe engaged with gay liberation and were inspired by it. They admired the way the growing gay movement was forging a positive, proud identity, and they appreciated some of the strategies the movement deployed. Barsøe wrote in *Handi-Kamp* that "there is something amazingly strong and confirming in the way gay men, through their language, try to fight self-oppression. They say (as we wrote in the last issue of *Handi-Kamp*): 'It's Good to be Gay.' Among members of the Youth Circle and people with muscular dystrophy, I have heard something similar, even if it is more like a joke. They say: 'It's Sexy to Be Slack' [*Det er smukt at være slapt*]."[62] In a later issue of *Handi-Kamp* a group calling themselves "revolting women" (*klamme kvinder*) discussed how they could eroticize the disabled body.[63] Several articles by men proposed that men with disabilities were often the best lovers "because they can't deliver the big physical performances, but instead expend their time and energy on caresses, closeness and tenderness."[64]

The issue of prostitution was raised numerous times. Discussion tended to divide along gender lines, with men insisting that prostitution, like pornography, was "part of ordinary male sexuality and so also of handicapped men's sexuality," and with women expressing reservations.[65] But sex workers were interviewed sympathetically (one reported that the biggest difficulty in having disabled clients was facing the disapproval of people who cared for them).[66] And even women who were critical of prostitution rallied when three politicians from the Socialist Party wrote a newspaper article saying that anyone who claimed that prostitution was necessary because disabled people needed it was mistaken: handicapped people, the Socialist Party members wrote, do not need prostitutes, because they "have a more genuine understanding [*en lødigere opfattelse*] of sex than many 'normal' people."[67]

Birgitte Bjørkman from *Handi-Kamp*'s editorial collective responded by wondering what a "more genuine understanding of sexuality" might mean, exactly. The reason more disabled people did not use the services of prostitutes, Bjørkman suggested, was because of negative attitudes toward disabled people's sexuality and because of the often insurmountable obstacles that society places before them to be able to explore that sexuality. To claim that disabled people have a "more genuine understanding of sexuality" was patronizing. "Might that not become a myth that certainly will not benefit anyone who is handicapped?" she asked. Instead of dilating about the supposedly higher moral rectitude of people with disabilities, Bjørkman advised concerned members of the Socialist Party to devote some of their time and energy to demystifying prostitution and developing policies that could facilitate more fulfilling sexual lives for disabled men and women.[68]

In addition to participating in discussions about sex in the pages of *Handi-Kamp*, activists associated with the journal formed a cabaret group they called the Crutch Ensemble (Krykensemblen). For twelve years this group produced and performed radio shows and cabarets, some of which were shown on national television, that satirized charity and the kind of condescending benevolence expressed through the proclamation of gimmicky events like "Disability Year" ("Use your strength for a common cause—ditch the Disability Year," they sang).

Sexuality was a recurring theme in the Crutch Ensemble's productions. The song "You Are My Venus" had a young man serenading a woman in a wheelchair with lines like, "Everything I ever thought would make my heart go thump / is nothing compared to what happens when I see your lovely hump" (*Alt hvad jeg tro'de om vild stimulans / må vige når jeg sanser din pukkels glans*). The group also produced catchy slogans, such as,

> Do you long all the time for total orgasms?
> The solution, then, is a partner who spasms.
>
> (*Drømmer De tit om totalorgasmer?*
> *Så er sagen en partner med spasmer.*)

and

> Has your wife gotten a little too big?
> Try someone with MS—lean as a twig.
>
> (*Hvis deres kone er blevet lidt for trind?*
> *Så skynd Dem og find en med muskelsvind.*)[69]

The performances of the Crutch Ensemble were reviewed favorably, both by the disability press and the mainstream media. The radio reviewer in *Politiken*, one of Denmark's largest daily newspapers, particularly loved the slo-

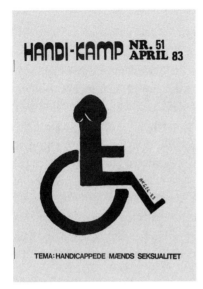
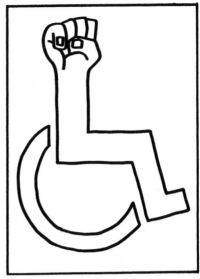

2.1 (*left*) Cover image from the Danish *Handi-Kamp*, no. 51 (April 1983), themed issue on "Handicapped Men's Sexuality"; artist Aksel Knudsen.

2.2 (*right*) Image from the Swedish *A.H. Bulletin* (*A.H.-Bulletinen*, no. 3 [1972]); artist Per Wickenberg.

gans. She called them "stinging" (*revyens skarpeste*) and praised the cabaret as a "perfect example of satire . . . a powerful response to the kinds of cute stories and modern slang terms that insult handicapped people of every kind."[70]

In Sweden, the progressive young activists associated with Anti-Handicapp also formed a theater troupe that toured schools and group homes in the south of the country. But, again, unlike their Danish counterparts, they never highlighted sex. Their play *Nutcakes* (*Nötkakor*) criticized charity and mocked the idea that disabled people were radically different from nondisabled people. Another play, *Knutte the Cripple* (*Knutte Krympling*), related the tale of a factory worker who loses his hand in a workplace accident and becomes despondent until he realizes that he can channel his unhappiness and anger into fighting the capitalist system that caused his disability in the first place. The play was serialized as a comic strip in *A.H. Bulletin*, and there one can follow Knutte as he comes upon a large group of similarly one-handed men and women standing in front of the government Employment Office.

"What are you doing here?" he asks them.

"We tried to get work and got nothing," they answer. "Now we're really beginning to see the need for the Socialist Revolution!"[71]

Denmark and the Road to *Guidelines about Sexuality—Regardless of Handicap*

While Danish disability rights activists were discussing sex and highlighting the sexual entitlements of disabled women and men in *Handi-Kamp* and in sketches and songs produced by the Crutch Ensemble, Niels Erik Bank-Mikkelsen continued pressing ahead with his efforts to get helpers who worked with disabled adults to find respectful ways of engaging with their sexuality. In 1972 Bank-Mikkelsen ordered State Services for the Feebleminded's section on education to start working with the question of sexual rights. One of the first things the education section did was recruit three teachers who for various reasons they already knew were interested in that issue. One of them was thirty-six-year-old Jørgen Buttenschøn, the man who went on to become one of Denmark's most important advocates for the sexual rights of people with disabilities.

Buttenschøn was originally a teacher who happened to get his first job in a school for young people with intellectual impairments. In an article in which he describes the origins of his engagement with the issue of disability and sexuality, he recounts that when he began working in the school he was horrified to observe the ways in which the students' sexuality was actively repressed and punished by the teachers and other staff members. He soon discovered that these responses were the result of prejudice, ignorance, and insecurity, and together with some younger colleagues he began to develop ways to try to change this. Eventually Buttenschøn became the school's principal. At the State Services for the Feebleminded, his job was to develop educational material and methods that would help facilitate the sexuality of people with intellectual disabilities. Consequently, in 1973, Buttenschøn organized three conferences on sexuality and disability in different parts of the country. The conferences were intended to create networks among staff who worked in institutions and group homes.[72]

The first conference was a success, and while planning the next one, Buttenschøn met Karsten Løt, another schoolteacher who worked with adults with intellectual disabilities. Løt was to become Buttenschøn's closest colleague for the rest of his career. The two men collaborated for more than thirty-five years, developing courses and teaching materials for both people with intellectual disabilities and the people who work with and care for them.[73]

Inspired by Bank-Mikkelsen's "six commandments," which made it clear that it was a duty of people who worked in group homes to engage with the sexuality of individuals who lived there, Buttenschøn, who was universally known as "But" (pronounced *Boot*), developed a four-step strategy that he and Løt began to present in courses to social workers and teachers in October 1974. In its original version, "But's 4-step plan" (*But's 4 trins plan*), as this strategy came to be known, recommended that helpers should

1. establish, in cases when a disabled individual seems frustrated, if that frustration might be related to sexuality;
2. if it is, develop an educational plan to help the individual;
3. have the plan approved by a staff council (*personaleråd*) so that the helper will not be isolated and will know that he or she had the backing of other members of staff;
4. have the plan approved by the parents of the person to be assisted.[74]

This last step urging parental approval proved the most controversial, interestingly enough because the parental advocacy organization National Association for the Well-Being of the Feebleminded (LEV, the organization that had so influenced Bank-Mikkelsen) objected. Parents involved in LEV argued that informing mothers and fathers about the sexual behavior of their children would infringe on the integrity of their children, who were adults with the right to a private life. As a result of those criticisms, the Board of Social Services decided to change that last step into one that omitted mention of parents and instead called for the plan to be approved by the disabled individual himself or herself.

In 1986 the issue of sexuality reached the Danish national parliament. The reason for this was because a thirty-one-year-old man named Jørgen Lenger had been elected, two years previously, as a Member of Parliament for the tiny Left Socialist Party (Venstresocialisterne). Lenger, who like such advocates as Niels Erik Bank-Mikkelsen, Jørgen Buttenschøn, and Karsten Løt had no disability himself, was an important disability rights activist. He had worked with disability issues for the municipal board in Århus for more than ten years, and was the civil servant who had been given the historic task of calculating the exact amount of money that the pioneering young man in Århus who first moved out of the institution would receive from the municipality. Lenger later became a long-serving head of development at the Muscular Dystrophy Foundation (Muskelsvindfonden).

Lenger's election to parliament resulted in the Left Socialist Party highlighting questions related to disability. And after holding a series of meetings with disability activists to discuss their needs and demands, Lenger prepared a bill that was submitted jointly in February 1986 by all five Left Socialist Party Members of Parliament. The bill consisted of fourteen separate proposals, the most far-reaching being a suggestion to amend the Assistance Act of 1974 so that the "Århus arrangement" would be binding for all municipalities. It proposed to clarify the exact nature of the reimbursement that people with disabilities were eligible for, and it proposed reforms concerning pensions for people with disabilities, the scope of their choice regarding living arrangements, and the accessibility of the House of Parliament itself.

Sexuality was one of the proposals on that list. And not only was sexuality specifically mentioned, but it was the subject of three separate recommendations. Lenger's party proposed that the government should (1) develop guidelines concerning sexual education and training of people who lived in institutions; (2) investigate whether sexual education for people with disabilities, and assisting them in other ways with their sexuality, would be prosecutable under the existing Penal Code; and (3) present a plan for how sexual counseling for people with disabilities might be expanded and improved.[75]

A large majority in parliament was in favor of the proposal. Of nine parties represented, all except the right-wing populist Progress Party (Fremskridtspartiet) and the Christian People's Party (Kristeligt Folkeparti) expressed their support. A conservative MP said that it was difficult to legislate for everything, but since "it is a human right to have a good sexual life," she supported the proposal.[76] The proposal was never actually voted on; it was referred to the Standing Committee on Social Affairs (Socialudvalget), which recommended that the Ministry of Social Affairs act on it. And so, the minister of social affairs directed the National Board of Social Services (Socialstyrelsen) to prepare a report that would lay the groundwork for carrying out the proposal's three recommendations.

Under Bank-Mikkelsen, the National Board of Social Services had of course already been working with these questions for years, and the report requested by the minister of social affairs was ready eight months later, in October of that same year.

Titled "National Board of Social Services' investigation of the need for improvements regarding the possibilities for handicapped people's sexual life" ("Socialstyrelsens undersøgelse af behovet for forbedringer af handicappedes muligheder for seksualliv"), the report is a remarkable document. Considering that it is an official memorandum from a government department, its empathy and passion are startling.[77] The report is direct and graphic. Citing cases that had been collected in the mid-1980s by Buttenschøn, Løt, and Lasse

Bjarne Pedersen, a social worker who worked with people with intellectual impairments, it emphasizes the brutal cruelty meted out to people with disabilities simply because they expressed an interest in sex. One case it cites is the following:

A now 39-year old mentally retarded resident in an institution [*psykisk udviklingshæmmet beboer*], who came as a 10-year old and was at the time dependent and tidy, has since 16 years of age tried to masturbate, but never managed to do so to ejaculation [*uden at få sædafgang*].

The problem was dealt with by using restraints [*fiksering*]. Later, when that didn't help because he was able to free himself from the restraints, he was given female hormones. At age 22, he was given the white cut [*det hvide snit*, i.e., a lobotomy; the term is a reference to the white tissue that was severed in the brain's frontal lobes], but after half a year's time the result wore off and he began to masturbate again, without ejaculation.

Became increasingly untidy [*urenlig*] and aggressive.

At age 24 was lobotomized for the second time, and the effect of that intervention also wore off quickly. Electroshock treatment was tried, but this had no positive effect either.

At 25 he was lobotomized again for the third time, without any real effect. As a 26 year old he was still violent.[78]

The report consistently foregrounds experiences of individuals like this man. In a section in which it illustrates the kinds of situations that actually exist in institutions and group homes, the report asks readers to consider cases like the following:

A retarded resident with a conspicuous appearance [*et åndssvag beboer med påfaldende udseende*] has expressed the wish to have a relationship with a girl in the normal way. Desires contact with a prostitute but isn't, himself, capable of finding addresses, telephone numbers, etc. Is it permissible for staff to help this person come into contact with a prostitute who they know from experience is considerate toward the handicapped?

Two mentally retarded individuals try to have intercourse but are unable to understand how to do it. Can staff help them without being prosecuted under Section 232 of the penal code that regulates indecency [*blufærdighedskrænkelse*]? May the staff in a corresponding situation help two physically handicapped people have intercourse if they can't manage to do it on their own?

Using examples like these, the report drives home its message that there is an urgent need for measures to improve the possibilities for people with disabilities to have a sexual life. National guidelines that allow helpers to engage with the sexual lives of people with disabilities without fear of reprisal are essential, the report concluded. Such guidelines, it said, should be aimed at sexuality's affirmative dimensions. Instead of prohibitions, the guidelines should contain general directions. They should assist helpers in figuring out the principle of least possible intervention so that they would not impose more than was needed. And help should not just be perfunctory or geared toward mechanical sex aids—it should allow discussions and knowledge about emotions and feelings, and it should recommend ways to "tactfully establish contact with prostitutes." The special needs of women also need to be considered, the report continued, specifying those needs as "foreplay, etc."

The report also stressed the need to clarify, once and for all, the legal consequences of assisting people with disabilities to have a sex life. It concluded that authoritative statements were needed from both the Ministry of Justice and the attorney general (Rigsadvokaten) before the matter could be laid to rest. And finally, the report recommended that the government work out a plan for how it was going to expand sexual education and counseling services for people with disabilities. Such a specialized service existed only in one place, in Århus, the epicenter of *Handi-Kamp* activism. The report recommended that such services be spread throughout the country.

The Board of Social Services' report produced an immediate response. Upon reading it, the minister of social affairs instructed the board to begin preparing guidelines for how staff who worked in institutions and group homes could address the sexuality of people with disabilities. The board appointed a reference group consisting of professionals like Jørgen Buttenschøn and Karsten Løt, representatives from the parental organization LEV, and two people from the National Association of Cripples (Landsforeningen af Vanføre). (Niels Erik Bank-Mikkelsen had retired from the Board of Social Services several years earlier, in 1982, so he was no longer involved.) Drafts produced in consultation with those experts were then coordinated with advice from lawyers at the Ministry of Justice.

On 10 February 1989 the Board of Social Services presented its guidelines in a document titled *Guidelines about Sexuality—Regardless of Handicap* (*Vejledning om seksualitet—uanset handicap*; hereafter, *Guidelines*).

A thirty-four-page brochure, the *Guidelines* document consisted of ten short, mostly 1–2 page chapters (with rubrics like "Is the sexuality of people with a handicap different?" and "How can one help the intellectually handicapped?"); an eight-page bibliography of films, articles, and books of relevance to the topic; and a seven-page appendix of laws pertaining to sexual abuse, together with statements from both the Ministry of Justice and the attorney general that finally established that sexual education and practices that helped disabled adults with "sexual training" (*seksualoplæring*) were not, in themselves, criminal acts. Those statements were the conclusive legal response to Gunnar Wad's old threat to prosecute staff members who engaged with the sexuality of disabled adults, and they laid the legal groundwork that was essential for staff working with people with disabilities to intervene and help them have a sexual life.

We will discuss the content of the *Guidelines* document in the following chapter, where we illustrate the details of how sexual assistance actually occurs in practice. But in light of the way the issue of sexuality and disability came to be discussed in Sweden, two things in particular stand out and deserve mention here. The first is the explicit acknowledgment that people with disabilities have a sexuality. "Sexuality is an integrated part of the personality of every person," the *Guidelines* document begins, "and that includes people with a handicap."[79]

The second notable feature of the *Guidelines* document is the assertion that the active intervention of caring others may sometimes be necessary to ensure that the sexual lives of people with disabilities might be able to take form and be filled with content. Like the earlier report from the National Board of Social Services that resulted in the *Guidelines*—and sometimes using language taken verbatim from that report—the *Guidelines* document focuses on the most challenging cases. It is primarily concerned with people who were either born with impairments or acquired them at an early age. It discusses how children with disabilities do not always have the same possibilities as nondisabled children to move, play, and develop. The physical and emotional changes they experience when they enter puberty are frequently not engaged with by parents and others, who have a tendency to be overprotective, in ways that make it difficult for disabled children to participate in activities that will help them understand their bodies and their relationships with others.

Because people who grow up with disabilities have life experiences that differ from those of nondisabled people, helpers who work with and care for them cannot just sit around and wait for them to raise issues pertaining to sexuality, thinking that, if they do not, it means they have no sexual feelings or needs. Instead, helpers "should, with knowledge, affirmative attitudes, and *active behavior* [*aktiv adfærd*] in relation to the handicapped individual, tackle issues regarding sexuality" (emphasis added).[80] This should always be well-anchored in staff discussions, and it can be done through sexual education aimed at showing people how they can be sexual regardless of their disability, through conversations and exercises aimed at bolstering self-confidence and by following the modified version of Jørgen Buttenschøn's four-step strategy (the one in which parents were not included in the process and the plan for assistance was approved by the person being assisted). It should also be done, sometimes, and crucially, through "more direct assistance in the form of demonstrations or physical assistance" (*mere direkte støtte i form af demonstration eller fysisk støtte*).[81]

The precise content and character of that "physical assistance" and of the "sexual training," which the Ministry of Justice and the attorney general declared were not abuse, was one of the main areas of focus for one of the direct consequences of the *Guidelines* document; namely, the formation of a certification program for social workers and other staff who worked with people with disabilities and wanted to learn how to engage with issues pertaining to their sexuality. This program, called sexual advisor education (*seksualvej-lederuddannelse*), was what resulted from the Board of Social Services' recommendations about sexual counseling. The idea presented in the board's report was to expand the number of counseling centers, using the one in the town of Århus as a model. That never happened, but what developed instead was a course, run by Jørgen Buttenschøn and Karsten Løt, that helped an entire generation of social workers who worked with people with disabilities figure out what things like "physical assistance" and "sexual training" can actually mean in practice.

Sweden and the Road to "Individual Vibrator Adaptation for Woman Who Can Only Move Her Head"

The single most important difference between the way that issues about sexuality and disability came to be handled in Denmark and Sweden was in the kind of disabilities that were focused on by the people who came to engage themselves in those questions. As we have seen, in Denmark, women and men with physical disabilities debated sex robustly. Those discussions included considerations of how the sexual desires and needs of people with significant physical impairments might be engaged. One article, for example, discussed the experiences of some of the group's members who lived in institutions (*plejehjem*) where no sex life was possible. One man with muscular dystrophy suggested that the hospital should fire half of the cleaners and hire prostitutes instead, since "mental hygiene is more important than hygiene."[82] At the same time, individuals like Niels Erik Bank-Mikkelsen, Jørgen Buttenschøn, and the staff at Mose Allé school, who worked with adults who had intellectual disabilities, insisted that people with significant impairments must be the starting point for—rather than the forgotten shadow of or the abject exception to—discussions about sexuality.

All these reformers clearly perceived that for many people with impairments independence in itself was of limited value. Giving someone "one's own room, a key, and the right to be alone with one's visitors," as Swedish Gunnel Enby had argued, might be a fine solution for some people, but it would solve nothing for those who need active, empathetic intervention from knowledgeable, caring helpers in order to be able to understand sexuality and develop it in affirmative ways. The whole point of formulating guidelines regulating such engagement was to ensure that it could occur in open, respectful, nonexploitative, and nonabusive ways.

In Sweden, the people who engaged themselves in questions of sexuality and disability from the 1960s onward did not concern themselves with the kinds of individuals with intellectual impairments who were the focus of Bank-Mikkelsen's and Buttenschøn's reformist efforts. Like the Danish *Handi-Kamp* activists, Swedish reformers were almost exclusively concerned with physical disabilities. But unlike those Danish activists, the Swedes' focus was on rehabilitation and on people who had acquired disabilities, such as spinal cord injuries or disabilities resulting from degenerative conditions like multiple sclerosis. Karl Grunewald, who worked only with people with intellectual disabilities, was an exception to this, but as his later actions (which we will have more to say about in the next chapter) clearly demonstrated, his philosophy regarding sexuality and disability was pretty much summed up by the advice he offered parents at the end of the Apollonia meeting: "Don't burden [disabled people] with your own understandings, don't theorize, and don't poke around in things they haven't asked for your help with."

We have already mentioned Inger Nordqvist's work and how it was limited to trying to improve conditions for adults who had physical disabilities or mobility impairments. Besides Nordqvist, only one other key figure in Sweden active during this time deserves special mention: a physician in Stockholm named Claes Hultling. In 1984, shortly before his wedding, Hultling suffered a diving accident that left him paralyzed from the chest down. Prior to his injury, Hultling had worked as an anesthesiologist. After the accident, he and a neurologist colleague, Richard Levi, toured the United States and Australia to learn more about the rehabilitation of people who had suffered spinal cord injuries.

Five years later, in 1989, Hultling and Levi founded the Spinalis rehabilitation clinic just outside Stockholm. A feature of the clinic for which Hultling is well known is his insistence that sexuality is a crucial part of disabled people's lives. The Spinalis rehabilitation program includes sexual rehabilitation. In a 2003 television interview, Hultling recounted how, after working with men with spinal cord injuries, he grew so tired of trying out different erection aids on a gurney in a hospital room that he ordered a special room set up.

> I decorated it with a really nice Hästen bed, with a canopy and a little refrigerator and stereo, and dimmer and everything. The idea was that I would be able to try out sex aids with couples, and also that I could use it to check on semen analysis and that sort of thing. But first and foremost, it was a sex room. And so I called it the "Fuck Room" [*Knullrummet*]. But that was too much for the staff. I put up a sign outside the door, "Fuck Room," but the staff screwed it off the door and put it in my desk.[83]

Hultling has conducted research on sexuality and fertility in men with spinal cord injuries and was, himself, the first person in the country with his kind of spinal cord injury to father a child through in vitro fertilization. One of his primary areas of research interest is parenthood. "There is no single therapeutic intervention that has a more positive effect or influence on a young paraplegic man than to inspect his own sperm in the microscope," he told us. He compared looking at one's own sperm as a paraplegic to winning ten million kronor in the lottery.

Claes Hultling's insistence that sexuality is part of a disabled person's life and that resources spent on rehabilitation should include sexual rehabilitation has made him an important figure among people with acquired disabilities as well as among occupational therapists, counselors, and others who work with rehabilitation. But Hultling's interest and his influence in Sweden have remained largely confined to his target group, which is people like him— men and women who have suffered a spinal cord injury but who had experienced, because they were not disabled from birth, the same kinds of socialization as most other people in society. Such people are also articulate—they normally have verbal language and can make demands. Furthermore, they are people who either already have a partner or can conceivably find one on their own with little assistance, and certainly with no assistance from any third party, such as a personal assistant.

As happened in Denmark, the question of sex and disability eventually reached the national parliament in Sweden. But when it did, the discussion occurred in a very different register. In January 1985 two Members of Parliament from the Communist Party (Vänsterpartiet kommunisterna) proposed an initiative concerning sexuality and disability.

Like what happened in Denmark, the initiative in Sweden arose less from party politics than from one individual's engagement with sexual politics: the MP who drafted the motions, Margó Ingvardsson, had always been involved with sexual education, and five years later (during which time she left the Communist Party and became a Social Democrat), she became the executive director of the Swedish Association for Sexuality Education (Riksförbundet för Sexuell Upplysning, RFSU). The initiative that Ingvardsson and one of her colleagues proposed in parliament was about subsidized sex aids for people with disabilities. The justification for the proposal asserted that sex aids, like other assistive aids, can "extend the capacities" (*komplettera den egna förmågan*) of people with disabilities. However, the proposal said, sex aids are available to disabled people only through porn shops and mail-order catalogues. That situation needed to be remedied. The proposal, therefore, was to add sex aids to the list of assistive devices to disabled people that are subsidized by the state. If sex aids were subsidized, Ingvardsson and her colleague argued, doctors would feel more comfortable talking about them, and people with disabilities would feel more comfortable requesting and obtaining them.

The two MPs also proposed a second, related initiative, this one requiring all rehabilitation clinics to make sure that at least one employee is knowledgeable about sexuality, disability, and sex aids.[84]

These motions were sent to the Standing Committees on Social Affairs (Socialutskottet) and Social Insurance (Socialförsäkringsutskottet) for discussion. The Committee on Social Affairs recommended that the second proposal be dismissed because rehabilitation clinics ought to have the right to decide for themselves what personnel they needed. And besides, it was pointed out, there was already a person whose salary was paid by the state to coordinate information on sex and disability, namely, Inger Nordqvist.[85]

The first proposal, though, to subsidize sexual aids in the same way the state subsidized other assistive devices, was sent out for comment and evaluation to the country's two largest disability organizations,[86] the National Board of Social Health and Welfare and the Handicap Institute (a new government agency, to which Inger Nordqvist and her work had been transferred in 1980). Interestingly, the responses from disability organizations were tepid. This lack of enthusiasm partly reflected the disengagement of such organizations in the question of sexuality generally. But it also expressed an anxiety shared by many disabled people (Gunnel Enby, for example, raised it in *We Must Be Allowed to Love*), that any special consideration of the sexuality of people with disabilities amounted to a condescending proclamation that disabled people were unable to find partners in a "normal" manner. The National Association of the Handicapped (DHR) flatly rejected the idea that sex aids for people with disabilities should be a special concern of the state. Since people with disabilities could purchase such products just like anyone else, they wrote, there was no need for any special state intervention.[87]

Inger Nordqvist, perhaps unsurprisingly, was of a different view. On behalf of the Handicap Institute for which she now worked, she formulated a response that urged a broader investigation of the issue. It was not enough to say that that sex aids were available for purchase, Nordqvist wrote, because "mail-order companies' catalogues contain devices used in sadomasochist sexual relations, which further strengthens the feelings of being deviant in people who suffer from neurological injuries."[88]

The result of the responses received by the government was that the deputy minister of social affairs commissioned the Handicap Institute— which in practice meant Inger Nordqvist—to investigate the issue further and write a report on sex aids.[89] While Nordqvist was busy working on this report, however, the same minister who appointed her appointed *another* commission to research the question of assistive technologies, more generally, for people with disabilities. The Assistive Devices Commission consisted of eleven people, was given a generous budget, and was awarded the status of being included in what are called Official Government Inquiries (Statens Offentliga Utredningar). There was no contact or collaboration between Nordqvist's inquiry and the Assistive Devices Commission.

The Assistive Devices Commission published its results in 1989, one year after Nordqvist had finished and delivered her report. In one sentence, the commission mentions that Nordqvist's report had been passed on to them (they ignored it), and in another clause, toward the end of their text, they note that the Handicap Institute was running a project about "relations and sexuality."[90] That was the extent of what the commission had to say about sexuality in their 263-page report and 342 pages of appendices.

Such neglect in an official report whose explicit purpose was to improve the living conditions for people with disabilities is striking—and typical. Since the 1950s a number of government-appointed commissions in Sweden had produced reports that were crucial in gradually laying the groundwork for the comprehensive social insurance system that characterizes the country today. From the Invalid Care Commission of 1951, which presented its proposals in a 340-page report, to the Handicap Commission of 1965, which published five smaller reports and one final report about the participation in cultural life of people with disabilities (a total of 890 pages), to the Handicap Commission of 1989, which published fourteen reports of various length, totaling 2,492 pages, virtually no dimension of disabled people's lives was left unexamined by government commissions.[91]

Except sexuality.

There was, however, Inger Nordqvist's inquiry. To complete her investigation, Nordqvist gathered a twelve-person reference group consisting of sexologists and people appointed by disability organizations like the National Association of the Handicapped. She sent out a questionnaire asking doctors whether they had ever prescribed a sexual aid to anyone with a disability and, if so, whether it worked. She went on a month-long fact-finding mission to California, Texas, and New York to learn about new methods in sexual rehabilitation.

After two years of work Nordqvist was ready with her results and conclusions. Unlike the main report of the Assistive Devices Commission, which was published in a handsome volume embossed with the imprimatur of "Official Government Inquiry," Inger Nordqvist's report was never actually printed. It was typed on a typewriter, presumably by Nordqvist herself, and bound by her Handicap Institute as two booklets (the report and the appendices), with a cartoon drawing on the covers. The result looked unofficial and amateurish. The report itself listed a number of conclusions, including the recommendation that individuals who had disabilities that influenced their ability to function sexually be given free sexual aids. But the contrast between Nordqvist's hermitical battle for subsidized sexual aids and the coordinated, collaborative activities that were taking place at the same time across the Öresund sound in Denmark was absolute.

Whereas Danes, in 1988, were busy devising guidelines that emphasized the need for broad engagement with the sexuality of people with disabilities, Inger Nordqvist's primary recommendation, besides subsidized sex aids, was to keep the issue of sex and disability medicalized, bureaucratized, and under the control of specially educated authorities. She urged the creation

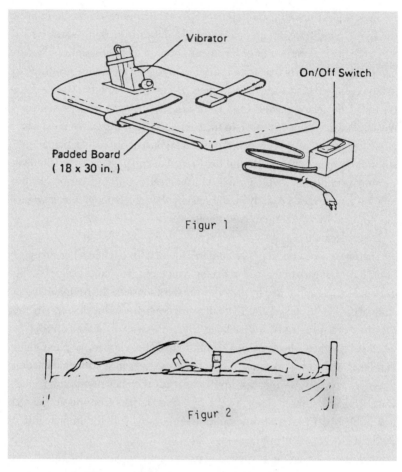

Vibrator

On/Off Switch

Padded Board
(18 x 30 in.)

Figur 1

Figur 2

2.3 "Individual vibrator adaptation for woman who can only move her head." From Inger Nordqvist, *Utredning om hjälpmedel i sexuallivet för män och kvinnor med funktionshinder* (Bromma: Handikappinstitutet, 1988), 57.

of a cadre of specialists (*ordinatörer*) to be educated by sexologists and by her. These specialists would be responsible for deciding whether or not individuals with disabilities were entitled to sexual aids. Those decisions, she proposed, would be based on "diagnostic reports [*utredningar*] on the reasons for the sexual difficulties experienced by each individual."[92] The kinds of sexual aids the specialists would be able to prescribe were illustrated in the appendices of her report. These occur complete with drawings, names ("KG Anal," "Impoex," "Vibrator Vagina Best"), descriptions of which kinds of sexual problems for which the aids are most appropriate ("men with spinal cord injuries," "rheumatism"), and Nordqvist's own evaluations of their effectiveness ("Vibrator's weight, 3 pounds (ca. 1.5 kg), necessitates hand strength in order to be used").[93]

In only one brief section of her report does Inger Nordqvist indicate an awareness of the existence of the kinds of people who had been at the center of Danish discussions of sex and disability from the start: the people who, for a variety of reasons, needed practical assistance to understand their sexuality, engage in erotic relationships, and experience sexual pleasure. Inger Nordqvist mentions such people in two sentences. She concedes that they are "in principle, a large group."[94] However, rather than consider the implications that such a large group of disabled adults might have for her intractable focus on sex aids, as opposed to other forms of engagement, her solution to the problem that such individuals present was to build special sex aids especially for them. She illustrates one under the rubric "Individual vibrator adaptation for woman who can only move her head."

Nowhere in Nordqvist's report is there even the faintest clue about the kinds of discussions that might precede an "adaptation" like this: of how a woman who can only move her head would ever come to express an interest in such a contraption; of who would build or procure it; of how and to whom the woman would indicate that she wanted to use it; of who would prepare the apparatus, undress the woman, and position her on it; of who would monitor that it worked; of who would clean up afterward. Those questions—the actual practices of engagement and assistance that so occupied the Danes—are nowhere considered in Nordqvist's report.

Instead, in an image that is a concentration of everything that came to characterize the Swedish approach to sexuality and disability, we are presented with a disembodied mechanical aid and a passive, faceless figure: controlled, undemanding, isolated, and alone.

CHAPTER 3 :: how to impede and how to facilitate
the erotic lives of people with disabilities

As we explained in the introductory chapter, Don did not conduct ethnographic fieldwork in Sweden. We wanted to understand "best practices"—
that is, we wanted to document situations where the erotic feelings and
sexual lives of people with disabilities were acknowledged and facilitated,
not ignored and impeded. And we could find no one in Sweden who
could suggest a single group home anywhere in the country that had policies and practices resembling anything we found in Denmark. What this
means is that if you are a person with a disability in Sweden who needs
help to engage in sexual activity, and you do not have a partner who can
help you, the chances are very great that you will never be able to have a
sexual life.

Any erotic desire you wish to express will likely be dealt with in one of
three ways: it will be ignored, disciplined, or classified as a problem and
then passed on to someone who others think may know how to handle it.
That person, in turn, will pass on "the problem" to someone else, and so
on, with the result that "the problem" will likely end up being dealt with
by the final arbiter either pretending it has been solved (that is, by ignor-

ing it) or by disciplining the adult whose actions constitute the perceived problem.

How Sexuality Is Ignored

Here is an example of how the sexuality of a person with a severe impairment is ignored. Viktoria is a young woman in her early twenties who is employed by a Swedish county as a personal assistant. She told the following story. One of the people she cares for is a young man who has what she referred to, using the English expression, as "locked-in syndrome." She explained that this means that he is "clear in the head, but he is completely paralyzed from top to bottom and he can't move anything, he can't say a word and the only thing he can move is his eyelids." She said he can communicate by moving his eyes: to signal "yes" he looks up; for "no," he looks down.

This young man has his room covered with posters and pictures of Marilyn Monroe. "You know," Viktoria said, "those pretty pictures where you see her cleavage, and you see a lot. He lies there and looks up at those pictures." Viktoria said the young man also communicates by making bellowing sounds when something displeases him. And when he likes something, he laughs: "Whenever we watch a film together he smiles, and he laughs as soon as someone kisses someone else. And as soon as any kind of sex scene appears on television, he laughs and laughs."

Every week this young man has a visit from a masseur. Viktoria has noticed that the man obviously enjoys the visits and the physical contact with the masseur—"it's not the kind of massage where the masseur pounds and digs; it's more a massage where he touches him and strokes his back. I can see that that is the thing he likes most. It must be just the fact that he gets that kind of physical closeness with somebody." Having witnessed the massage sessions and the young man's reaction to them, Viktoria surmises that he has feelings in his body. And, she said, "I can't imagine that he doesn't have feelings of attraction for people. But he can't say anything. And it's very frustrating; what can we do? We can't ask him."

"Why can't you ask him?" Don asked Viktoria.

"We are ordered not to talk about sex," she replied. "We're not allowed to discuss anything that is too private—that's the way it is formulated. We can't ask about anything private. If they want to tell me about it, that's OK."

And she laughed. "But come on," she said. "How is this man supposed to tell me about anything private?"

How Sexuality Is Disciplined

One example of how the sexuality of people with disabilities is disciplined in Sweden can be found in the advice that is given to deal with a situation in which a man gets an erection during a bath or when one is changing his trousers or his diaper. One woman recounted that, "in the surgery clinic in Uppsala, there was a new nursing assistant who came into the staff room all out of breath and flustered. 'Oh, this, this, this thing, these erections. It's stressful [*jobbigt*] when it stands up.'

"And the head nurse looked at her and said, 'Just take the palm of your hand and hit it at the base. It'll lie down.'"

Another woman who worked in a rehabilitation center said the advice she was given in such situations was to press the nail of her middle finger against the inside of her thumb and flick the offending penis with a quick painful strike. A third woman who worked as a personal assistant told us that the advice passed along the grapevine to her was, "If you're washing a man and he gets an erection, you press the nerve and it goes down. You grip it right under the head, under the ridge, and press with two fingers." This maneuver has a name that many people who work with disabled men apparently know. The name is, *penisdödargreppet*, "the penis-killer grip."

Another example of how sexuality is disciplined is taken from an ethnographic study of a Norwegian group home for people with intellectual disabilities—but from everything we have learned, the same kinds of discussions and practices occur in many similar group homes in Sweden. Anthropologist Marit Sundet observed that the staff in the group home she worked in regarded sexuality as something they had no real competence to deal with or even discuss. They also regarded the residents' sexuality as fundamentally different from their own. The staff's own sexuality, Sundet says, was perceived by them to be "natural, but private." The sexuality of the people who lived in the group home, on the other hand, was seen as "unnatural, but public."[1]

The residents' sexuality was "unnatural" because the staff couldn't figure out its character. They thought that most residents didn't understand sexual intercourse or that they couldn't or didn't want to experience it. One female resident who did have sex with different men worried the staff. Even though there was no evidence that the woman did not welcome the visitors she received in her room, individual staff members thought she was probably being used by the men, and they discussed whether and how they should stop the visits.[2]

The sexuality of the group home's residents was "public" partly because they had virtually no privacy. They had rooms of their own but they frequently left their doors open or unlocked, and members of the staff just as frequently walked into their rooms whenever they felt like it (which is how staff discovered that the woman just mentioned was having sex with the men who visited her). Some residents also masturbated in the public spaces, or they used sexualized language. These actions provoked reprimands from the staff.

The staff avoided speaking about sexuality, says Sundet, because they considered it an "intimate topic that they didn't want to get involved in [blande med] in their jobs." The absence of any serious discussion about sexuality led the staff in the group home to define the residents' sexuality partly in terms of their own moral convictions and partly in terms of problems that needed to be solved.[3] The solutions to those problems tended to be either direct reprimands or aversion techniques that Sundet labels "taming" (dressere).[4]

Sundet describes the case of one male resident who rubbed his crotch and sometimes began to masturbate in the communal living room. The staff handled this by having everyone agree to ask him, whenever they saw him rubbing his crotch in the living room, whether he wanted to remain with the others or continue what he was doing—in which case he had to go to his room. He usually indicated that he wanted to continue and so would be ordered to go to his room. Sundet observed that dealing with the young man's actions in this way created a situation where not only did he quickly learn how to get staff members to pay attention to him whenever he wanted but also the staff, instead of helping the young man be more social, instead, in practice, habitually encouraged him to go off and masturbate.[5]

How the Buck Gets Passed on Sexual Problems

Finally, here is an example of how "the problem" of disabled people's sexuality gets passed on to experts who pass it on to others, and so on, until "the problem" is resolved either by ignoring it or by disciplining the person who is the cause of the problem. In Sweden, there is a cadre of professionals who are educated to work with people with disabilities, and with individuals who have sexual problems. In addition to people like doctors and psychologists, there are social workers (kuratorer or socialarbetare) who counsel people with disabilities and help them navigate the social welfare bureaucracy; there are physical therapists (sjukgymnaster) who help heal physical injuries and rehabilitate bodies; sexologists (sexologer) who specialize in helping individuals improve the physical aspects of sexual lives, with advice about vacuum pumps, medical interventions, or mechanical aids; and there are occupational therapists (*arbetsterapeuter*) who help devise solutions to practical problems like how one can get into bed after an accident or how one can eat by oneself if one has limited mobility in one's arms.

Most of the people who work in these different professions are told during their studies that in order to meet the needs of the people who will seek them out for help they have to have a holistic perspective (*helhetsperspektiv*)—that is, they need to know something about the many different fields of expertise that are relevant to assisting people with disabilities. In practice, though, each group becomes specialized in particular areas. Whenever anyone who comes to them for help needs assistance with anything outside their specific area of expertise, they pass them on to others who have other specializations.

In this web of specializations, many kinds of sexual issues that concern people with disabilities fall between the cracks. Krister Andersson is an occupational therapist, one of the very few in the country who has also completed nearly a year's worth of courses in sexology. He explained how the buck constantly gets passed in Sweden. Most professionals who meet individuals with disabilities decline to raise sexual issues at all, he said. His colleagues avoid talking about sex with disabled people because they define it as a private concern that has nothing to do with them. Sex may sometimes arise in conversations with individuals who have recently acquired a disability, such as a broken neck, because one of the first things that many of those people wonder is whether they will ever be able to have sex again. For people with spinal cord injuries there is counseling, literature, and physical therapy available to help them regain some of their previous sexual functionality, particularly at places like the Spinalis rehabilitation clinic that we mentioned in the previous chapter. But conversations about sex with individuals who have congenital disabilities, such as cerebral palsy or intellectual impairments, occur only very rarely.[6]

Whenever anybody with a disability does raise the issue of sex with a professional they see frequently and have come to trust—a physical therapist or an occupational therapist, for example—a typical response is to refer that person to a sexologist for help. Andersson explained:

> So they'll be sent to a sexologist, who won't have the vaguest idea what to do, because it isn't a sexological problem:
> "Does your vagina work right? Is there lubrication?"
> "Yeah."

"Does your penis work? Do you get erections?"

"Yeah."

"Well then, how do you think I can help you?"

"Because it isn't working."

"Well that's another problem. Talk to a physical therapist or your occupational therapist."

"But you see?" Andersson said, "That person's physical therapist or occupational therapist is the one who sent the poor guy or the poor woman to the sexologist in the first place."

Because Andersson both is an occupational therapist and has studied some sexology, he gets called to group homes to devise interventions on issues that involve sex. Most cases involve staff wanting to pass onto him a problem they don't want to deal with themselves. He recounted a time he was called to a group home for people with intellectual disabilities and mobility impairments. He traveled there and met the director, and they had the following conversation:

"Yeah, we have a man who masturbates at the dinner table, and it's a problem that has to be solved."

"Wait a minute. Does it hurt him when he does it?"

"What?"

"Does he hurt himself when he masturbates? Does he use a knife or some kind of implement?"

"No . . ."

"What does he use?"

"He uses his hand."

"Does he look like he's enjoying himself?"

"Yeah . . ."

"Well then it isn't a sexual problem. He seems to manage perfectly well."

"Yes, but it's a problem."

"Yeah, but it's a social problem."

"You mean you think we're the ones who have to solve it?!"

"They wanted me to make him stop," Andersson said, "because they didn't want to have to deal with it." Andersson told Don that the subtext of the entire visit was, "You're the one who has to do this because we don't want to touch it; we don't even want to have to say the word 'dick' [*snopp*]."

"Don't Wake the Sleeping Bear"

When Swedish professionals, social workers, and caregivers discuss the sexuality of significantly disabled individuals, two phrases tend to come up frequently. The first is the proverb "Don't wake the sleeping bear" (*Väck inte den björn som sover*). The second is the adage "If I don't do anything, at least I haven't done anything wrong" (*Om jag inte gör något så har jag i alla fall inte gjort något fel*).

The first of these two sayings is the Swedish equivalent of the English-language proverb "Let sleeping dogs lie"—don't draw attention to something that isn't seeking it. Here the idea is that disabled people's sexuality is not something that necessarily naturally expresses itself. This might be because the person with the disability either doesn't understand that he or she has erotic desire, or because the desire the person may have is satisfied in ways that do not involve genital eroticism, such as by hugging, holding hands, or by giving people kisses on the cheek. In cases like these, for anybody to raise the issue of sexuality—for example, in educational programs, group discussions, or private conversations—is to project his or her own sexuality onto a sexually innocent individual and thereby risk awakening in that person an unasked-for desire that can manifest in unforeseen, unhappy, and possibly even uncontrollable ways.

The belief that the sexuality of people with congenital disabilities is like a sleeping bear best left unperturbed is an old one—and one that is far from limited to Sweden. In the debates of the 1960s and 1970s in Denmark that ultimately led to the adoption of the *Guidelines about Sexuality—Regardless of Handicap*, opposition to social workers involving themselves in the sexuality of people with intellectual impairments frequently invoked "sleeping bear" reasoning, even if critics did not use the Swedish proverb. In 1969, in the professional journal *Civil Servant Magazine* (*Funktionærbladet*), for example, the director of an institution for people with intellectual impairments expressed shock that the staff at Mose Allé school had publicly raised the issue of how one might help intellectually disabled people masturbate. "I don't believe that we can just assume that the severely feebleminded's sexual needs are like the retarded's or the normal's [*at den dybt åndssvages seksuelbehov er lig den debiles eller normales*]," he wrote. "If we now try to force onto the severely mentally feebleminded [*påføre den dybt åndssvage*] an unwanted sexual relationship, don't we let loose forces that can't be controlled . . . ?"[7]

In the same issue of that journal, another director of an institution, S. Jørgensen, addressed the issue of masturbation with these words: "In the more than 20 years that I have worked with the feebleminded, I have never been confronted with pupils who haven't been able to find another form of satisfaction. (And if they haven't, I doubt that they have the need.) . . . If pupils can't eat by themselves, they get fed. That is quite simply a necessity so that they can live. But if the same group can't learn to masturbate themselves, it is definitely not a condition of life that they should be taught how to do it."[8]

We saw in the previous chapter that these kinds of objections to exposing people with intellectual impairments to sexual education and counseling were vigorously contested in Denmark by engaged individuals like Niels Erik Bank-Mikkelsen, Jørgen Buttenschøn, and the authors of the 1968 open letter from the Mose Allé school. During the course of the 1970s and 1980s those more progressive voices won the day. The belief that talking about sex with intellectually impaired people constituted an unsavory projection at best and a form of sexual abuse at worst came to be replaced with the conviction that sexual education was important even for people with intellectual impairments and that assistance in discovering activities like masturbation could be both permissible and desirable.

It would not be too much of an exaggeration to say that, on this point, Sweden today is where Denmark was forty years ago. Among individuals who work with people with disabilities in Sweden there is a widespread view that sex is best not considered or discussed with a disabled person unless that person has explicitly raised the topic, either through questions or comments or through some unmistakable and usually unacceptable action, like masturbation at the dining table or an attempt to feel up a staff member. As in Marit Sundet's Norwegian study that we discussed earlier, in Sweden there is a pervasive sense that the sexual drives of congenitally disabled adults— especially adults with intellectual impairments—are different from those of nondisabled people. For the most part, they are considered infantile. But once stirred, they can be volatile and difficult to control.

Social work researcher Lotta Löfgren-Mårtenson has documented how staff members who accompany young adults with intellectual impairments to evening dances staged especially for them (dances that always start at 7 PM and end promptly three hours later at 10 PM, in well-lit venues, with no alcoholic beverages on offer) survey the dancing couples and intervene if they observe that certain couples are dancing together for too long, for example, by going up to them and telling them it is time for a coffee break. They are tolerant of hugging or cuddling on the dance floor or in the surrounding area, but more overt behavior often leads to what Löfgren-Mårtenson calls "distracting maneuvers" or to reprimands. This surveillance and policing, she says, is grounded partly in an uncertainty about what kinds of sexual activities young people with intellectual impairments are actually capable of, and partly out of a concern that any form of sexual activity might be unwanted, or not fully understood, by the participants. This results in a default attitude that sexual activity should be prevented, "just in case" (*utifall att*).[9]

This perception of intellectually disabled people's sexuality as innocent and vulnerable determines the resistance encountered by anyone wishing to discuss sexuality or educate them about it. The Swedish sexologist Margareta Nordeman told us about an argument she had over this issue in the mid-1990s with prominent Swedish experts on disability. Nordeman was at a conference on disability and spoke about the films she was making with the support of the Swedish Association for Sexuality Education (RFSU) about masturbation for women and men with intellectual disabilities. These films, which we discuss in detail in the next chapter, consist of three scenes in which a nondisabled man masturbates to orgasm and three scenes where a nondisabled woman does the same thing. Nordeman said the response to her presentation was scathing. One of the experts snapped at her, "If they can't masturbate themselves, that means they don't need it, and it's something that no one under any circumstances should get involved with [*det ska man över huvud taget inte lägga sig i*]."

"But if a person can't feed themselves, and we see that the person has the possibility to learn how to eat, isn't it our responsibility to try to help that person?" Nordeman asked her critic.

Invoking a version of the same argument that the Danish director S. Jørgensen had used in his letter to the journal *Civil Servant Magazine* twenty-five years earlier, this man replied, "Yeah, yeah, but there's a difference. Masturbation is private."

"If I Don't Do Anything, at Least I Haven't Done Anything Wrong"

The second formulation that occurs very frequently in Sweden when sex and disability is discussed among personal assistants and others who work with disabled adults is the mantra "If I don't do anything, at least I haven't done anything wrong." The attitude encapsulated by this adage is related to the "just in case" perception that allowing or facilitating sex is potentially harmful to people with disabilities because they may not understand the implications of sexual activity. Rather than offer any help to understand those implications, it is better not to do anything, "just in case." The "not doing anything" part of the "If I don't do anything . . ." formulation is misleading, however, because personal assistants, staff in group homes, and others who use the phrase do not actually do nothing. The "nothing" they believe themselves to be doing is actually "something," usually something that discourages sex or impedes it. This can take the form of interrupting an intertwined couple on the dance floor and telling them it is time for a coffee break, or it can be as simple as following instructions not to raise the topic of sexuality with someone who might want to discuss it, as in the case with personal assistant Viktoria and the man with "locked-in syndrome" who likes Marilyn Monroe.

"Not doing anything" has many other manifestations—from refusing to insert a pornographic DVD into a DVD player to declining to assist a couple with mobility impairments who need help to lie together and caress each other. "Not doing anything" is grounded, again, in uncertainty over whether disabled people really understand sexuality or whether one has really understood what the disabled person wants in regard to his or her sexuality. But, significantly, it is also grounded in fear. This heavily affect-laden word was mentioned with surprising frequency in the discussions about sex and disability we had with people in Sweden. Social workers and experts spoke of themselves and others as being afraid to even broach the topic of sex with disabled adults, let alone offer them any assistance. A few people suggested that the fear they observed was a general anxiety about sexuality. "I think that Swedish society is undeveloped when it comes to sexuality," one Swedish sexologist told us. "We think we're free from prejudices, but we're afraid of something. I don't think things are the way they are because people are stupid. I think they're the way they are because sexuality involves strong forces that we don't know how to deal with." A Swedish occupational therapist who had experience working in both Sweden and Denmark said that she had reflected many times on how Swedes seem to have a "naked fear" (*hudlös rädsla*) when it comes to talking about intimate matters—a fear she says she did not encounter in Denmark.

Most others we spoke with identified the fear that they said characterized Swedish attitudes toward sexuality and disability as having two root causes. The first is a worry that one's colleagues will talk if one pays attention to the erotic lives of the disabled people one works with. The second, related, reason for the fear is the concern that any attention to the sexuality of people with disabilities can easily be interpreted as sexual abuse.

In a conversation about sex and disability with four social workers who work in a health clinic that provides information and counseling about sexuality for young people (*ungdomsmottagning*), one of the staff members commented, "Everyone's so afraid of doing something wrong" (*så rädda att göra fel*). Her co-worker elaborated,

> Well that's because of the general hysteria, you know, that someone is going to report one. So obviously one gets afraid that one has contributed to something that suddenly gets seen as being wrong. Then I turn into a shit [*då blir ju jag en skit*], and one doesn't want that. You do something that you agree on and that you thought was right and then it goes wrong and then I become a dirty old git who has behaved badly [*en snuskmänniska som har betett mig illa*]. I can really understand why people don't do anything; I really can.

This fear that if one engages with a disabled person's sexuality one will be seen by others as a "dirty old git" was mentioned by many others we spoke to. A counselor in the south of Sweden who specializes in sexuality and disability told us, "We're so terribly afraid [*frukstansvärt rädda*]. . . . I think it might have something to do with the fact that people have personal difficulty with it, you know? But I don't think that's the biggest reason. The biggest reason is that I think that people are afraid of what others will say, you know, like, 'Why is he doing this?'"

The fear also surfaced in a discussion with Bettan, a Swede with a disability who earns part of her living by giving public lectures about what it means to live with a disability. Bettan described a talk she had given just a few weeks previously at a company that employs personal assistants for disabled people. She is friends with the woman who owns this company, and her friend had asked Bettan to come and talk to the employees about sexuality. Nearly thirty people turned up, and Bettan led a group discussion focused on sexual situations that might arise in their work—for example, disabled couples who might want help to be able to lie together or a person needing assistance who goes out to a club and wants to come home with someone he or she met there.

Bettan chuckled when she described what happened. "Moral panic broke out," she said. "People started shouting. 'No way in hell would I ever help anyone with sex; that's my damn boundary, and I'd never . . .'" She said people insisted that anyone who did assist disabled people with sex must be a *pervo* (pervert) or a *snusk* (dirty old git). "What kind of turn on do they get out of helping them?" several of those present demanded to know.

Bettan said she told the assistants that she thought it was unfortunate they were so worked up, and so adamant, about the issue because the tone they set made it impossible to have a reasoned discussion. "I hope you all understand," she said, "that you've now raised the bar so high that if there is anybody sitting here who might think differently than those of you who are talking, they aren't going to say a word, because you've all already defined them as perverts."

And that is exactly what happened. The group reached the consensus that anything having to do with sex was beyond the bounds of personal assistance and that anyone who had another viewpoint was disgusting (*skitäcklig*).

Bettan told this story wearily because, she said, she was used to that reaction whenever she spoke in situations like that about sex. But Bettan was also used to individuals in the audience coming up to her after her talks to have a private conversation. Those individuals are the ones silenced by the overheated public discussion. The usual pattern, she said, is that someone approaches her after her talk and starts talking about how inspiring they thought she was. If the person sticks around, as soon as others are out of hearing, Bettan has learned that she should ask him or her if there was anything in particular in what she said that resonated with his or her experiences. "And then it comes out," she told Don.

> Like I had one guy who told me that he worked for a young woman, twenty-five or twenty-six, something like that. And she expressed erotic feelings [*hon uttryckte en kåthet*] when she lay in bed. "I feel all tingly." And they discussed it, or talked about it in some way, and she said to him, "If you would just rub me there on top of the blanket, just nicely, I wouldn't have anything against it. But I understand if you don't want to do it." He said, "I don't have a problem with it."

Bettan said that what this young man wants—what everyone who comes up to her to confide stories like this wants—is confirmation that they are *not* the disgusting perverts that the disapproving chorus of the group discussion they have just listened to has decided they must be. And sensing the shame and the guilt that the people who come up to her after these discussions are trying to work through, Bettan is usually happy to bestow her blessing, as a kind of tiny reward for noticing that disabled people have an erotic life. She sometimes asks questions that she thinks the person seeking her benediction might want to consider. In the case of the man rubbing the young woman nicely through the blanket, for example, she asked him whether there were any feelings involved. Could it be that the woman was in love with him?

"No, I don't think so," the young man answered.

"How do you know?"

"That's something you know."

Answers like that worry Bettan, because she regards them as troubling evidence that people like this young man have no support at their workplace or probably anywhere else. They are isolated and alone, which makes them deeply vulnerable should anything go wrong. A young man like this, she told Don, is in real danger. "He is walking a fine line. He is in a real risk zone. If what he was doing ever became public it would be a story about how he was sexually abusing that woman. What he described to me wasn't even in the ballpark of sexual abuse. But that's not how it would go down if it became public."

Sexual abuse is the ominous greasy haze that hangs over relationships between people with disabilities and the individuals who assist them. Non-disabled helpers, especially male helpers, are very vulnerable to charges of sexual abuse. Helpers and caregivers do of course sometimes sexually abuse the people they are paid to assist. How much this happens is hard to know—statistics are difficult to come by and unreliable, and from what is known, it seems that disabled women are far more likely to be subjected to abuse at the hand of their husbands or their relatives than from paid service providers.[10] But regardless of actual occurrence, the widespread perception that people with congenital disabilities are childlike and innocent with regard to sex means that they, like children, are imagined to be inherently vulnerable to sexual predation by those who care for them.

People with disabilities—especially, again, men—also come under fire. Every year men with disabilities are fined in Swedish courts for sexually harassing or abusing the female personal assistants who work with them. A typical story, this one reported in the newspaper *Örnsköldsviks Allehanda* in 2010, looks like this:

PERSONAL ASSISTANTS SEXUALLY ABUSED
Part of the job as a personal assistant was to massage the wheelchair-borne man's back. The daily massage often ended with sexual approaches and intimate actions by the man. Four female assistants reported him to

the police in the end, and now he has been found guilty in Ångerman-land's county court of sexual abuse. . . .

During the trial, the man denied having committed any crime. He explained the fact that his hand moved up and down during the massages by saying that he has spasms in his back, neck, and arms. The county court found the man to be guilty of sexual abuse. However, the court's chairman [lagman], Peter Svedberg, dissented. He believed that it couldn't be ruled out that the man moved involuntarily and spastically because of his disability. The penalty was a hefty 100 daily fines à 200 kr. [= 20,000 kronor or US$3,000]. In addition, the man was ordered to pay each of the four plaintiffs 5,000 kronor [US$750] in damages.[11]

Sexual harassment and abuse of workers by people with disabilities is also a topic that gets ventilated on websites like personligassistent.com, which has a discussion board where people who work as personal assistants for disabled people ask questions and comment on their jobs. Sexual harassment comes up in these discussions in relation to

- telephone sex ("My wife works as a personal assistant, and today she was subjected to something that I think is completely twisted [förryckt]! The person she assists had loud telephone sex, and he used something that vibrated for TWENTY minutes! My poor wife is completely devastated [knäckt] and feels like she's been subjected to an attack. She sat on the other side of the room; a wall separated them, that was all.")
- looking at pornographic magazines ("I think there's some kind of prosthetic aid that can turn pages. Otherwise maybe there's some kind of cover you can put the porn magazine in so that the assistant can turn the pages without having to see it.")
- watching pornographic films ("It can actually be regarded as sexual harassment or sexual abuse to have a porn film on a volume so high that someone else can hear it.")
- unwanted comments or behavior ("The person I assist has begun touching me [småta på mig] every now and again. Takes the opportunity to stroke my back when I help put on trousers, comes and puts an arm around me sometimes, etc.")

Also common are disputes over things like pornographic images in the disabled person's home. An occupational therapist we interviewed told a story of how he once helped a young man with cerebral palsy, at the young man's suggestion, cut out pictures of female genitalia from pornographic magazines and paste them on the buttons of a remote control he used to change the channel on his television and perform a number of other functions. This created an uproar among the personal assistants who cared for the young man. They complained that they were being sexually harassed by being exposed to offensive sexual images in their workplace. That their workplace happened to be the young man's home was considered to be beside the point. The conflict only ended when the young man succumbed to the pressure and asked the occupational therapist to draw bikini bottoms on all of the pictures.

That so much anxiety and conflict can arise over issues like these is a result of the fact that there are almost never any clear-cut policies regarding what helpers or personal assistants can or cannot do in regard to sexuality. Löfgren-Mårtenson reports that a main reason why staff members actively intervene in situations where two young people with intellectual impairments are alone is because "they don't really know what rules apply, and they're uncertain about whether they're even allowed to leave a young person with an intellectual impairment alone with someone else. The uncertainty is especially intense when it comes to situations that are potentially sexual." And so they distract or lead them away from each another, "just in case."[12]

A senior-level manager at a large company that hires personal assistants for people with disabilities told us that in 2009 her company was phoned up by a Swedish television program that wanted to arrange a discussion about sexuality and disability. They asked if the company could send someone to talk about its policy regarding sex. The phone call "was a real hot potato," this manager told us:

> Everyone kept passing it on to someone else. Finally the call ended up with a colleague who was interested in the whole question but who never got any kind of response whenever she tried to talk about it.
>
> So at a staff meeting she said, "Yeah, we can go on television and talk about our policy." But the whole problem was that when they rang and asked us, we realized that we didn't have any policy.
>
> "Oh yes, we have a policy," she said.
>
> "Oh?" and everyone looked around at each other like big question marks.
>
> "We have an ostrich policy. We stick our heads in the sand and pretend like we don't see or hear any of these questions."

Swedish social work researcher Julia Bahner confirms that this kind of "ostrich policy" is the rule in Sweden. There is little or no information about sexuality for people who work as personal assistants. The job is badly paid and has low status; people who do it receive little or no training; and the only courses ever offered to develop any skills are courses that focus on things like how to lift people safely or how to perform emergency first aid. How can personal assistants be expected to deal with issues of sexuality in a professional manner, Bahner asks, "when there is no profession to seek guidance from?"[13]

If policies regarding sexuality do exist, they emphasize avoiding the topic, except when it comes to teaching women to say "no" to sex. The instructions that Viktoria, the young woman who worked as a personal assistant to the man with "locked-in syndrome," received from her employer—that sexuality is "private" and not an appropriate topic for discussion—is an example of the most common kind of guidelines that helpers receive in Sweden. People who work with and assist disabled adults are encouraged not to notice or discuss signs of sexual expression. When Viktoria told her boss she wasn't sure how to handle the fact that one of the young men she assisted got erections when she washed him, she was instructed to "just ignore it. Pretend it isn't happening."

Karin, a personal assistant interviewed by Julia Bahner, talked about how she used to accompany a man she assisted to the local swimming pool. She noticed that he greatly enjoyed looking at the young women in bikinis, but she told Bahner that she "didn't experience this as anything sexual because of his severe impairments."[14] This enforced pattern of not-noticing sexuality, of not-seeing it, of not-talking about it, of pretending that it doesn't exist makes it virtually impossible for personal assistants or staff members in a group home to discuss sexuality, even among themselves. This leads to the isolation of anyone who does notice it, which can lead, in turn, to suspicions of prurient interest or perversion if that person decides to engage with it in any way or attempts to get others to take notice of it too. Needless to say, staff resistance to acknowledging the sexuality of the people they assist also makes it difficult or impossible for residents of a group home, or an adult who has personal assistants, to raise the topic in a way that does not immediately risk being heard as an infringement or an abuse.

Swedish ethnologist Åse Linder interviewed four female staff members who worked in a group home for adults with slight intellectual impairments in a suburb of Stockholm. She asked the women if they could give her any examples of times they brought up the issue of sexuality with residents of the group home and discussed it in a positive way. The response to her question was that the women did not see it as their job to talk about sex because sex, they told her, is private. But they did actively raise the issue when they saw things they didn't approve of. A staff member told Linder, "One woman here was an easy target for men. Men from outside the group home. And in that case, you know, we told her about AIDS and that she shouldn't pick up unknown men or let herself be seduced by them [*lockas av dem*]. It was like, we had to take a stand." Linder concludes from stories like this that the only sexuality that ever actually got talked about in the group home she studied seemed to be sex that residents were told they should protect themselves against.

"Negative sexuality," she calls it.[15]

In Another Part of Köping

If the picture we have been painting of sex and disability in Sweden appears bleak, it is perhaps important to say at this point that it is not the case that expressions of intimacy between people with disabilities are completely impossible. Relationships and even sex can occur. But they can only occur under certain conditions. The nature of those conditions is clearly glimpsed in a Swedish reality series titled *In Another Part of Köping* (*I en annan del av Köping*). The titular Köping (pronounced "Shupping") is a small town of about eighteen thousand people located an hour-and-a-half's drive from the capital city, Stockholm. The series first aired in 2007 and continued for two more seasons, in 2008 and 2010. It describes itself as follows:

> A group home. Four friends. A series about dreams and longing.
> *In Another Part of Köping* is about longing, love, and dreams [*längtan, kärlek och drömmar*]. But also about worries and disappointments and about the anxiety that one can feel before a dance in the town square [*Folkets Park*]. About how important it is to win even if you're just bowling for fun, about how much and how intensely one can long for one's mother sometimes. And about the dream of at some point finding Mr. Right [*den rätte*].[16]

The four friends mentioned in the description are three men (ages twenty-five, thirty-three, and forty-four when the first season was produced) and one woman (thirty-three years old) who live together in a group home for people with intellectual impairments. The exact nature of their impairments is never discussed, and this is one of the features of the series that critics and viewers liked—the show focuses on the protagonists' personalities rather than their disabilities. The youngest of the four, though, obviously has Down syndrome. This young man is also the only one of the group who has no real verbal language. The other three are verbally articulate, and they are also mobile, though the woman uses a walker.

The program follows these four co-residents during the summer months. It shows them doing things like eating dinner together in their group home, going on a bus trip to Stockholm with other disabled adults, having coffee with their parents, celebrating one another's birthdays, bowling, and going to dances for people with disabilities arranged by the county where they live. Each program is about twenty-two minutes long, and each season consists of six episodes that aired once a week. *In Another Part of Köping* was extremely popular. Several episodes were seen by more than a million viewers (that is, one in nine people in the country), and the first season was awarded a Kristallen, the Swedish equivalent of an Emmy Award, in the categories of best documentary and best program.

In Another Part of Köping is narrated by Linda Hammar, the sole female in the group. Linda is a chubby woman with short hair and big glasses who is indefatigably happy. She punctuates virtually every sentence she utters with laughter. Much of the charm of the series is Linda's unflappable good cheer, and much of the dramatic tension is generated by her search for love: the "longing, love, and dreams" mentioned in the series' description are mostly hers. "The thing I think about most these days is probably guys [*killar*]," Linda informs viewers early on in the first episode. "It's been a bit messy [*lite struligt*] on that front lately."

During the course of the first season, Linda decides that she is in love with her fellow housemate, Mats, after she has a dream in which they are a couple. She informs Mats that she is in love with (*kär i*) him, and then she announces to her fellow housemates, her parents, and everyone else she meets that she and Mats are together. Mats—a gentle, John Goodman–sized thirty-three-year-old man—acquiesces to Linda's decision, and the two become acknowledged by others as a couple. This relationship is one of the main narrative arcs of the entire first and second seasons (the other is Mats's efforts to get a driving license). It is given very little air time in the third season, perhaps because it apparently never ended up amounting to much. Mats is clearly much more interested in the car he ends up buying than in Linda, and the few third-season scenes that show the couple alone together highlight Mats's discomfort and Linda's dissatisfaction more than they depict any feelings of romance or love.

But whether or not it was ultimately a source of satisfaction for either of them, the way that Linda and Mats's relationship is portrayed in the series is iconic of the form that a romantic relationship for people with disabilities is permitted to take in Sweden. Both Mats and Linda are charismatic and verbally articulate. They can clearly state their likes and dislikes. Even though Linda uses a walker, both she and Mats are also mobile. Neither of them expresses a desire to have any kind of erotic or romantic relationship with someone who is not disabled. Mats is not a man of many words, and he says little about his relationship with Linda. But Linda is prolix, and the way she giggles excitedly and happily announces to anyone who will listen that she has a boyfriend has the effect of making her sound more like a preadolescent girl reveling in a first crush than a thirty-three-year-old adult woman talking about a romantic partner.[17] This ingenuousness frames Linda and Mats's relationship as innocent and cute—and probably asexual.[18]

In Another Part of Köping plays up "longing, love and dreams," but it plays down sex. There are a couple of brief scenes at various points in the series of people with disabilities giving each other pecks on the mouth in public spaces, like well-lit dance floors and communal living rooms. And once, in the final program of the second season, Linda gives Mats a brief kiss on the lips, and they are shown sitting on a sofa watching television and holding hands before she leaves to go back to her room. But sex is not explored as a topic, and whether Linda and Mats actually have sexual relations is never made clear—indeed, whether they even are in a relationship is left ambiguous in the third season. But even if they do have sex, it is apparent that they do not need a third person's assistance to be able to manage an erotic life. The topic of pregnancy and parenthood is never mentioned.

Verbal articulateness, mobility, restricting desire so that it is directed only at members of one's own group, innocuous public displays of affection, little or no sex (and in any case no sex that would involve assistance from a staff member or helper), and no talk of parenthood. These are the features that characterize a permissible and acceptable kind of romantic relationship for people with congenital disabilities in Sweden.

Facilitating Sexuality in Denmark

Let us contrast Linda and Mats from *In Another Part of Köping* with another couple about their same age, this one living in Denmark.

Steen is a young man in his early thirties with alert blue eyes and a pronounced overbite. Born with a neurological problem that resulted in paralysis from the neck down, Steen is also spastic, on the autism spectrum (he is obsessive about certain things, like having newspapers stacked in a particular order), and he is deaf. He has no verbal language and cannot use sign language either, since he is not able to move his hands. However, Steen understands sign language, and he communicates his desires by making sounds that are modulations of the syllable, "uh." Caregivers and staff members in the group home where he has lived for many years interpret these sounds by asking him yes/no questions, either through sign language, if they know it, or by pointing to a small square of paper taped to the arm of Steen's wheelchair. The paper, about half the size of a postcard, is divided into five rows, each of which contains eight squares. Inside each square is a letter, or, in the bottom rows, a number from 1–10. So the first row reads A, B, C, D, and so on, to H. Below that, the next row starts with I, J, K, and so on. When Steen makes it clear by uttering an "uh" sound that he has something he wants to communicate, his helper will put a finger on the "A" and move, letter by letter, down the row and onto the next until Steen makes another sound, indicating that the helper's finger has hit upon the correct first letter of the word he is thinking of. Then the helper goes back to "A" and starts over again, until coming upon the second letter.

This goes on until the helper successfully says the word that Steen has in mind. At that point, the helper will start to ask more yes/no questions, hoping to discover what it is that Steen wants to communicate, going back to the square for more spelling out in cases where it is still not clear what Steen wants to say.

Steen has a girlfriend named Marianne. Marianne lives in another group home. She and Steen met at the activity center where both of them spend most of their days. Marianne is forty years old, has a Liza Minnelli haircut, and always wears orange. She has an intellectual disability, is deaf and nearly blind. She has no verbal language, though she can sign, and she understands the sign language of others, if they make the signs against her cupped hands so that she can feel them.

Steen and Marianne have been a couple for six years. They see each other daily at the activity center, and once every six weeks the staff at Steen's group home arrange their schedules so that Marianne can come over, spend the evening, and sleep over in Steen's bed. Those evenings are romantic ones, and Steen always makes sure that the staff has purchased a bottle of rosé wine, which Marianne drinks through a straw and he through a tube with one end inserted into the glass and the other end clipped to his collar, as they enjoy their dinner together at the group home's dining table. Marianne is much more mobile than Steen, but she also requires help to do a number of things. The staff at Steen's group home are willing to assist her, even though her presence means more work for them, since they also have to perform all their usual tasks, such as feeding all the residents, and getting them into bed in the evening and out of bed in the morning.

Steen and Marianne in Denmark are very different from Linda and Mats in Sweden. Both couples live in group homes, but parallels end there. Whereas Linda and Mats are verbally articulate, neither Steen nor Marianne has verbal language. Communication with both of them requires patience and time. Whereas Linda and Mats are mobile, Steen has extremely restricted mobility and requires help to do almost everything—eat, dress, bathe, get into and out of his wheelchair, into and out of bed, and so on. While Linda and Mats could clearly express their desire to be a couple, Steen and Marianne had to depend on others to recognize that they wanted to be a couple and to make the arrangements that allow them to spend time alone together. And whereas any sex engaged in by Linda and Mats is their private concern, in the case of Steen and Marianne, whole staff schedules get arranged so that the couple can spend a romantic evening together in the same bed.

Don asked Lene, a social worker at Steen's group home who knows sign language and who has the closest contact with him, how his relationship with Marianne came about.

"Steen used to be together with another woman," Lene said.

He's very attractive as a boyfriend because he's smart. If anyone thinks, "Steen just sits there in his wheelchair and doesn't know anything," then they don't know him. He's very popular. And he was together with a woman at his activity center named Ulla. They were engaged, in fact. But Ulla ended up not wanting Steen. She wouldn't make arrangements to see him, she never came to visit him, she didn't want to kiss him; she just wasn't interested. It created a lot of problems; everyone at the activity center got involved. They tried to get them to agree, "Well you're engaged, you can kiss each other good morning, you can kiss goodbye." Because otherwise Steen just sat there all day and stared at her. He couldn't concentrate on anything else. But she was not interested.

Finally, we started talking to him. We can't refuse to call her if he wants us to. We can't say to him, "No, I don't want to call her again because she doesn't want to arrange a time to meet you." So if he wanted us to call, we called. But she always just refused to make arrangements to meet him outside the activity center. So we spoke to him and said, "Steen, she doesn't want to. You need to find another girlfriend. You know we'll support you but we can't make her do anything she doesn't want to do. We can't tell Ulla that she has to meet you. Ulla doesn't want to meet you. We can call her, but she doesn't want to meet you." He just kept getting refused, time and time again. And finally they agreed that they weren't engaged anymore.

So a little while after that we get a call from the activity center that Steen and Marianne were a couple. The staff saw them kissing, and they seemed to like one another. The social workers who work there know us all, and we know the social workers who work at Marianne's group home. So we started talking about what we could do to support their relationship and make it work. What kind of framework could we establish that would allow them to be together outside the activity center? Because we spoke to both Steen and Marianne, and they were clear that that is what they wanted. Steen is really good about communicating what he wants. If he wants to make arrangements to see someone or do something with someone, he lets you know, and he makes sure he is understood and gets what he wants.

So I called the social workers at Marianne's group home and started a conversation with them about what needs to happen so that they can spend time together outside the activity center. It isn't all that easy. Marianne's group home won't let Steen come over without a helper. They're dealing with budget cuts, just like us and everyone else, and they often only have one staff member in the house. And they say that if something happens in the house then they can't be there for Steen and Marianne. We tell them they don't need to be there for them. We would just like it if Steen could go home with Marianne after the activity center, just to spend a few hours with her there. But they say no, they won't allow him there without a helper.

So we're still a bit upset about that, you might say. But we decided to support them. So Marianne came here with her social worker, and we got to know her. I remember that I wrote up a sixty-page memo during those visits: What happens when Marianne is here? What kind of help does she need? How would the evening be set up? If there are any problems, who do I contact? You have to prepare a written plan for what needs to happen so that it will all work. Because Marianne can get testy and do things. Like once she arrived and Steen wasn't here. And suddenly she was gone—she'd taken the bus into town or something. But there we are standing there, not knowing where she is. Who's responsible when something like that happens?

That's the sort of thing we needed to sort out. So we talked a lot among ourselves, social workers. Here we talked about it in staff meetings—Are we willing to this? What are we willing to do? Who is willing to do what? Where is it best that they sleep? Should they sleep in the physical therapy room? In Steen's bed? How should the bed be prepared? How should Steen be placed in the bed? What works best? All that discussion wasn't going on behind the backs of Steen and Marianne. It was to support them by making sure that we could accommodate them in an optimal way.

And so we tried it the first time. We got Steen ready for bed, and we put him in bed, and then we left the room and let Marianne get herself ready afterward. And so they spent the night together. And since then we've had a running dialogue with them. Does it work? Is anything wrong?

Don asked Lene if there had been any problems with the arrangements that had been worked out to accommodate Steen and Marianne.

"Not as far as supporting their relationship is concerned," she answered.

But we have had a few problems because Marianne has trouble understanding. Once she disappeared with Steen. He was in his manual wheelchair and she just left with him, without saying anything. Poof, she was gone. She took him down to the petrol station to buy chocolate. She crossed that busy street—can you imagine, deaf, and with her vision? And Steen in his wheelchair. He couldn't say anything. We were hysterical. It's not that Steen can't go out. He's an adult; he can do what he wants. But she can't just disappear with him.

So we say to her, "You can't do this [det duger bare ikke]. You can't do it. If you do it again we're calling a taxi to take you back to where you live because we can't accept this." And then the howling begins, and the tears, and the "No, no, I'll be good, I won't do it again." And that's how we work.

I talk to the social workers who work at her group home, and they talk to her, because Marianne has to hear it again and again and again before she understands. And we repeat it all again when she is here next time. So we've had those kinds of problems, since her impairment makes it hard for her to understand some things. And so sometimes she does things that we can't accept.

Sexual Advisors and the *Guidelines about Sexuality—Regardless of Handicap*

The fact that Steen and Marianne are recognized as a couple, and the fact that they receive support from a variety of social workers and other helpers to actually *be* a couple, is illustrative of everything that differentiates Denmark from Sweden in this context. The active role taken by staff members who not only notice that Steen and Marianne seem to like each other but who then also make a point of talking to them, and to one another, in order to plan ways for the couple to be able to spend time together outside the activity center—this kind of interested, engaged, professional involvement in the social and erotic lives of individuals with disabilities is decidedly not an instance of "If I don't do anything, at least I haven't done something wrong." If anything, Lene and her colleagues' engagement in Steen's and Marianne's lives can be summarized the opposite way: "If I don't do anything, then I *have* done something wrong."

What is it about Denmark that fosters such a vastly different attitude from the one that prevails in Sweden?

In the previous chapter we discussed some of the historical reasons that have led Denmark and Sweden down two very different paths when it comes to policies and practices regarding sexuality and disability. Cultural and ideological differences between the two countries are also a factor, and we will discuss some of those later. But two practical factors in particular permit and facilitate the kind of engagement that Lene describes in relation to Steen and Marianne.

The first of these factors is the existence of a corps of social workers who have studied to obtain a special certification in the area of sexuality and disability. The course that leads to this certification was established in 1990 and was led until only a few years ago by the pioneering sexual rights activists Jørgen Buttenschøn and Karsten Løt. The course consists of twenty full days of meetings and coursework spread over one-and-a-half years. During that time, students read materials on sexuality and on disability, they complete practical assignments, and they initiate projects at their places of work that they later discuss and have critiqued when they meet together as a study group. The course results in certification as a "sexual advisor" (*seksualvejleder*; the verb *vejlede* means to "advise" or "supervise" in the sense of guiding and offering counsel and support). There are currently nearly four hundred certified sexual advisors in Denmark, and since 2010 two more diploma programs have been instituted, one in Copenhagen and one in Hans Christian Andersen's birthplace, the town of Odense.

If one or more social workers with certification as sexual advisors work in a group home, that home is likely to have open and progressive policies regarding sexuality. For example, while Lene, who talked about Steen and Marianne, is not a trained sexual advisor, the woman who directs the group home where she works is. Over the years that director has used her training as a sexual advisor to promote discussions about sexuality among residents in the group home, among staff members, and between residents and staff. The fruits of those efforts and discussions have led to both an awareness that the significantly impaired residents of the group home, like Steen, have a sexuality, and to a willingness on the part of the permanent staff to help residents understand and explore their erotic desires. Sexual advisors take the initiative to provide information and education. They make practical arrangements to accommodate sex between disabled lovers. They help people with mobility impairments pleasure themselves. And they provide assistance to individuals who want to contact sex workers—a topic we will discuss in detail in chapter 5.

The second concrete factor that differentiates Denmark from Sweden when it comes to an engagement with the sexual lives of people with disabilities is the existence of the set of national guidelines that advises people who work with disabled individuals on how to think about and engage with their sexuality. These are the *Guidelines about Sexuality—Regardless of Handicap* (*Vejledning om seksualitet—uanset handicap*; hereafter *Guidelines*) discussed in chapter 2. We noted there that this document first appeared in 1989. It was expanded and slightly revised in 2001, and again, just recently, in 2012. The 2012 revision was substantial, and we will discuss it toward the end of this book, in chapter 6. Here though, we will focus on the 2001 version of the *Guidelines*, partly because that was the version that was in effect when we did the fieldwork for this study, in 2011, and also because the most recent version of the *Guidelines* needs to be understood in relation to the version that preceded it.

The *Guidelines* document regulates the conduct of social workers and others who work in service housing and are employed in the public sector. It applies to people who work in group homes, homes for senior citizens, and service flats. The document does not explicitly regulate the conduct of personal assistants who are hired privately by individual persons with disabilities. Their conduct in relation to sexuality is not regulated at all, a situation that is identical to the one in Sweden.

The *Guidelines* document begins with an assertion that "people with a reduced physical or psychological functionality [*mennesker med nedsat fysisk eller psykisk funktionsevne*] have the same basic needs and rights as other people." It then goes on to state the following:

> A significant goal with a social intervention is to improve an individual's social and personal functionality and their possibilities to develop. The intervention shall also help improve the individual's possibility to develop his or her own life by assisting with, among other things, contact and being together with others. This context includes the question of support and help in connection with sexuality.
>
> In the UN Standard Rules for Equalization of Opportunities for People with Disabilities (rule 9), it is emphasized that people with reduced functional ability shall have the possibility [*skal have mulighed*] to be able to experience their own sexuality and have sexual relationships with other people, and that they, in accordance with this, shall be supported through legislation and relevant counseling.[19]

There are several things to note in these formulations. The first is that "sexuality," as the word is used here, clearly does not just mean that people have the ontological right to be a certain kind of person. The document is not only declaring that people have a right to be straight or gay or whatever. The document addresses sexuality as *sex*—that is, as an activity and as a relation. Note also that the document formulates entitlement to a sex life not as what in political philosophy is called a negative liberty—that is, it doesn't just say "We're not going to stop you from trying to have sex by putting obstacles in your way." The *Guidelines* formulate sexuality as a positive entitlement: it says that the individual "*shall have the possibility* to experience their own sexuality and have sexual relationships with other people." This is a profound difference. An analogy would be the difference between saying "We're not going to hinder you from learning to read" and "We're going to provide you with opportunities to learn to read."

This difference is all the more significant because the Danish text is either a mistranslation or a deliberate reformulation of the United Nations document that it cites. Rule 9 of the UN Standard Rules for Equalization of Opportunities for People with Disabilities discusses sexuality in negative terms: "Persons with disabilities must not be denied the opportunity to experience their sexuality, have sexual relationships and experience parenthood," it says.[20] The authors of the Danish *Guidelines* document changed that negative formulation to a positive one—the passive admonition not to hinder ("must not be denied") becomes an active encouragement to facilitate and to help ("shall have the possibility").

What follows this introduction in the *Guidelines* are forty pages that provide explicit instructions that clarify what helpers are prohibited from doing, what they may do, and what they are obligated to do in regard to the sexuality of the women and men they assist. This tripartite dimensionality is important. The *Guidelines* do not just say what people who work with individuals with disabilities are forbidden to do or are allowed to do. They also state what they *must* do. This is crucial.

Activities that are explicitly prohibited in the *Guidelines* are sex between a helper and a person with a disability; providing sexual assistance to a person who has indicated—verbally or nonverbally—that he or she does not want it; and any form of sexual assistance with children under the age of fifteen.

What is permitted in terms of sexual assistance are the following:

- Assistance can be provided in learning how to masturbate (*Der må ydes hjælp til oplæring til onani*).
- Assistance can be provided to persons who wish to have sexual relations with one another (*Der må ydes hjælp til personer, der ønsker samleje med hinanden*).
- Assistance can be provided to contact a prostitute (*Der må ydes hjælp til at kontakte en prostitueret*).[21]

But even while these activities are allowed, the *Guidelines* also explicitly state that nobody can be commanded to do any of this. In other words, it is not the case that if you work in a group home your supervisor can order you to go into Rasmus's or Anna's room and help either of them masturbate. The way this is formulated in the document is as follows: "A helper should be aware that he or she should be able to counsel and support an individual in relation to sexuality. However, a helper may not be ordered by his or her workplace to help an individual learn to practice sex. If a person needs assistance to practice sex, then *the helper, however, does have the duty to see to it that another helper or a qualified expert is referred to that person*" (emphasis added).[22]

So while one cannot be ordered to provide sexual assistance for a person with disabilities, one has an obligation, if that person desires sexual assistance, to make sure that she or he gets the assistance they want. Notice where the locus of responsibility is placed: it is not up to the person with a disability to keep on asking until she or he eventually perhaps finds someone who is willing to help buy her a vibrator or roll a condom onto his penis. The person with a disability only has to ask once, and the helper she or he asks is then responsible for seeing to it that she or he gets the assistance: if the helper does not have the expertise or the time to help, or if she or he thinks the whole idea of sex and disability is too problematic to deal with, then it is *that person's* responsibility to find someone else who can help.

The *Guidelines* document is the cornerstone to everything that happens in Denmark regarding the sexuality of people with disabilities. While most people with significant disabilities have not read and do not even know about the document, all sexual advisors are familiar with it, since it provides the practical and ethical basis of their profession. They use the document to justify the interventions they devise to discuss sexuality, educate people, and actively facilitate sex—for example, masturbation or sexual contact between a significantly disabled couple.

Sexual Facilitation in Practice

How does this happen in practice? How is it possible to facilitate something like masturbation without actually engaging in sex with the person one is assisting?

In Sweden, discussions about sexuality and disability run aground on questions like that. No one seems able to imagine that it is possible to facilitate sex for a disabled person without either contacting a prostitute, who would have sex with that person (which would mean engaging in a criminal activity in Sweden, since purchasing sexual services or helping someone purchase sexual services is illegal there) or, barring that, by actually sexually servicing the person being assisted—acting, in other words, like the young male helper who assists the woman he works for by rubbing her privates through a blanket. Even individuals in Sweden who recognize and lament the fact that adults with disabilities are impeded from having sex do not consider that helping them have sex could involve something other than prostitution or sexual servicing. That those two options are the only conceivable ones for sexual facilitation is the direct cause of what Bettan called the "moral panic" that invariably arises whenever sex and disability are discussed in public.

Danes are more imaginative. Here is an example of how it is possible to assist a disabled person to have sex without having sex with her. Helle is a young woman in her late twenties who lives in a group home for adults with cerebral palsy. Helle has no verbal language. The only part of her body in which she has even limited movement is her head. Helle communicates with her eyes, by smiling and making a variety of sounds, and also with the help of a laser strapped to her head that she can use to point to symbols on what is known as a Bliss board (named after the creator of the symbols, Karl Blitz, who fled Nazi Germany and changed his name to Charles Bliss). The following is a plan of action (*handleplan*) for Helle, handwritten by a sexual advisor who works as a social worker in Helle's group home.

PLAN OF ACTION FOR HELLE RASMUSSEN
Helle would like help in positioning her sex aid. Helle is laid naked on her bed. A large mirror is placed at one end of Helle's bed, so that she can see herself. A pillow under her knees, legs spread. Put lubricant on the sex aid and on her privates. Place the sex aid on her privates. The helper asks Helle how long she would like to lie alone, 5 min. or 10 min. or 15 min. Helle will nod at the exact number of minutes she wants. The helper goes back in when the agreed upon minutes are up and asks Helle if she is done. If she says no, ask again how much longer Helle would like to lie in bed. When Helle is finished, wash the sex aid and ask Helle if everything is OK.

The following is another example of this kind of plan of action, this time for a man in his early thirties whose cerebral palsy is so severe that he cannot control any of his limbs:

PLAN OF ACTION FOR LARS AND SEX AIDS
[*SEKSUELHJÆLPEMIDDEL*]
Lars gets laid in his bed with his head slightly raised.

Lars has his diaper removed and he lies with an undershirt and naked from the waist down. Lars gets the cord to his call buzzer in his hand.

Rub lubricant or some other cream on Lars's penis, put his vibrator between his legs and put his penis in it. Turn on the vibrator and ask him which speed he would like. Come to an agreement with Lars about when to come back in to his room if he doesn't buzz for help.

When Lars is finished, take the vibrator and wash it clean with soap and water.

Put the vibrator on Lars's desk to charge. Next time one is at work and sees that the vibrator is lying on the desk, put it in the box that is in the big basket in the bedroom.

"Plans of action" like these are made possible by the *Guidelines* document because the *Guidelines* make it clear that persons with a disability are entitled not just to a sexuality, but to sex, and they obligate helpers to be observant about sex and to provide or find someone who can provide help to anyone who expresses a desire for such help. These plans of action break down a sexual activity like masturbation into its component acts, in a way that allows a helper to facilitate sex without performing it or without intruding any more than necessary on the privacy of the person who needs the help to have sex. They exemplify a fundamental feature of the help sexual advisors provide: they help individuals have sex, but they do not *have sex* with them—in fact, they are explicitly prohibited by the *Guidelines* document from doing so. So sexual advisors who facilitate the erotic lives of adults with disabilities are not sex workers or sex surrogates. They are social workers with special training and competence.

One reason sexual advisors give for writing contracts like these is that they help guard against abuse—on both sides. If a contract like this exists, the person with a disability has grounds for saying "You transgressed our agreement" if the helper does something not in the agreement. And the person providing the help knows exactly what she or he is agreeing to—she or he can also refuse to do anything beyond what is made explicit in the agreement.

Plans of action like these are not public documents. They are not part of a resident's file in the way his or her medical needs might be. Instead, they are agreements between a resident and a particular sexual advisor, or some other staff member who is willing to assist, and they are kept with the sexual advisor or staff member. If the person receiving assistance ever wanted a copy of such an agreement, they would be given one. What *is* public knowledge among full-time staff in a group home is that particular staff members assist some residents to have an erotic life. This is discussed in staff meetings. So everyone working in Helle's group home, for example, would know that Helle relies on the sexual advisor who wrote her plan of action, and perhaps several other staff members as well, for assistance with sex. But the details of that assistance—exactly what it consists of, when and how often it occurs—are not known by others.

Agreements like the ones with Helle and Lars come about through conversations with staff members of group homes, who often take an active role in talking about sex. They organize discussion groups in which men and women sit together in same-sex gatherings and talk about sex, relationships, love, jealousy, contraception, parenthood, and anything else they want to talk about concerning their intimate lives. Several group homes also stage role playing, where people with disabilities act out scenarios—such as how one manages a situation like seeing that one's boyfriend wants to dance with someone else, or where one feels attracted to someone but does not know what to do. This role playing leads to group discussions like the following, which occurred during a two-hour meeting in a group home for adults with intellectual disabilities. The meeting took place in the group home's gym, which doubled as a dance hall and a general meeting space. Large folding tables were set up, pizzas were ordered, big bottles of Fanta were opened, and the atmosphere was happy and convivial. Separate men's and women's groups had been meeting once a month all year long, and this meeting was the final gathering before the summer holidays. The participants in both groups were gathered together, and the staff members who ran the groups engaged everyone in role playing and discussions about sex and relationships.

After a role play and a discussion about whether it is OK to have sex with one's partner if the partner doesn't want to (it isn't), Johan, a male staff member asked, "If you don't have a partner, who may you have sex with? Can one borrow Helene's boyfriend?" (Helene is a young woman who lives in the group home and who had just talked about her boyfriend.)

"With yourself," several people answered.

"That you can always do," said Johan. "Can you have sex with yourself if you have a partner?"

"No," came the response from several residents.

Johan looked at a raised hand and said, "Max. Max has an opinion on this."

"I have an opinion," said Max. "Yes, you can."

"Yes."

"There's not a problem with that."

Sigurd, another resident in his late twenties, who had been expressing conservative views on sexuality all evening, said, "That may be, but it isn't normal."

"Yes, it is," corrected Johan. "It is normal."

Sigurd: It's not normal to do it with yourself so much.

Johan: Do you know what we mean when we say "do it with yourself"?

Sigurd: Not when you have a partner, no.

Johan: Do you understand what it means, to have sex with yourself?

Sigurd: I understand.

Johan: What does it mean?

Sigurd: It's when you do it yourself.

Johan: Yeah . . .

Sigurd: For example, masturbation.

Johan: That's right.

At this point, Henrik, another staff member, said, "So what happens if your partner only wants to have sex once a night and you want to have it twice? Can't you do it yourself the second time?"

Yeses and Nos answered this question in equal measure.

"Would it embarrass your partner?" Henrik asked.

Sigurd answered again, "Yes, if your partner saw it."

"And if you went into the bathroom and did it?"

"Yuk."

"Sigurd, that's your feelings about it," said Henrik. "And that's fine. But there is nothing in the law that says one can't do it. One can do it if one wants to."

"That may be," said Sigurd, "But it's disgusting" (*pisse ulækkert*).

"That's your view. But one can do it."

In addition to ongoing discussions and role playing about sexuality, some group homes in Denmark also have written policy documents about sexuality that are handed out or read aloud to anyone who moves in. An example of such a document is the following, printed on a piece of folded A-4 paper and illustrated with photocopied black-and-white photographs of a man in a wheelchair kissing a woman wearing lingerie, and drawings of dildos, vibrators, vacuum pumps, and silicone vaginas in a can:

SEXUAL POLITICS OF (NAME OF GROUP HOME)

All people are sexual beings and have the right to a sexual life.

It is important that personal boundaries and freedom are always respected. This applies to residents as well as to staff.

Everything that is not against the law is permitted—with an important limitation: that those partners who have sexual relations both consent, and that they engage in their sexuality privately.

If one person in a couple asks for help, or if we can see that a person who can't express him- or herself is being abused, or is in danger, then we don't just have the right; we have the duty to intervene.

Residents who can manage their own sexual needs have the right to do so, in a private space.

If residents ask, staff will help with counseling and the procurement of sex aids, or they will refer the resident to a sexual advisor. Residents must purchase sex aids themselves if a subvention cannot be obtained.

Sexuality is a private arena that the staff respect. Individual residents' sexuality is not discussed, therefore, in staff meetings, etc. unless the resident has requested that it be.

Staff are obliged to wash and clean used sex aids for residents.

Staff will not tolerate sexual harassment. If this occurs, the resident will be made aware that limits have been transgressed. If the sexual harassment continues, a sexual advisor will be asked to meet with staff and the resident to work out a solution.

Documents like this, together with discussion groups and role playing sessions, contribute to an atmosphere that makes it clear to residents that sexuality is a possible and acceptable topic of discussion. This, in turn, permits both residents and staff to broach the subject of sex with individuals, some of whom have never discussed sexuality before in their lives. When Ingrid, a twenty-six-year-old woman with cerebral palsy, moved into the group home she now lives in five years ago, she received a brochure like the one just quoted. This led her to ask a staff member about sex. "I didn't know I had a sexuality," she told Don. "We had had some lessons about sex in the school for the handicapped I went to, but it was talk about how we had uteruses and would get menstruation. I didn't know I had a sexuality. So when I got here, I asked, and they told me, 'Yes, you do, and you can receive help to explore it if you want, and there is a lot of different kinds of sex aids that are available.' I was really happy [*rigtig glad*] to learn that, because I didn't know."

In cases where sex arises as a topic and a sexual advisor is not absolutely certain that he or she has completely understood the wishes of the person asking for assistance—because that person has no verbal language, for example—then another staff member, who ideally but not necessarily is one who also has undergone training as a sexual advisor, will be called in. That individual will be asked to sit together with the person requesting assistance and the sexual advisor who is agreeing to provide it. The sexual advisor will ask the person requesting assistance to repeat his or her requests, and the third person will be asked to confirm the sexual advisor's understanding of the requests. In the rare cases where neither staff member feels certain that they are able to understand exactly what the disabled person wants, they will do nothing until they are able to talk with the person more and feel confident that they do understand.

Written agreements can also be prepared when couples are assisted. Recall that Lene talked about how she wrote a sixty-page document in preparation for Marianne's overnight visit with Steen. That document does not describe sexual activity, since Steen and Marianne—who has no mobility limitations—are capable of having sex without assistance. But the document does include details such as how Steen was to be laid in his bed, how many pillows should be in the bed, and how high the bed should be raised so that Marianne is able to get into and out of it.

A couple that needs assistance to be able to develop intimacy and have sex is helped in concrete ways. A young man and a sexual advisor who assists him in intimate situations with his girlfriend talked about how the assistance developed over time. The man, David, is in his midthirties. He is not able to control his limbs and he has a speech impairment. His girlfriend at the time he recounts, Lisa, had no verbal language and also was unable to control her limbs. The sexual advisor, Trine, is a social worker in her forties who works in David's group home and has known him for many years. Trine explained:

> You have to create a framework. You have to be a little creative. So I suggested to David and Lisa, what would you think about lying together on an air mattress? Because I thought that we could blow up an air mattress and put it on the floor, and that way they could lie close together safely. If they fell off the air mattress they wouldn't really hurt themselves. And they could lie close together and look at one another and kiss each other if they wanted to because their faces would be close together.
>
> At first all this was with their clothes on. And we would take Lisa home and make a new arrangement for when she would come back here. Because she always came here. In the group home she lived in, she only had a small room, whereas David has this big two-room apartment here. And Lisa wanted to come here more and more often.

"It developed [*det tog mere og mere form*], I'd say," said David.

"Yeah, their relationship developed."

"And we kept seeing each other, and so it got to the point where we wrote a paper so that nothing would transgress our boundaries."

"Yeah, a plan of action," said Trine.

David continued, "It's important that the person who helps is also clear about their boundaries. And so we eventually got to the point where we lay naked together, and in the end we had sex together."

"With assistance from a helper?" Don asked.

"Yeah. But a helper is just there to help, not to do anything sexual. They helped us to lie in positions that we wanted to lie in."

"And we had written that down," said Trine.

"And then they left the room."

Don asked David how he felt about having help with something as intimate as sex. He answered that he didn't think it was such a big deal. "People have been close to my body all my life," he said. "I've been washed and dressed and fed and everything since I can remember. Help with sex isn't that different. And being able to have a sexuality and being able to explore my sexuality has made me a whole person. It's a part of a person, I think, that one has a right to regardless of who you are. And I believe that anything is possible, as long as you have the right framework and the right helper to help you."

Don asked Trine how she felt about being that helper. "When I help," she said,

> I have a kind of force field that I activate because I also have to look out for myself. I have this kind of force field that I imagine surrounds me, and I come into the room and help them with the kinds of things that we've talked about and have written down. I go out and then I come back, and back and forth like that. I don't say anything when I come in. I tell them at the beginning that I'm not going to say anything. I tell them that because I don't want them to think that me not talking to them is because I am disapproving or in a bad mood. But when I come in, I read them, I look, and I try to sense whether it's all OK or not. A lot of the help is about reading the situation, helping them with what they want, and keeping quiet as you go in and out.

Contrasting Countries

Just as it would be misleading to suggest that people with disabilities never have sex in Sweden, it would be equally misleading to give the impression that Denmark is an erotic utopia for people with disabilities. People with disabilities in Denmark, as well as the individuals who work with them, are the first to point out that there are many group homes and other places in the country where the sexuality of people with disabilities is not only not facilitated—it is not even acknowledged.

One social worker who was training to become a sexual advisor told us that staff in the group home for people with mobility and intellectual impairments where she has worked for the past ten years are very hesitant to discuss sexuality. Many of her colleagues refuse to acknowledge that the residents have any sexual feelings or desires. One particularly unhappy outcome of this, she said, was that the sexual assault of a woman by another resident who lived in a nearby group home went unreported because nobody knew quite how to deal with it. The social worker's realization that there was no language in the group home to discuss sexuality—for either the staff or the residents—was one of the reasons she applied to complete a sexual advisor certification course.

So while there are many group homes in Denmark where people with disabilities do not receive any help in discovering, initiating, or sustaining a sexual life—"no arms, no cake" (*ingen arme, ingen kage*) is the way one sexual advisor described such places, using a Danish proverb—and while there are many individuals who work with people with impairments who are unwilling to even consider that those people might have sexual desires, Demark differs crucially from Sweden because of the existence of the *Guidelines about Sexuality—Regardless of Handicap*. The *Guidelines* document is not a law; it is only a set of recommendations. But its existence mandates the development of attitudes, policies, and practices that acknowledge and support disabled adults' entitlement to a sexual life. The *Guidelines* is the reason why Denmark has sexual advisors. And anyone who knows about the document can use it as a tool to argue for respect and assistance. It can be used to try to change an unhappy situation into something better.

Sweden, as we have pointed out, lacks anything resembling the *Guidelines*. We discussed the historical reasons for this difference in the previous chapter. But another key reason behind the absence of guidelines relating to sexuality is the pervasive insistence in Sweden that sexuality is "private." This insistence is tinged with the memory of the shameful history of institutionalization that still casts a shadow over how disabled people are treated in society. Until as recently as the 1970s, when the large institutions began to be dismantled, people with disabilities had nothing even approximating a private life. Gunnel Enby's 1972 memoir, *We Must Be Allowed to Love*, recounted her life in the institution in which she was raised during the 1950s and 1960s. Independence or privacy was unthinkable. "Let us describe what it was like to be young and handicapped in an institution," she wrote. "How it felt to be put to bed in the afternoon in the summer when the sun was shining on the hospital walls and it felt pretty good to be alive. The angst that tore at one's chest that made one want to cry out to everybody that here we lie, put to bed for the night at 7 o'clock, when the young people in town are just getting ready to go out."[23]

In the institution where she grew up, Enby wrote, "one ate on schedule, was washed on schedule, was turned on one's side for the night and given one's medication, sleeping pills and drugs."[24] There was no such thing as privacy: "One isn't allowed to have any personal belongings in the room, except for a photograph and the usual toiletry items. The staff walk in and out without knocking, and one is often forced to share one's room with other patients—rooms that at any rate can't be locked."[25]

Given a disturbing, oppressive and still fresh historical legacy like this— one that of course is far from exclusive to Sweden—it is understandable that issues of privacy should resonate powerfully for people with disabilities and everyone involved with them, and that the right of disabled people to have a private life should be treated with the utmost respect. In Sweden, however, "privacy" tends to be invoked at precisely the moment when helpers might be called upon to do something positive or helpful in relation to the sexual lives of disabled people. The point of insisting that sexuality is private seems to be not so much about accommodating or facilitating a private life as ensuring that such a life never emerges.

Maintaining that sexuality is private would appear, on the surface, to express respect for the integrity of people with disabilities. Upon closer examination, however, privacy seems to function, in Sweden, more as a shield or a fence to demarcate an area beyond the bounds of engagement. This defensive and silencing use of the notion of privacy is evident in everything from the instructions personal assistant Viktoria received to not mention anything sexual to the man with "locked-in syndrome"—because sex is private—to the response of the staff members interviewed by Åse Linder, who told her they did not see it as part of their jobs to raise the issue of sex with the residents with whom they worked—because sex is private.

The way privacy is invoked in Sweden to discourage engagement with the erotic lives of people with disabilities is summed up in a particularly distilled form in a review of the masturbation technique films scripted by the sexologist Margareta Nordeman that we mentioned earlier. The films, which came out in 1996, have been used in Denmark, Norway, and Finland, Nordeman told us. They have even been dubbed into Japanese. But they were shot dead in the water in Sweden. As soon as they appeared they were reviewed in *Intra*, a respected journal for people who work professionally with individuals with intellectual impairments. The two editors of *Intra*—one of whom was none other than Karl Grunewald, the august head of the Bureau for Handicap Issues who opened the Apollonia conference on sexuality discussed in the previous chapter—excoriated the films. Grunewald and his coeditor called them "vulgar and indiscreet" (*vulgär och oblyg*). They wrote that Nordeman and the Swedish Association for Sexuality Education that financed the films were "clueless" (*aningslös*), and they asserted that allowing intellectually disabled people to watch the films could easily be considered a form of sexual abuse. The editors ended their review with these forbidding words:

> It is obvious that an intellectually impaired person [*den utvecklingsstörde*] has the right to his or her own sex life. The form that such a life takes is none of the staff or anyone else's business as long as it isn't directly offensive for others. In that case, the person can require help to close the door and protect his or her private life. Because at the end of the day, that is what this is about: that everyone has the right to a private life, and other people's well-meaning advice and meddlesome guidance [*beskäftiga handledningar*] is often more harmful than it is beneficial.

"The right to a private life" has a very specific, and very circumscribed, meaning here. For adults with disabilities, it means the right to hide sexuality, to shut it up behind closed doors, out of sight and beyond the awareness of anyone else. For individuals who work with disabled adults, "the right to a private life" means that any attempt to offer advice, guidance, or assistance is not just "meddlesome"; most likely it is "more harmful than . . . beneficial." Privacy, in this understanding of sexuality, implies "don't get involved." It signifies "back off." It means—and the editors actually use this word in their text—"halt."[26]

The notion of privacy also comes up in Denmark when disability and sexuality is discussed, for example, in the "Sexual Politics" brochures handed out to new residents in some group homes as part of their welcome package of information. But in Denmark, labeling sexuality as private does not shield it with the same forbidding armor that barbs the Swedish usage. Danish social workers and others use the word to mean "out of public view," as in "Residents who can manage their own sexual needs have the right to do so, in a private space." It also means confidential, as in "Individual residents' sexuality is not discussed, therefore, in staff meetings, etc. unless the resident has requested that it be." What it does not mean is "back off" or "halt." Referring to sexuality as private in Denmark does not consign it to the frozen outer limits of engagement. On the contrary, it configures a space of respect in which particular forms of engagement can occur.

This space is mutually constructed between helpers and people with disabilities, even in cases where the person with a disability is quite significantly impaired. The plan of action worked out to help Helle explore sexual pleasure, for example, was a collaboration between Helle, who has no verbal language, and the sexual advisor who helps her. That woman had long conversations with Helle to determine what kind of sex aid she wanted, and she helped Helle try out several before they settled on the ones Helle liked best. The sexual advisor added some details to the plan of action that Helle had not thought of herself—the instruction that a large mirror be placed at the foot of the bed so that Helle could see her whole body was the sexual advisor's idea, because from many years of experience working with people who had spent their entire lives in beds and in wheelchairs, she knew that someone like Helle had likely never actually viewed her entire body naked.

In Denmark, the ones who usually take the initiative to discuss sex are the people employed to work with disabled people. They take this initiative because they know that many adults with disabilities have received little sexual education—at most they might at one point have heard the kind of uterus-and-menstruation anatomy lesson mentioned by Ingrid. Individuals who work with people with disabilities also know it is unlikely that many of them will have heard much about sex from the parents who cared for them before they came to live in the group home. Ingrid's surprise to discover as a twenty-one-year-old adult that she even had a sexuality is not an uncommon occurrence among women and men with congenital impairments.

With little concrete knowledge about sex and no language to broach or explore the topic, people with severe congenital impairments are hardly in a position to start a conversation about it, particularly if they sense that the topic is distasteful to, or taboo among, the people employed to assist them. In such a context, Swedish instructions to personal assistants and group home staff not to talk about sex because it is private, and because the form that a disabled person's sexual life takes is nobody's business, are directives that effectively smother sex under the guise of respecting its private nature.

Women and men with disabilities who require assistance to understand interpersonal relations or perform activities like move, bathe, and eat often define privacy and respect differently from the people who formulate and follow the rules about such things in Sweden. Recall David, who didn't think it was such a big deal to ask for help with sex because as far back as he can remember he has always had people fussing with his body. Privacy in the sense demanded by individuals like the editors of *Intra* magazine is an impossibility for David or his partner Lisa. They need assistance to undress, to get into bed, to position their bodies, to tidy up afterward. To insist that all this is private and, therefore, beyond the bounds of assistance is not to do nothing, as the adage that is so popular among Swedish helpers would have it. On the contrary, declining to assist in cases like this is a purposeful undertaking that actively deprives people like David and Lisa of the possibility to experience an erotic life. David is adamant that such a deprivation is not defensible. "Being able to have a sexuality and being able to explore my sexuality has made me a whole person," he says, expressing a sentiment that few adults—disabled or nondisabled—could contest, deny, or condemn.

For nondisabled people to recognize not only that people with significant physical and intellectual impairments may have erotic desires but, also, that they require assistance to be able to understand, explore, and express those desires is to do something important. It is to recognize both a fundamental sameness but also, just as important, a crucial, irreducible difference. The space between that familiar sameness and the in-many-ways unknowable difference is the space of ethics. It is the space that creates the possibility for a statement like this, which is printed on a piece of paper and handed to everyone whom Marcus, a thirty-eight-year-old Danish man with cerebral palsy, interviews for a position as his personal assistant.

SEXUALITY
Sexuality can be difficult to deal with, not least because of your own boundaries and norms. It's incredibly important in this area to be completely clear about what you want or don't want. To begin with, it's important for me to say that you will not be asked to do more than you are used to doing in the rest of your work. For example, you might sometimes be asked to go and rent a DVD film. That DVD might sometimes be a porn film.

You know that I use a uridome that you will put on every morning and take off every evening [a uridome is like a condom with adhesive glue on the inside, with a plastic tube coming out the tip. The condom is rolled onto the penis and the tube is attached to a plastic bag that is strapped to Marcus's calf, where it collects urine]. When it comes to sex, it will be a condom that you will be asked to put on. If I have my partner [kæreste] over, it might happen that you will put me in bed like you usually do, and then put on a condom instead of a uridome, and then position us like we want to be positioned. Or maybe you'll just go.

My partner can usually manage on his/her own [klare sig selv] or is accompanied by a helper. If we need help with the sexual act itself, we'll get someone from outside—this is not something you will be asked to do.

If I go to a brothel, this is what usually happens: You drive me to the brothel and help me up on the bed, maybe unbutton my pants and take them off, and then you go on a long walk—we can manage the rest.

I hope, and you can understand this from what you are reading here, that you won't have to do any more than you usually do in the course of a normal day. Of course you will be asked to wash my privates, but you would do that anyway in the course of a day.

I want to stress that I expect you to be able to do the things I mention here if you are hired. If not, you need to tell me and we have to talk about it. But I want to be honest, and I advise you not to take the job in that case because, if you do, we can end up transgressing your boundaries.

Finally, I want to say that it's no fun asking for help with these kinds of intimate things, but I do because sexuality is a need [et behov] for me—just as it is for you.

CHAPTER 4 :: shifting boundaries

It's natural that sex is private, intimate. One normally doesn't root around in people's sex life. But in the caring professions one "steps over" many boundaries: one washes people's privates for example. And it's also important to even see sexual needs and problems. —Swedish sexologist Birgitta Hulter

It's the sex that is the problem. If they fall in love and *don't* have sex, then it's generally really cute and charming. But if they're going to get involved with all that messy stuff, then it's, "Uh oh, wait a minute ..." It's not so cute anymore. There's a clear boundary, between being in love without sexuality, being in love with sexuality, and just sexuality—well, that last one is completely out of the question. —Swedish female staff member who works with young people with intellectual disabilities

If you have the understanding and the education and you know how important it is to be able to experience one's sexuality, as a person, then you work out the boundaries. You aren't their sexual partner, you're not there to satisfy them sexually. Your job is to help them have sex if they want help. —Danish sexual advisor Jeannette Bramming

Boundaries are important when it comes to sexuality and disability. They are a source of continual consideration, consternation, and negotiation. Concern about boundaries arises in relation to public and private, permissible and forbidden, care and abuse, sex and reproduction. Some of the concern is practical: When does washing someone's privates cross a boundary and become something else? At what point do I tell my personal assistants that I want to have a sex life? Some is professional: Can I help someone to masturbate without becoming involved in the act myself? Can I intervene in a relationship that looks to me like it is making one of the partners unhappy? And some is moral: Is it defensible to encourage a young woman who wants children to have herself sterilized?

A main reason why boundaries are forever pondered, discussed, and debated in relation to sexuality and disability is because people with disabilities, by their very existence, confound boundaries—and redefine them. The boundaries between ability and inability, between language and communication, between understanding and misunderstanding, between helplessness and independence, between intimacy and distance—all these, and many others besides, are challenged, blurred, crossed, and reconfigured by individuals with different kinds of intellectual and physical impairments. They are also transgressed by people who care for and work with people with disabilities. Many parents of disabled adults, for example, are much more involved in the sexual lives of their children than they ever imagined they would be, or would like to be.

Sexuality itself also crosses and reconfigures boundaries. The exploration and fulfillment of erotic desire involve reaching out beyond the self to engage with others—be this in real life or in fantasy. In this sense, sexuality—even when it is solitary—is always social. The American literature scholar Teresa de Lauretis once famously observed that it takes two women to make a lesbian.[1] This is an insight about desire and connection that applies to any form of erotics. You are never alone when you have sex.

The Boundary between Private and Public

The combination of bodies with impairments that require assistance to understand or to move, with an activity that by its very nature blurs and transgresses boundaries, is what makes the sexual lives of people with disabilities such a profound challenge, both for people with disabilities and those who assist them. Demarcating limits that allow for assistance while still preserving integrity and dignity is a challenge for people with disabilities. In a widely cited article from 1991 about how disability rights activism tends to disavow the existence and needs of profoundly disabled individuals, the artist Cheryl Marie Wade wrote that there is a fundamental difference between disabled people who need assistance to perform basic activities and everyone else who does not. "To put it bluntly—because this is as blunt as it gets," Wade wrote,

> we must have our asses cleaned after we shit and pee. Or we have others' fingers inserted into our rectums to assist shitting. Or we have tubes of plastic inserted inside us to assist peeing or we have re-routed anuses and pissers so we do it all into bags attached to our bodies.
>
> These blunt, crude realities. Our daily lives. Yeah, I know it ain't exactly sexy. Not the images we're trying to get across these days.
>
> The difference between those of us who need attendants and those who don't is the difference between those who know privacy and those who don't. We rarely talk about these things, and when we do the realities are usually disguised in generic language and gimp humor. Because, let's face it: we have great shame about this need. This need that only babies and the "broken" have.
>
> And because this shame is so deep, and because it is perpetuated even by our movement when we emphasize only the able-ness of our beings, we buy into that language that lies about us and becomes part of our movement, and our movement dances over the surface of our real lives by spending all its precious energy on bus access while millions of us don't get out of bed or get by with inadequate personal care. Because we don't want to say this need that shames us out loud in front of people who have no understanding of the unprivate universe we live in, even if that person is a disabled sister or brother. We don't want to say out loud a basic truth: that we have no place in our bodies (other than our imaginations) that is private.
>
> And yes, this makes us different than you who have privacy of body. Yes, this is a profound difference. And as long as we allow our shame to silence us, it will remain a profound difference.[2]

The "profound difference" that Wade describes necessitates a variety of coping strategies by people who, like her, need assistance with intimate activities like bathing, going to the toilet, or shaving one's privates. A common strategy that many adults in this situation adopt is to try to allow only same-sex help. For heterosexual women and men, being assisted by a person of the same sex helps to mute any latent sexual undertones that might arise if the person helping you clean yourself after a visit to the toilet were someone of the opposite sex. Another strategy is to do one's best to limit the number of people who help one to four or five individuals with whom one feels comfortable and trusts. This can work if one hires one's own personal assistants, but if one lives in a group home, it is difficult, partly because there are larger numbers of staff—most of them female—and partly because a permanent staff member may go on holiday or parental leave, or get sick, with the result that his or her position will get filled for a while with a replacement who may be a total stranger.

During assistance with intimate matters, many people with significant physical disabilities describe a kind of out-of-body dissociation that allows them to accept the help they receive without feeling violated. "I shut down," one woman with cerebral palsy told us. "I get into this state where I don't care. I don't think about the fact that someone is touching me. I think about what I need to do at work, or something like that. I just shut down that part of me."

It is not difficult to imagine that this kind of dissociative behavior, coupled with the sense of shame that Cheryl Wade describes so starkly, has consequences for whether people with significant impairments feel they can ask for assistance with their erotic lives. Many simply never do, either because they don't know that they can, or how they can. The authors of the book *The Sexual Politics of Disability* sum up the situation succinctly when they observe, "Many disabled people who want to employ personal assistants who will facilitate their sexual needs find themselves with no one to turn to for advice. Individuals must carefully tread this path, often with a sense of frustration and dread or fear of rejection. It is not surprising that many disabled people live with desires and unmet needs for fear of losing essential care."[3]

If individuals do ask for help, they risk being flatly refused. One Danish man with cerebral palsy told us that together with his first girlfriend, Beate, who also had cerebral palsy, he had hit on a method that might allow them to have intercourse.

> The plan was that I would be strapped into the hydraulic lift, and I would control it with the remote control to be able to move close to her. That way, we wouldn't have to have much help—just help with getting us undressed and positioned so that I was in the lift and she was on the bed and I had

the remote in my hand. I couldn't lay on top of Beate—her body couldn't manage that. So we thought that trying the lift would be a good way to try to do it.

But the plan was never put into action. The man's assistant refused to put a condom on him.

He told me this when I was on my way out to the car to go to Beate and do it. "I don't think I can put a condom on you," he said. It was a little late in the game at that point to try to find another solution. There was no one else I could ask. This was in the beginning of the AIDS epidemic, and I had heard that a condom was really important. So it never happened.

Keeping Sex Out of the Public Domain

In addition to being relevant to ministrations around disabled people's bodies, the boundary between private and public is an issue also in relation to space. The instance where this issue of space is most commonly directly confronted is when individuals—usually, but not exclusively, men—engage in some behavior that thrusts sexuality into what many consider to be the public domain. The behavior can be linguistic—using vulgar and sexualized words at the communal dinner table or in public spaces like buses or shopping malls. It can be inappropriate touching—like what a personal assistant in the previous chapter described in a complaint that the person being assisted "takes the opportunity to stroke my back when I help put on trousers, comes and puts an arm around me sometimes." Or it can be the archetypal behavior that inevitably gets mentioned, sooner or later, whenever the topic of sexuality and disability comes up for discussion—the fact that many men with physical impairments get erections when they are bathed and that some men with intellectual impairments masturbate in public.

Anxiety around sex appearing in public has different consequences for people with physical impairments and people with intellectual impairments. The difference, simply put, is that people with physical impairments are easier to ignore. If they have restricted mobility and little or no verbal language, the chance that their sexuality will disturb public decorum is small. Men may get noticed by staff or personal assistants because they get erections when they are bathed, and some of them come to express their sexuality by defecating as often as they can because being cleaned afterward is the only time their privates get touched. But erections can be ignored or flattened with a flick of a finger or the "penis-killer grip," and excessive defecation can be punished by reprimands and threats, or by neglecting or "forgetting" to clean it.

Women with profound physical impairments and little or no verbal language can be utterly ignored. They might also develop an erotic life that centers on anal release, but the likelihood that such behavior will be identified as having anything to do with sexuality is small, and it will also be disciplined by the staff members or personal assistants confronted with it.

Men and women with intellectual disabilities are harder to ignore, to the extent that they can speak and are mobile. The fact that they can touch their own bodies and move around freely makes their sexuality much more difficult to disregard or control. Unmistakable manifestations of sexuality can make sudden appearances in the communal living room, the local park, or the corner grocery store. The difficult-to-contain sexuality of some people with intellectual impairments is the reason why most discussion about congenital disability and sexuality arises from engagement with intellectual disability. It is not mere coincidence that the driving forces that eventually led to the adoption of the Danish *Guidelines about Sexuality—Regardless of Handicap* were individuals like Niels Erik Bank-Mikkelsen and Jørgen Buttenschøn, whose careers had been spent working with adults with intellectual impairments.

The concern that occupies everyone who works with individuals with disabilities is how to get them to appreciate that sex is private. Conveying this message is not always a simple matter, especially when people live in a milieu like a group home, whose very structure and organization blurs the boundary between (private) home for the residents and (public) workplace for the staff and assistants employed there.

Cheryl Wade's insistence that individuals with severe impairments live in a profoundly different world from that inhabited by non-disabled people or people with less restricting impairments needs to be tempered with a realization that even many individuals with disabilities who do not require assistance with the kinds of things she does live in what she calls an "unprivate universe."

The lack of privacy for people with disabilities is a theme that emerges in most writing about personal assistance and group homes. In her study of young people with intellectual disabilities who go to dances organized by their county, Lotta Löfgren-Mårtenson describes how "school life, work life and social life for people with intellectual impairments is organized by other people to such a large extent that the boundary between public and private is erased. Even when young people or adults with intellectual impairments do something 'privately,' there are always a large number of adults around them."[4] She quotes the director of a group home who told her, "Nobody is more under surveillance, nobody gets watched more than people who are intellectually impaired! Other people know everything, 24 hours a day, what you are doing and when you go to the toilet and everything else. It's a bit much, I think sometimes."[5] A man who organized activities like the dances for young people with intellectual disabilities agreed. "It's always the case that whenever they do anything, there is *always* staff who come with them and don't allow them to just disappear. If anyone is gone for more than 5–10 minutes, someone is going to start wondering, 'What are they up to now?' And they go and check, right away."[6]

There are several consequences to this constant surveillance and lack of privacy. One is that it often wears young people down and makes them docile and less resistant than nondisabled young people might be to the demands of parents, staff, and other adults. Some young people complain about it—one young woman lamented to Löfgren-Mårtenson that she could never be alone with her boyfriend: "Mama won't let us be alone, because she thinks we'll get up to something naughty [*busigt*]. And the staff won't let us be alone either."[7]

But the more common reaction seems to be acquiescence. A sexual advisor in Denmark told Don that she hated the fact that most of the disabled people she worked with didn't seem to mind that they had no privacy. "Sometimes you're in a hurry—I do it myself—and you knock on a resident's door and just walk in," she said. "I can't get them to lock their doors. It's impossible. So a private life—they don't have one. Many of them have lived in institutions their whole lives, so they're used to people coming and going all the time, you know? My biggest wish is that one day I'll knock on someone's door and the person inside will say, 'No, you can't come in.' I'd be like, '*Yes!*'"

Another consequence of the absence of privacy is that it can lead some people with disabilities who live in group homes to become surreptitious and deceptive in order to try to find some private space that is not accessible to helpers or staff. This tactic usually backfires and results only in intensified surveillance ("What are they up to now?"). It can lead to a situation where the disabled person ends up defining his or her home as a public space. Hence, privacy and the opportunity to do things like masturbate are sought in places where no staff are around to interfere, like parks or playgrounds.

A third consequence of never having any privacy is that many people with disabilities who live in group homes end up either never really learning about, or overly caring about, what others identify as the public/private divide. A staff member in a Danish group home for people with cerebral palsy who require a great deal of help told Don

> Sometimes it's difficult for residents to differentiate between when we are with them and when we aren't with them. For example, it sometimes happens that if one of them is watching a porn film and having a good time, and we knock on his door, the person just continues having a wank, even if he answers and tells us to "Come in." Like that. Sometimes modesty is a bit lacking. Or if I'm helping someone put on a porn film, I can look over and see the guy already beginning to masturbate before I even leave the room, you know?
>
> When that happens, I say to them, "You know what? I'd really appreciate it if you wait until I leave. This is your private life. I should not be involved in it like this."
>
> "Huh? Oh, yeah, OK."
>
> But that's how it is. They sometimes get so focused on what they really want to do that they just stop noticing that someone is standing there beside them.

"Masturbation Techniques for Women and Men"

Situations like these engender efforts to instill in people with disabilities an understanding and appreciation of social decorum and the public/private divide. Many times these efforts are punitive. Löfgren-Mårtenson observed an instance at one of the dances she attended when a young man and young woman with intellectual disabilities lay down together on the stage in the dance hall. The reaction to this was immediate. "A woman in her fifties comes up to them and tells them to sit up. When they do, she keeps standing near them, keeping an eye on what they do."[8]

But there are also gentler and more respectful ways of helping people understand that they should not have sex in public. One particularly inventive solution to a seemingly unmanageable problem involved a young man with intellectual impairments in Denmark who insisted on masturbating at the edge of a highway. Every day this young man managed to elude staff members at his group home, turning up by the side of the highway and prompting near accidents and outraged calls to the local police. Desperate, the staff called in a sexual advisor for advice. The woman who came to help managed to figure out that what the young man found exciting was the sound of the traffic. At her suggestion, the staff recorded a video of the highway at the site where the young man liked to stand, and they gave the video to him, telling him that whenever he felt like looking at cars and touching himself, he could do so—in his room, with the sound up and the door closed. Problem solved.

An especially ambitious pedagogical effort to instruct disabled adults about sexuality and its place in relation to the private/public divide was the production of two Swedish films made with the explicit goal of teaching people with intellectual impairments how to masturbate. The films—the same ones Karl Grunewald and his coeditor of *Intra* so objected to—have the says-what's-in-the-tin titles of *Masturbation Techniques for Men* (*Onaniteknik för män*) and *Masturbation Techniques for Women* (*Onaniteknik för kvinnor*). As we mentioned in the previous chapter, the films were made in 1996 by the Swedish Association for Sexuality Education (RFSU), under the direction of sexologist Margareta Nordeman.[9] Nordeman told us that the idea for the films was hers. She said that at every group home or activity center she went to and lectured about sexuality, the problem of masturbation came up and nobody seemed to know how to talk about it or what to do about it. She completely understood why.

"It's not something that we sit around and talk about, generally, with our friends or with anybody," she said. "It's a really tabooed area. I don't sit and say to someone, 'When did you last masturbate, and how do you do it, and can I get a few tips from you?'" From these experiences, Nordeman reasoned that a short how-to film that simply showed a person masturbating would be useful to people with intellectual disabilities.

Each of the two films, for which she wrote the script, begins with an on-camera speaker—in the film for women, it is Nordeman herself—who briefly explains what the films will be about. What follows this introductory speech are three, 3–5 minute scenes in which the same person (that is, the same man in the film for men, the same woman in the one for women) masturbates: first on a bed, then in a bathroom, and finally back on the bed, this time using a sex aid.

The film for men begins with a midbody shot of a bearded man in his late fifties wearing round glasses and a black sweater. The background is a plain beige wall. The man looks straight into the camera and speaks in a deep theatrical baritone. He pauses dramatically as he intones slowly, "You are now going to see three different ways [pause] a man can satisfy himself [pause] sexually [pause]. It's called 'to masturbate' [pause]. Or, 'to wank' [*runka*]."

He continues, saying it is normal to masturbate and that there are differ-ent words for male genitalia—"*penis* [pause], *snopp* [wiener, pause], *och kuk* [and dick]," the word he will use in the rest of the film. The speaker explains that when one "wanks" one usually ejaculates (*man brukar få utlösning*) and that when this happens a fluid comes out of "the little opening at the tip of the dick." He then says that viewers will be shown three different ways to mas-turbate. The man we will see, he says, "we can call Anders."

White text against a black background announces "1. In the bedroom." This cuts to a shot of a sparsely and rather dourly furnished bedroom (framed lithographs, straight-backed chairs). The camera is inside, pointed at the door. The speaker's voice-over says, "Anders sat and was talking to his friends in the living room, when he felt like he was horny [*kåt*]. He felt that his dick began to get hard. And for that reason, he got up and left."

The male actor, "Anders," enters the room, fully clothed. He is a lean man with a receding hairline who looks to be in his midforties. Anders closes the door behind him, and the camera zooms in on his hands as he turns the key to lock the door and then turns the handle to make certain that the door has indeed locked. The speaker says in voice-over, "Anders comes into his room and closes the door. He wants to be alone."

Anders crosses the room and briefly looks out a window, then turns to face the bed in the middle of the room. He undresses and lies on the bed naked. He starts to touch his penis. Narrating Anders's actions, the speaker says, "He takes his dick in his hand and feels how it gets harder. He grips it firmly [*han tar ett stadigt tag*] with his whole hand. He likes to hold it pretty hard. But it shouldn't hurt. He strokes it up and down, and after a while, faster." The camera alternates between long shots of Anders's whole body and close-ups of his face and of his hands and penis. Anders is silent throughout this act. His eyes are either closed or looking down at his penis.

A minute after Anders starts masturbating, the speaker announces, "Soon Anders will ejaculate [*snart får Anders utlösning*]. And he will make sure that it sprays [*sprutar*] on his chest and his stomach." At that, Anders ejaculates (on his chest and his stomach), moaning slightly as he does so. "He is satis-fied," the speaker declares, as Anders leans back on his pillows. The speaker continues, again narrating what we see Anders doing. "After a little while, he takes toilet paper that he has on the floor. And he wipes himself off." The scene ends with Anders, having wiped himself and clutching the toilet paper, standing up from the bed and going to look out the window. The camera zooms to the back of Anders's head, blurs, and cuts.

This scene is followed by "2. In the bathroom." The same man, this time wearing only a pair of white jockey shorts, enters a bathroom, locks the door, and sits down on the toilet. There he once again masturbates to orgasm, this time with the help of a little tube of lubricant he has brought with him. The voice-over narration again gives instructions about how this should be managed: "When the ejaculation is about to happen, Anders bends forward so that his dick points downward into the toilet, and he lets the cum [*satsen*] go there." When Anders is finished, he cleans himself with toilet paper and flushes it down the toilet. He gets up, puts his underwear back on, and leaves.

The third scene is back in the same bedroom as the first scene, but this time Anders walks over to a dresser and takes out of a drawer a pink machine the size and shape of a small drill. Instead of a drill bit, it has a round suction cup that looks like something one might use to buff a car. Anyone who had read Inger Nordqvist's 1988 report on sex aids for men and women with disabilities would recognize the machine as the muscle vibrator called Relax, sold by RFSU, sponsors of the film.[10] The man plugs his Relax buffer into the wall, turns it on, sits on the corner of his bed facing the camera, and proceeds to rub it over his penis. He then lies down on his back and continues rubbing in silence. The only sound heard is the mechanical hum of the machine.[11]

As in the other two scenes, the narrator explains what Anders is doing: "and with one hand, he presses his dick against the plate that is vibrating." Again, the speaker also issues instructions about how Anders should conduct himself when he ejaculates: "He's spread a towel under him on the bed so that the cum won't get onto the sheet and be sticky and cause stains. He doesn't want anyone to be involved with his sex life [*Han vill inte att nån ska ha med hans sexliv att göra*]." After Anders has ejaculated, he once again cleans himself off—this time with the towel he has been lying on. He continues to lie on the bed with his eyes closed and the towel draped over his privates.

At this point the film cuts back to a close-up of the black-clad baritone who says that we have now seen three ways to masturbate but that the viewer should experiment to find the ways it feels best for him. The viewer is reminded that masturbation is something that one does in private—"at home or in a bathroom"—and that one needs to think about one's hygiene, "both for your own sake and so that others will think that you smell good."

"Take care of yourself," are the final words of the film, "and discover your body's possibilities to feel lust and satisfaction."

The three scenes for women are similar in setting and staging. The actress who appears in all three scenes, "Anna," is a fleshy woman who looks to be in her midthirties. Like Anders, Anna is businesslike and brisk when she masturbates. She uses no visual stimulation, and the whole act is over in only a couple of minutes. Anna never looks at the camera—while she pleasures herself her eyes are always closed. Her scenes contain slightly more vocalization, such as the intake of breath and soft moaning, perhaps because this is the only way to convey that she has achieved orgasm. In the bathroom scene, instead of sitting on the toilet, Anna sits on the edge of a bathtub and stimulates herself with water from a showerhead. And instead of the Relax machine she uses a white plastic vibrating dildo. There are no instructions for Anna to clean up after herself or to put a towel under her body so that her sheets don't get soiled and so that no one will know she has a sex life. And the narration, by Margareta Nordeman, is more plainspoken and much less dramatic than the King Lear cadences declaimed by the man who narrates the films featuring Anders.

These are daring films—far too daring for some. As we explained in the previous chapter, they were scaldingly reviewed by Karl Grunewald, who wrote that to show the films to intellectually disabled people would be a form of sexual abuse. Nordeman told us that this attack effectively killed the films in Sweden; they were never used there. They are known in Denmark, though, and some sexual advisors told us that they sometimes use clips from them when they advise young people with intellectual disabilities about masturbation. Others told us that they can't use the films because the actors are too old, especially the male actor. "Nobody wants to see someone in his father's generation sit on a toilet and have a wank," one sexual advisor said tartly.

That the *Masturbation Techniques* films were made in Sweden is no coincidence. They are a 1990s manifestation of a tradition of sexual education for the masses stretching back to the 1930s and pioneered by the Swedish Association for Sexuality Education, which produced the films. This education has always been characterized by a combination of pedagogical instruction, frank sexual images, and exuberant admonitions to pay attention to one's health and hygiene.[12]

The masturbation films made in 1996 are also the direct descendants of another cinematic representation of sex and disability, this one from the 1970 Swedish film *More from the Language of Love* (*Mera ur kärlekens språk*). That film was a sequel to the enormously successful *The Language of Love* (*Kärlekens språk*), which made headlines around the world—and, subsequently, a great deal of money—when, in 1969, it was seized by U.S. customs officials and declared to be obscene. Both the original film and its sequel are framed as sex education documentaries. In both films, psychologists, sexologists, doctors, and representatives of minority groups who speak about particular sexual issues sit smoking and drinking tea in the living room of Inge and Sten Hegeler, a Danish couple who were well known throughout Scandinavia as the authors of books and advice columns about sex. The conversations about sex are interspersed with "educational" scenes, such as a gynecologist inserting a diaphragm into a woman's cervix and couples having sex.

The first *Language of Love* film depicted what today would be called vanilla sex—young, white heterosexual couples having gentle intercourse to the strumming of a baroque guitar. The second film tried to cash in on the success of the first, and it raised the bar by discussing and depicting more audacious sexuality: homosexuality, transvestism, live sex shows, old people—and the sexuality of people with physical disabilities. That latter kind of sexuality is illustrated by a scene that, even when judged by the liberated standards of the swinging sixties, is difficult to regard as anything other than surreal.

The scene follows a conversation in Inge and Sten's living room in which a young blind man tells the couple that he wishes that sexual education for blind people could involve a tactile component—one in which blind people could actually feel the bodies of a member of the opposite sex in order to "see" him or her.[13] This cuts to a scene that Inge Hegeler's voice-over tells us is a staging of how the young blind man, and the sexologists, think that blind people should be taught about sex.

The camera shows a bare classroom. Six teenage students, five boys and one girl, sit around a table with their backs to the camera. In front of the classroom, facing the camera, stand a man and a woman in their twenties. Both are naked. Another teenage girl—clearly a classmate of the seated students—is standing in front of the man, and a male classmate stands in front of the woman. Dressed in clinical white and standing slightly to the side is a revered Swedish sexologist named Maj-Briht Bergström-Walan: a small, busy woman with a no-nonsense newsreel voice, then in her forties.

Bergström-Walan announces crisply to the classroom, "We're now going to determine the bodily differences between a man and a woman."

She tells the boy and girl to lift up their hands and feel the hair of the model in front of them. They are then instructed to move their hands down to the models' faces—all the while guided by Bergström-Walan's monologue: "Jennifer, you feel how the man has beard growth. That is one of the secondary sex traits."

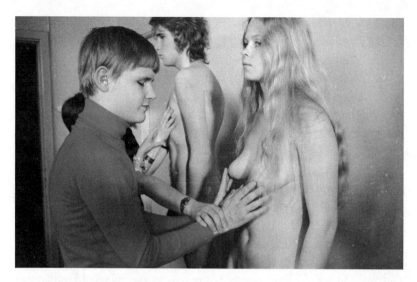

4.1 Still from *More from the Language of Love* (*Mera ur kärlekens språk*), 1970.
© www.klubbsuper8.com.

The camera follows the movement of the teenagers' hands as they travel down to the shoulders and to the chest. "Rolf feels the breasts of a woman," explains the sexologist. "You feel how round they are. If you move your fingers forward to the nipples," she says, reaching her hand over to press the young man's fingers into their target, "you feel that they are bigger and more pronounced than a man's."

After skimming down along the hips, and across the stomach, the students reach the models' genitals. Bergström-Walan guides the female student's hands to clasp the man's flaccid penis. "You feel, Jennifer, how much hair the man has," she says. "And you feel his penis here." She tells the young man, Rolf, that "inside that vulva you feel, there are two labial folds, the outer and the inner. And up at the top there is a little organ called the clitoris. You can feel it there, right?"

A scene like this furthered the international reputation Sweden had already acquired in the 1950s, when it became the first country in the world to provide mandatory sex education in schools, as a sexually enlightened and progressive place. And certainly the plainspoken language, the absence of prudery about showing naked bodies, and the willingness even to discuss an issue like disability and sexuality is remarkable, even today—even if the setup, again, is decidedly weird (as well as, these days, probably illegal in most places).

Notice, however, that even though the scene in the blind school occurs in a film titled *More from the Language of Love*, it is not about love; it is about anatomy. Bergström-Walan, the stern sexologist, does not talk to the blind students she directs about relationships or emotions: she wants them to know what pubic hair feels like. The entire scene is played out in utter, somber seriousness. Nobody laughs or cracks a joke at the absurdity of young students crowding around two naked models in front of a classroom and feeling them up, and both models stand straight and stiff, looking off dutifully into the horizon or shutting their eyes as young people half their age fondle testicles, roll back foreskin, and separate labia.

The *Masturbation Techniques* films made twenty-six years later to instruct women and men with intellectual disabilities how to pleasure themselves continue this earnest pedagogical tradition. Even though they are about a sexual act, the films are not about sexuality as a social and relational practice. They do not depict sex as an activity that connects one to others and provides an opportunity for sharing and engagement. On the contrary, sex in those depictions is not appreciably different from the sex portrayed in Inger Nordqvist's image of the "Individual vibrator adaptation for woman who can only move her head." It is a rather dour, monastic activity that takes place alone, behind securely locked doors, quickly, in silence, with minimal movement, without any assistance from anyone else, and seemingly without relating to anyone else.

Here is where the absence in those films of any hint that a person might use erotic images or pornographic films as part of a masturbatory experience becomes telling. As is the repeated insistence in the sequences with the male actor that one needs to clean up after oneself, that one needs to have toilet paper beside the bed to wipe oneself off with, that one should point one's penis downward into the toilet and ejaculate there, that one needs to use a towel "so that the cum won't get onto the sheet and be sticky and cause stains."

These instructions are presented as tips to help the disabled person ensure that he maintains some privacy. ("He doesn't want anyone to be involved with his sex life.") But the pedantic detail in which the instructions are phrased and depicted, and their recurrence in the films, seems to have less to do with privacy and more to do with erasure. Sex should not only be private, the films seem to say—it should be invisible.

These details suggest that the Swedish *Masturbation Techniques* films are just as much for the benefit of staff members as they are for people with intellectual disabilities. Even as the films instruct intellectually disabled adults how to masturbate, they reassure the staff who work in group homes and activity centers that issues relating to sexuality and disability can be resolved in a way that does not have to involve them. If the lessons offered in the film are learned well enough by their intended audience, staff and assistants will never have to deal with sex. They won't even have to be aware that it ever occurs at all.

Not even by being confronted by a sticky stain on a sheet.

The Boundary between Work and Intimacy

Whether or not people who help disabled adults want to get involved with their erotic lives, it often happens that they do. Stains sometimes do appear on sheets, couples lay down together on a stage, penises become erect during a shower. Staff members in group homes and personal assistants who work in the apartments of people with disabilities are also sometimes confronted by other evidence that the people they assist have sex lives.

While living in the room of a young man who is a resident in a Danish group home for people with cerebral palsy (the room's usual occupant was away on holiday), Don's first sight waking up every morning was the beach ball bosoms and spread, shaved pubis of Galina, a beckoning brunette whose glossy poster the young man had had a helper tape to the wall that faced his bed. This same young man had a series of manicured beaver shots as the screen saver on his computer. A young man in another group home for adults with cerebral palsy had had helpers decorate the walls of his bedroom with six carefully selected centerfolds that displayed the qualities (long blonde hair, pert breasts) he found most desirable. In a group home for adults with intellectual disabilities, a young man had papered the side of a bookcase with choice girl-of-the-week centerfolds (Maja, Alice, Christina . . .) pulled out of a weekly scandal magazine called See and Hear (Se og Hør). The bookcase faces his bed, which was strewn with the teddy bears and plush puppy dogs that (also) comfort him at night.

Danish helpers say they have no problems with pictures like these. "It can be a little embarrassing when you're sitting there with someone from the technology center and they're repairing some problem with his computer," a female staff member told Don when he asked her what she thought of the pornographic images in the room he was occupying. "But it's his home; it's his choice. He does what he wants." Helpers even work with the residents of group homes to display evidence of their sexuality in mischievous ways. One sexual advisor, for example, was delighted to have discovered a little

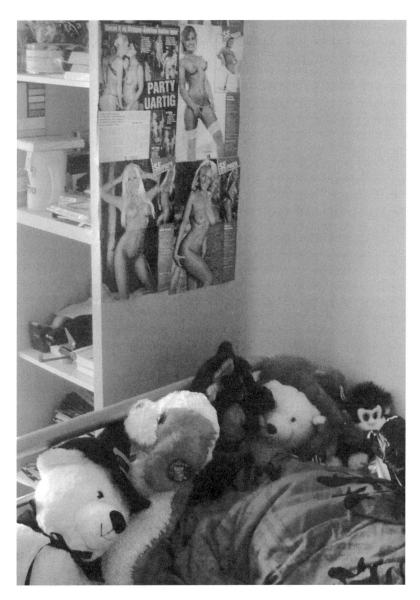

4.2 Objects of affection and comfort.

Japanese vibrator that looked exactly like a Russian matryoshka doll. She recommended it to many of the disabled women she advised because they didn't have to worry about hiding it. "When grandmother comes for a visit, she can't see what it is," the sexual advisor chuckled, turning one on and holding it up for Don to feel as it hummed cunningly.

Swedish helpers have decidedly more ambivalent responses to evidence of sex. While there surely must be assistants and staff members who do not mind things like displays of pornography in residents' rooms, the actions of many helpers suggest that expressions of sexuality are not greeted with equanimity. In the previous chapter we described what happened when an occupational therapist helped a young man with cerebral palsy paste photographs of vulvas on the buttons of his remote control. The staff complained, and the images were given fig leaf bikini bottoms. We also saw how the website personligassistent.com airs complaints from assistants who feel they are being harassed by being made to help the people they assist turn the pages of a pornographic magazine or even to hear a pornographic film. ("It can actually be regarded as sexual harassment or sexual abuse to have a porn film on a volume so high that someone else can hear it.")

Other examples of this same phenomenon include an article in the Swedish trade union magazine *Municipal Worker* (*Kommunalarbetaren*), which reports that upon discovering that the person she assisted had pornographic magazines, a personal assistant packed them up in boxes and carried them down to the cellar; and the case we mentioned in the introduction where helpers refused to lift a disabled woman because they perceived that she found the action of being lifted pleasurable.[14] Even ostensibly progressive engagements with the sexuality of disabled adults contain caveats. For example, in a document from 2006 titled "Staff's Role in Relation to the Sexuality of Adults with Disabilities" ("Personalens roll när det gäller vuxna brukares sexualitet"), one Swedish city instructs employees in service homes that "staff cannot forbid adults with disabilities from watching porn films. However, they can discuss porn with that person and tell them how things work 'in real life,' and they can suggest some other ('softer') film and perhaps limit the amount of time they can watch such films."[15]

Swedish personal assistants and group home staff who complain about being confronted with sexuality when they work with people with disabilities often invoke the country's Work Environment Act (Arbetsmiljölagen), which protects workers from sexual harassment in the workplace. This law is invoked in a similar way in discussions that have been occurring since 2000 about pornography in hotel rooms. In the early years of that decade, the feminist separatist lobbying group Roks (Riksorganisationen för kvinnojourer och tjejjourer i Sverige; National Organization of Shelters for Young and Adult Women) began a campaign that is ongoing to provide certification for "porn-free" hotels. This campaign was supported by a number of parliamentarians, union representatives, and journalists, and it ultimately led to several large organizations (including the National Defense Force, the city council of Stockholm, and the Kommunal (municipal workers') trade union, which has over six hundred thousand members) to declare that henceforth they would only book rooms in hotels that do not include pornography as an option on their pay-to-view cable channels.

A main reason for the campaign was the claim that pornography, by its very nature, is degrading to women and should not exist at all. But the "porn-free" hotel campaign goes further than this: it argues that pornography is particularly egregious in hotels because it creates a hostile work environment. Why? Because cleaning staff have to "wipe sperm off of television sets" (*torka av sperma från tv-rutor*). The tabloid newspaper *Aftonbladet* reported on the problem under the rubric "Cecilia quit: Wiping up sperm isn't a normal job."[16] An article in *Hotellrevyn*, a magazine for people employed in the hotel and restaurant industry, quoted a hotel receptionist who explained that the whole issue was a workplace environment problem. "Staff should not have to wipe sperm off TV sets."[17] A Member of Parliament who introduced a bill to provide everyone in parliament with a list of "porn-free" hotels wrote, "it's not permitted to destroy the furniture [in a hotel room]. Why should a hotel guest be allowed to make a pigsty out of a hotel room by spraying sperm all over it [*att svina ner inredningen genom att spruta sperma på den*]?"[18]

While it is conceivable that Swedish men who stay in hotels may be both more myopic and more fire-extinguishingly potent than males from other places around the world, it seems more likely that hyperbolic rhetoric like this is more an expression of a particular kind of refusal regarding sex than it is an accurate description of it. The refusal turns on an assertion that what is normally imagined to be a private space (in this case, a hotel room) is, in fact, a part of the public domain. Therefore, activities that occur in that space must comply with regulations that protect workers' rights (as opposed to, say, laws that protect a person's right to privacy).

This is the line of reasoning that personal assistants use when they complain about things like the existence of pornographic images in the rooms of the people with disabilities whom they assist. The space in which those images occur may be someone's home, they will concede, but it is also their workplace, and workplace environment legislation protects them against sexual harassment and sexual abuse.

In legal terms, the status of a disabled person's home is a grey zone, since it is both a private residence and a public workplace. Disabled people who use the services of companies who recruit personal assistants sign contracts with those companies ensuring that they will provide a "good work environment" (*god arbetsmiljö*) for the assistants who work in their home. If a person with a disability hires a personal assistant him- or herself, then he or she is the assistant's employer, which entails an entire catalogue of responsibilities and obligations in relation to the employee.[19] These complicated and ambiguous statuses make both the disabled person whose home it is, and the assistants or staff who work there, uncertain about what rights they may have and, consequently, what they can insist on or demand. This uncertainty usually impacts the person with the disability most heavily, since unlike a personal assistant, who can often quit a job that she or he finds unpleasant, or a company that recruits assistants, which can terminate a contract with a disabled person who proves too difficult, the disabled person has no choice but to seek assistance.[20] While some people with disabilities tenaciously defend their right to do what they want in their own homes, many others are compliant, and complaints by assistants or staff about things like pornography often result in outcomes like the one that followed from the vaginal photographs taped onto the remote control buttons. The wishes of the disabled person are overruled.

Infatuation and Love

Besides pornographic images in private rooms or apartments, another place where the boundary between work and sex often gets blurred is when infatuation or love starts to infuse a relationship between a disabled person and a helper.

This occurs frequently—an unsurprising fact given that many people with significant disabilities have limited social networks and that their most intense personal relationships often revolve around family members and the people who assist them in their day-to-day lives. It sometimes happens that relationships between people with disabilities and individuals who assist them blossom into romance. The physicist Steven Hawking's second wife had previously been his nurse and personal assistant, the book

The Sexual Politics of Disability informs readers.[21] That book also contains an autobiographical chapter by a man called Juniper, who writes about several affairs he had with various female assistants, all of whom apparently took the initiative to seduce him.[22] Both Danes and Swedes who work with people with disabilities told us a few stories about women and men who became couples as the result of one of them working as an assistant to the other.

Happy romances like those are heartwarming, but they also are the exceptions that prove the rule that the much more common scenario is that the person receiving assistance falls in love with one of the people providing the assistance, with predictably messy results. This situation is depicted with unflinching candor in the 2005 HBO documentary *39 Pounds of Love*, about a thirty-four-year-old American-Israeli man named Ami Ankilewitz who has a rare form of muscular dystrophy that has resulted in complete paralysis except for one finger of his left hand. The "39 pounds" of the title is a reference to Ankilewitz's weight. The film follows Ankilewitz and a few friends on a road trip across the United States to find the doctor who told his mother, when he was born, that he would not live to be older than six. This trip is set into motion by the "love" in the title: Ankilewitz's feelings for his twenty-one-year-old personal assistant, Christina.

"She bathes me, she feeds me, she scratches my nose when it itches," Ankilewitz's voice explains, as we see images of rose-haired, full-lipped Christina shampooing him, laughing with him, giving him playful kisses on the mouth. "She makes me laugh. She's been with me for two years. She's my caretaker. She's beautiful, young, alive. Her smile says it all. There's nothing in the world I want more than to be with her."

Ankilewitz makes these feelings explicit to Christina, and her response crushes him. She loves him as a friend, she says, but not "in the real meaning of the word." Devastated, he fires her as his personal assistant. And to try to get over his broken heart, he undertakes the American road trip that occupies the rest of the documentary.

Everybody loses in a situation like this. Ankilewitz feels rejected and betrayed; Christina feels misunderstood—plus she loses her job. This kind of outcome is the far more usual one when feelings of love enter the relationship between a disabled person and his or her personal assistant.

Attempting to keep these kinds of situations from arising or going too far is difficult. The kinds of contact that helpers have with young people and adults with significant impairments often necessitate intimate physical contact as well as, in many cases, long-term emotional bonds. The intensity of these relationships is often pleasurable in many ways for both the disabled person and the helper, but the very fact that it is pleasurable also makes it problematic.

Tension over pleasure was brought to a head in one of the group homes Don lived in when staff complained that one of the female residents with cerebral palsy always expressed enjoyment when the shower head used to wash her sprayed water on her privates. "Oh that feels nice," the woman would say. "Can't you do it a little more?" Some staff members were upset by this request. They felt as though the woman was using them sexually. The issue was raised at a staff meeting. The director of the group home, a certified sexual advisor, asked the individuals who complained, "Isn't it odd that we have no problem doing things to the residents that hurt them or make them feel bad? If they need insulin shots, we give them. If they need a catheter inserted, we insert it. No problem. But if someone gets a bit of pleasure out of being showered a little bit longer, we stop it. Why do we feel so bad about doing something that makes a resident feel good?"

A discussion ensued, and the meeting ended with an agreement among the staff that one was not really being exploited just because a resident enjoyed an activity like being showered. But everyone was also reminded that individual boundaries needed to be respected, and the director took the opportunity to raise the issue of masturbation with the female resident. She explained to her that it ought to be possible to find a way for her to masturbate herself, even though she had limited use of her arms. Together, they found a sex aid that they had mounted on the edge of a table at wheelchair height and that the female resident was able to control with the help of a button.

Discussions like this one, which articulate a problem and involve a number of people talking about it, are effective ways of both acknowledging the kinds of erotic tensions that may arise between helpers and the people they help and finding solutions that respect the integrity of everyone involved. In cases where discussions like this do not occur, at least four worst-case scenarios can arise.

One is that a helper acquiesces to the erotic desires of the person being assisted and agrees to perform some kind of sexual service, all the while convincing himself or herself that he or she is merely acting as a kind of charitable prosthesis. This is the situation that people like the young male assistant who helps the woman he works for achieve erotic satisfaction by rubbing her genitals on top of a blanket can find themselves in. A situation like this, as the Swedish woman who told Don the story pointed out, is liable to end very badly.

A second scenario is emotional blackmail. Helpers can foster dependency in people with disabilities and convince them that they have to remain in an unhappy or abusive relationship or else be deprived of all help and satisfaction. From the literature on sexual abuse and disability it seems clear that this kind of blackmail happens most frequently when the person helping the disabled individual is that person's partner or spouse. A 2011 Swedish booklet titled *Seldom Seen: Educational Material on Violence against Women with Disabilities* (*Sällan sedda: Utbildningsmaterial om våld mot kvinnor med funktionsnedsättning*) contains several examples of disabled women being coerced into staying in unsatisfactory relationships. Aside from threats to stop providing help, punishments in the cases mentioned include partners hiding wheelchairs or deserting blind spouses in unfamiliar surroundings. In one case, an angry husband suspended his wife in a hydraulic lift and abandoned her there.[23]

But blackmail can cut both ways. It does not escape the attention of some people with disabilities that helpers, too, are vulnerable. A counselor in Sweden who is often called in as a consultant to assist with issues involving disability told us a story of a young woman in her late twenties who had been in a traffic accident and was now in a wheelchair. She asked this counselor's advice about a situation she was beginning to regret and feel guilty about, but wasn't sure how to handle.

The circumstances involved the woman's relationship with several men she had met because they worked for the taxi company that had a contract with her county (*färdtjänst*) and that always sent drivers to pick her up when she needed to be taken anywhere. The woman was attracted to four of these drivers. She tried various ways of getting the men to come in to her apartment, but nothing worked. Then, she said, she figured out that all of them were interested in sailboats and sailing. A plan was hatched. The woman canvased the county where she lived and applied for many of the various governmental and NGO funds that are available to help disabled people travel with assistants and go on vacation. By pooling these resources, she managed to collect enough money for a weeklong sailing trip, for her and the four men, who had agreed to act as her assistants. "The four guys thought it was a great job," the counselor told us. "A week out sailing, right?"

> But her plan the whole time was that she would seduce them. And she succeeded with three of them. The fourth one didn't do anything; he was more professional. How she managed to seduce all three of them, who knows, but she managed it.

And so when the week was over, she wanted it all to continue. The problem was, they didn't. They must have realized that they'd made a mistake and the whole situation was not exactly a good one. And she told me that on weekends she would call one of them and say, "Why don't you come over to my place tonight?"

And the guy would say, "No, it's over, this can't continue, you have to stop this."

So she'd call the next one, who'd say the same thing. And when she'd called all three and none of them would come to her, then she began to get it, and so she started to threaten them. She's not clueless; she understands that if she wheels herself up to the authorities and tells them that those guys abused her, they'd be behind bars before they knew what hit them. And so one of them would always come to her in the end.

A third worst-case scenario that can occur in an attempt to negotiate the boundary between work and intimacy is public chastisement and humiliation. Lotta Löfgren-Mårtenson recounts what for her was a startling episode at one of the dances for young people with intellectual disabilities that she attended during her research. A young man who had become infatuated with her sat down on the floor in front of her when the dancing was over. What happened next happened swiftly: "The assistant is there in a second, and she tries to pull him up off the floor. He hides his face in his hands and starts to cry. I hear the assistant say, 'If you don't stop that right now we are *never* going to another dance again! She is a staff member and she can *not* be your girlfriend!'"[24]

Finally, the instability of the boundary between work and intimacy can result in staff members becoming so anxious about the possible sexual connotations of physical contact that they refuse to permit even nonsexual expressions of tenderness and affection. The sobering story we mentioned in the introduction, of the Swedish woman in the wheelchair whose helpers refused to lift her when they saw that she was aroused by being lifted, is an example of this kind of panicked attempt to keep work and intimacy strictly separated. Another example—this one with a happier ending—is recounted in the Danish documentary film *One Doesn't Have Words for It* (*Faktisk mangler man ord for det*). In the film, a mother named Käthe Piilmann describes how anxiety about intimacy led staff members of the group home where her son lives to deprive him of what she regarded as crucial human signs of affection.

Piilmann describes how her son Morten, a young man with Down syndrome, has always loved having people sit and stroke the palm of his hand, slowly and rhythmically.[25] The touch soothes him and can result in him entering a kind of pleasurable trance. A problem with this innocent touching arose once Morten entered puberty, because some staff members began to interpret the pleasure he derives from this touch as sexual. His mother says that when those staff members noticed that Morten had started to sink into bliss, they reacted brusquely. They pushed his hand away and got up and left him because they felt as though he had transgressed their boundaries and used them as a sexual object.

The staff members who objected to Morten's behavior mentioned it to his mother and expected her to do something about it. She was not sympathetic. "'You know what,'" she says she told the staff,

> "the ones who have the problem here are you. If you actually take care to notice what my son does, and then think about how you feel, you can certainly find a limit that you can set. You can sit and hold his hand but stop it when you see that his eyes begin to get all starry. Then you can stop and say to him, 'That's enough now.' And Morten accepts that because he doesn't suddenly get rejected really late in the game." I told them there's no reason why they can't allow him to have the pleasure of having his hand stroked. But that it could be stopped before it went too far. It's really not a problem. If you just are aware, you can say, "Now we're stopping."

The Boundary between Love and Sex

In another segment of *One Doesn't Have Words for It*, Käthe Piilmann describes how she dealt with the fact that Morten began masturbating in public—on buses, playgrounds, and in the living room of their house. She says she taught her son that whenever he felt like touching his privates he needed to go and lock himself in his room. She was firm, she said.

"I told him, 'Morten, you can't do this. I don't want this. Other people don't want this either. We don't like it. But you can gladly do this in your room.' I took him into his room and said 'And you can lock the door.' And I locked the door to show him how he could lock it himself, and then it was OK [*var det i orden*]."

Piilmann says she was careful to always respect that her son had locked the door to his bedroom or the toilet. She would always knock, and if the door was locked she would retreat. In this way, she says, Morten experienced a success—that he could control his environment in a way that allowed him some privacy.

This kind of intense maternal involvement is illustrative of how the parents of disabled children often find themselves having to become engaged in the sexuality of their children in ways they are not prepared for and that they often find deeply discomforting. And although having to deal with issues like public masturbation or fears of pregnancy is challenging and distressful for parents, most disturbing of all is the way that the love and the intense emotional and physical bonds that severely impaired children have with their parents—particularly, in most cases, their mothers—can transform as the child matures into an adult and begins to express an interest in sex. Especially in cases where the child has intellectual impairments, the boundary between care involving things like bathing, dressing, or going to the toilet, and erotic satisfaction, can become murky, sometimes putting the mother in an intolerable situation.

This infected dimension of care for a disabled child—particularly a disabled son—is a source of tremendous shame among mothers. In our experience, parents do not discuss this aspect of their child's sexuality with anybody, including with other parents of disabled children. One mother who is the exception to that rule, however, is a well-known Danish actress named Lone Hertz. In 1992 Hertz published *The Sisyphus Letters* (*Sisyfosbreve*), a memoir about raising and living with her son Tomas, who has severe autism. The book discusses struggles, breakthroughs, emotions, and relationships that will be familiar to many parents of children with significant disabilities. But a part of the book that makes it unique is Hertz's insistence on also discussing sexuality. She relates in some detail how the love between her and her son gradually came to be eroticized as Tomas grew older and entered adolescence. Their relationship reached a crisis point when Tomas, who at the time was sixteen or seventeen and twice her size, had an epileptic seizure in the middle of the night.

Hertz heard Tomas flailing about, and she rushed into his room, half-naked, throwing herself on her son's bed in order to help him like she had always done. "It's important to hold your arms," she writes, in the narrative mode of direct address to her son that she uses throughout the book, "so that the convulsions don't wrench your shoulders out of their sockets, and to wipe your mouth regularly so that you don't choke on your vomit. And to push all the blankets and pillows out of the way, so that they don't get drenched in pee when the convulsions wear off and your bladder becomes slack and empties. I'm always grateful when I succeed in doing that, especially if you don't defecate at the same time."

That night, Hertz continues,

you came out of it and became clear-minded sooner than you usually did. You pulled me down into bed so that I would lay with you and take care of you like I've always done in all the years of your convulsions—often they come back, several in a row. That night you wouldn't let me pull up a blanket around me, you kept pulling it off and throwing it out of the bed. I tried not to resist, because I was familiar with your mood swings that almost always followed right after a seizure. I feared them more than the convulsions. You became unpredictable and despotic. I needed to calm you down and not provoke you.

I tried to play, like it was a game of exchange, so I took *your* blanket, but the game didn't work. You made your darkest sound, a throaty howl that I felt was a warning. You took my arm and threw me up against the door, and you pressed up against me . . .

I had thrown my undershirt on, because this was very wrong, I knew that. I understood that. You stood there naked, with an erection, and touched yourself. Not violently, more like searchingly, innocently, like you were trying to find some answer there. You stood and looked at me, sat beside me and lay down on top of me. Like you were in doubt, like you were trying something out. I let you take charge and I tried to keep calm and collected, emotionless, to pretend that it wasn't me. But during all this I knew that unless I took control somehow, this would end very badly. You had so much strength and an enormous desperation. If nothing else, the whole thing would have ended very badly for *me*. I tried to tell myself that I was just imagining this, that you didn't have these wild feelings. That this wasn't really happening. That it wasn't you I was afraid of, I was afraid of my own apprehension. But that wasn't true. I *was* afraid of you, Tomas. It's pitiful to be afraid of your own child. I forced myself to be calm. I spoke calmly to you at the same time as I edged toward the door. And with an awkward kind of shrimplike flip, I was out in the corridor, where I tried to turn the key to the door. You ran after me with surprising energy, you grabbed the door so that I couldn't lock it. We pulled back and forth on the doorknob, like a parody, and you shrieked and roared, until I couldn't take it anymore. I don't know how I did it but suddenly I gave you a big push into the room, and I turned the key and pulled it out.

In the middle of all this horror, Tomas, the saddest part of all is perhaps an admission I have to make to myself that my work as an actress stayed with me, even in that "naked" situation that we were both in there. Despite the despair, I was cold-headed enough to think, in the middle of it all, that I really need to remember this, in case one day I should play a scene like "mother with a psychotic son."[26]

Here, and in several other places in *The Sisyphus Letters*, Lone Hertz discusses, with the kind of tough wryness she displays here, the anguish she felt in relation to her son's developing sexuality. She felt desperate as she came to understand that her son wanted to have sex with her, and she felt utterly forsaken as she realized that there simply was no one to whom she could turn for help or advice. In the mid-1980s, when Hertz was confronting Tomas's sexuality, Danish professionals were still uncertain about how to engage with the sexuality of people with significant disabilities. The *Guidelines about Sexuality—Regardless of Handicap* were just being formulated, and at the time there were as yet no certified sexual advisors who could offer a mother like Hertz any meaningful guidance about sex. In the end, she sought help in the only place she could imagine finding it—she helped Tomas purchase sexual services from a sex worker. That decision, and people's reactions to her writing about it, are discussed in the next chapter.

Lone Hertz may be unique in publicly airing some of the normally unspeakable issues that can arise between parents and their children who have significant impairments as the children enter puberty and begin to seek ways of understanding and expressing their erotic desires and needs. But Hertz is far from unique in having the kinds of experiences she describes.

Gull-Marie is a soft-spoken, matronly Swedish woman in her fifties. She has a son in his late teens who has been diagnosed with a condition she described as a combination of mental retardation and autism (*en utvecklingsstörning med autistiska drag*). She and Don had been talking about the differences between Sweden and Denmark, and Don had just mentioned that it did not seem to him that, in Sweden, parents were given much information or advice about disability and sexuality. This remark seemed to unleash something in Gull-Marie. She became flustered, and she spoke quickly, in a gush. "I think it's terrible, completely, awfully terrible [*jobbigt, helt frukstansvärt jobbigt*]," she said. "It's exactly like you say. When he was a teenager," she said, talking about her son, he started to masturbate everywhere. And it's hard as a mother. You move to a new neighborhood . . . he likes to be on the playground where children are. I went around and knocked on all the neighbors' doors and told them—because I thought it's better to be open about it. Then the parents won't be scared, anyway, and they'll come to me if anything happens.

I looked everywhere for help, everywhere. Doctors, everywhere, and everybody said the same thing: "We don't know what to do." Or else they said, "It'll pass when he's no longer a teenager."

But what was I supposed to do? I couldn't follow him around everywhere and guard him. He just disappears from home sometimes, and I don't know where he goes, and you can imagine, before I find him . . . I don't know what anyone has done to him, or what he has done to anyone, you know?

But then I talked to a sexologist—who was from Denmark, in fact—and she said, "Has he ever ejaculated?"

"I don't know," because I said that he can carry on for hours.

And she said, "You have to help him to ejaculate."

Gull-Marie paused here and looked at Don with an expression that was both plaintive and resigned.

It feels very strange to hear that as a mother, you know? But I went around and thought about it all the time and I thought, "I'll ask his brothers." He has two brothers who aren't disabled and I thought they could help him in the sauna or somewhere. They wouldn't. My husband wouldn't help him either.

So I thought, "Well, the only one left is me." I was so afraid—you know how it is here in Sweden with people phoning up the police and everything. And so I talked to him and I thought to myself, "Now, today, I'm going to do it."

On the day I thought that, he comes out of his room and says, "Mama, mama, this white stuff came out of my wiener [*snoppen*]."

And so I didn't have to do it.

Gull-Marie's story articulates a dilemma so sensitive and traumatic that it is hardly surprising that parents who share dimensions of her experience do not often talk about it, not even with one another. The love that a mother has for her child and the desire to keep him out of harm's way—and to keep him from harming others—becomes explicitly linked, in a situation like this, to satisfying him sexually.

The advice the Danish sexologist gave Gull-Marie is common in these kinds of contexts.[27] The theory behind the advice is that some young people with intellectual disabilities have a difficult time discovering on their own that masturbation can actually result in something pleasurable. "Many mentally retarded people [*udviklingshæmmede*] get afraid when they feel that it starts to tingle [*kilde*] and that sort of thing," one sexual advisor told us. "They think, 'What's going on?'" So they stop or they redirect their focus without ever understanding that manipulating their genitals can have a purpose and an endpoint.

Danish sexual advisors recommend that individuals who seem to have that problem be taught to masturbate. If this cannot be done through verbal counseling alone, then other methods are sometimes used—one sexual advisor said he has helped some men learn to masturbate by writing a plan of action that permits him to sit in the same bedroom with the person he is helping. The sexual advisor holds a dildo, which he strokes to demonstrate to the person learning to masturbate what to do. That person then imitates the advisor's actions on his own penis. Sexual advisors say that once individuals discover that masturbation has a purpose, they can be taught to go into their bedrooms or some other private space when they feel like obtaining sexual pleasure.

Unfortunately, when the individual who has the problem understanding masturbation does not live in a group home in which a Danish sexual advisor or someone else with knowledge of these issues is employed, the delivery of advice like "You have to help him to ejaculate" is often accompanied, as it was in Gull-Marie's case, with no further counseling or practical help. Mothers like Gull-Marie are left on their own.

In that situation, some mothers, like Gull-Marie, make the agonizing, risky (and illegal) decision to literally take things into their own hands and help their child by physically satisfying him herself. Gull-Marie, of course, was spared from having to complete the act she had steeled herself to perform because her son managed to figure out masturbation himself. But some mothers are not so lucky. In his memoir of how the Danish *Guidelines about Sexuality—Regardless of Handicap* came into being, sexual reformer Jørgen Buttenschøn recounts the following incident that occurred in the early 1970s:

> At a meeting of the NFPU [Nordic Association of Mental Retardation] in Uppsala, the director of an institution, Nadja Mac, delivered an open-hearted lecture, where she described, in very precise detail, the behav-

ior and the kinds of repressions and conflicts that could arise if a mentally retarded person [*et udviklingshæmmet menneske*] wasn't allowed to develop and learn practical methods to satisfy him- or herself. Nadja concluded her talk with a personal confession that both surprised and pleased many people in her Nordic audience. As I recall, this is what Nadja Mac said:

"At home in our institution we have a young man in late puberty. Every day when we want to begin different kinds of pedagogical exercises, he refuses to participate. He's so fixated by his erect genitals that he can't come away from them. He toils and pulls, but he can't manage to find a workable way to satisfy himself, and so his agitation persists. He's actually destroying himself.

"So one day I couldn't bear to watch this futile labor anymore, so I took him into the bathroom, put my hand on top of his hand, which I moved down to his penis. And with up and down movements, I showed him how a man can achieve an orgasm. Complete calm fell over the boy, and after that he quickly learned to service himself, and he learned how to do it discreetly and alone."[28]

Buttenschøn writes, "I still remember the silence in the lecture hall, how many people thought now the lecturer has transgressed a boundary, and according to Chief Physician Wad [i.e., Gunnar Wad, whom we discussed in chapter 2], she should be reported to the police. But no report was ever filed—maybe because Nadja Mac finished her lecture by saying: 'And that's how I taught my son to masturbate.'"

Nadja Mac could say something like this publicly only because of the distinct Scandinavian zeitgeist around sexuality that existed in the early 1970s, the fact that Danes were engaged in active discussions about intellectual disability and sexuality, and because of her own engagement with these issues, which was both personal and professional. It is unlikely that any mother today would publicly admit to providing her son with the kind of assistance Mac describes—indeed, it is unlikely that a mother *could* admit to that without inciting precisely the police intervention that Buttenschøn was relieved to see did not happen after Nadja Mac finished her speech and that Gull-Marie was concerned might happen if she had helped her son in the manner prescribed by the Danish sexologist and word of it ever got out.

What some mothers in Denmark do decide to do is publicly insist that their children's sexuality is not their responsibility. The director of a group home for adults with cerebral palsy remembers very clearly that one of her first encounters with the sexuality of people with disabilities occurred in 1988, when the group home where she still works was built and residents started moving in. The mother of one of the young men who moved in insisted on having a meeting with all the staff members. The director recalled,

> She sat there, the mother. And she says, "There's something I want to say to you all"—and we didn't even know one another, we had just all started together in this completely new group home. "One thing I want to say to you. My son has tried going to a prostitute, and it was good for him. You all need to damned well follow up on this." His mother said that. She slammed her hand down on the table and said that. And so we were all forced to figure this out, even though we didn't even know one another and we'd never even spoken about things like sexuality.

The director said the mother's insistence that the group home staff acknowledge her son's sexuality was the spark that led to conversations and to engagement with the sexuality of the residents.

> We began to develop some basic policies around sexuality. And then after about two years, the same woman's son got a girlfriend, who was also in a wheelchair. And they wanted to have sex. That was a bit difficult because they weren't able to do it by themselves, and at that time the idea that we might go in and help them was really new.
>
> And so in comes his mother again. And she says, "They want to have sex. Surely it can't be reasonable that I, his mother, should be the one to go into his room and lift them up onto and down from the hydraulic lift. That's your job. I don't want to know anything about it. Because I am his mother. I shouldn't have to have anything to do with this. But you should."

"She was fantastic," the director said of this cantankerous, plainspoken woman. "She was completely adamant." This adamant mother also illustrates the way that parents can use their status as parents to bring about change. The ingenuous argument that "surely it isn't reasonable" to expect a mother to get actively involved in her child's sex life is a difficult one to counter. It demonstrates the significant power that parents can have in contexts like these to compel others to take seriously the reality of their disabled child's sexuality and to devise ways of helping to facilitate an erotic life.

The Boundary between Affection and Abuse

Any book or pamphlet on sexuality directed at people who work with individuals with disabilities will almost inevitably contain at least one description of a situation like the following, from *When the Feeling Carries You Away,* by Margareta Nordeman:

> *Is Emma being abused by Hasse?*
>
> Emma is 29 years old and has a moderate developmental disability. She has a limited vocabulary and some ability to describe her feelings. Hasse is 43 years old and has a mild developmental disability. They work at the same sheltered workshop and that's where they met.
>
> Hasse openly shows that he likes Emma a lot, but it's harder to know what kind of feelings she has for him. She's fairly reserved [*inbunden*].
>
> It's clear, though, that she is happy when he comes up to her and gives her little hugs and kisses. The staff think that they are cute [*gulliga*] together and they encourage their contact, until one day when both of them have been missing for a while and the staff find them in the staff resting area, in the middle of having intercourse.[29]

The situation, which in Scandinavian contexts usually has exactly this dramaturgy—a younger woman with an intellectual disability having a relationship with an older man who often but not always also has an intellectual disability and who may or may not be taking advantage of her—is phrased as a dilemma, an example whose point is to get readers talking. What is the appropriate response from staff or personal assistants? Should they intervene or not? Why? How?

The boundary in question in an example like this is the boundary between a disabled adult's right to explore sexuality and relationships, even to the point of having bad sex and unhappy relationships, and caring others' responsibility to protect those adults from abuse. This boundary is a source of great frustration for people with disabilities, and of tremendous anxiety among parents and everyone else who works with or cares for individuals with significant disabilities. The frustration arises when people with disabilities feel they are being bossed around by helpers and parents, even though they are adults. And the anxiety comes from the helpers' and parents' fear that by leaving disabled adults to do what they want they might inadvertently facilitate or fail to put a stop to encounters or relationships that are nonconsensual or abusive. This apprehension about abuse focuses most intensely on women, especially on women with intellectual disabilities. But a general nimbus of unease hovers around the romantic relationships of most disabled adults.

Twenty-eight-year-old Pernille, for example, has no intellectual impairment. But she has cerebral palsy so intense that her speech is difficult to understand and her entire body needs to be restrained in order to control its spasticity. Raven-haired, attractive, and articulate, Pernille's first and, to date, only intimate relationship was with the driver of the short bus that picked her and several others up from their parents' houses every day to take them to the activity center where they spent their weekdays. At nineteen, Pernille fell in love with this man, who was fifteen years her senior.

Pernille's story about how she fell in love with the bus driver is romantic. She thought he was kind, she said, and he drove her to secluded places where the two of them could have long private conversations. The bus driver convinced Pernille that her parents were limiting her development and that she was capable of doing more than she thought she could. Her introduction to sex was with him ("I was like a frightened bird; I didn't know what sex was"), and she described that experience, and their subsequent relationship, wistfully and with warmth.

Pernille's description of her relationship with the bus driver stands in stark contrast to how people who know her talk about it. The relationship led to a break between Pernille and her parents—because they objected to the relationship, she moved out of their house and refused to have any contact with them for many years. The staff in the Danish group home where Pernille came to live told Don that they agreed with Pernille's parents. All the staff thought that the bus driver was a shady character. He was an unattractive man with a large potbelly whose only friends seemed to be young people with disabilities. He exhibited odd behavior, like insisting on sitting with Pernille whenever she went to the toilet, and on his Facebook page he posted nude photos of her. The staff couldn't stand him. They knew that Pernille's greatest desire was to have a relationship with someone who was not disabled (she told Don, "I really want to be together with someone who is normal. Someone who can make food and who can take me for drives and, to come right out and say it, someone who can have sex with me without a bunch of help or sex aids"). The staff were convinced that this was the only reason she accepted the bus driver.

Several staff members spoke to Pernille about what they saw as the bus driver's inappropriate behavior, but she was always unmoved. She did not find his company in the toilet strange at all, and she thought the naked photos were flattering. In the end, though, after being together for nearly five years, the bus driver left Pernille. She blames the staff at her group home for his departure. She is certain that their coldness toward the man and their opposition to the relationship soured it and succeeded in turning him against her.

Situations like this illustrate the kinds of conflicts and impasses that can occur when people with disabilities have erotic contact or romantic relations with others. Their physical and/or intellectual impairments are presumed by those who care for and work with them to increase their vulnerability, making them easy prey for anyone who might want to abuse them. But from the perspective of many people with disabilities, erotic relationships with others, even if they aren't perfect, can still be important and life-affirming. As the author of the Emma and Hasse example cited above observed, "There are a lot of [nondisabled] women and men who are exploited in their relationships and who, despite that, still carry on with them. . . . Even a person with an intellectual disability can think that a bad relationship is better than no relationship."[30]

There is an irreconcilable tension between the sexual self-determination of an adult with significant impairments and the desire of caregivers to protect that person from harm. The tension is not irresolvable, but one way it is often resolved, especially in Sweden, is through policies and practices that make intimate encounters difficult. This is the situation documented by Lotta Löfgren-Mårtenson in her work on the arranged dances for young people with intellectual disabilities that she observed. She saw that such dances are eagerly anticipated gatherings saturated with hope, desire, and longing. But they are structured so as to make the development of intimate relationships virtually impossible. They last for exactly three hours, starting at 7 PM and ending promptly at 10 PM. (One is reminded of Swedish writer Gunnel Enby's remark about how she and everyone living in her institution in the 1970s were put to bed "when the young people in town are just getting ready to go out.")[31] Soft drinks and coffee are the only beverages on offer, lights in the dance hall are turned up to the brightest setting, and behavior is policed. When the clock strikes 10, everyone is bustled back to the buses that brought them to the dance and are driven straight home. That anyone who participated in the dance might go home with someone they met there is unthinkable. "That idea is so foreign," one staff member of a group home told Löfgren-Mårtenson in broken syntax that expressed a kind of shock that it would ever occur to her to even ask him about such a possibility. "It's so new that I don't even know if I can . . . I can't imagine it would be possible. It's never happened. The ones who live in the group home live there. No one else can just come there. I don't even think we're allowed . . ."[32]

Events like the arranged dances resolve the tension between disabled adults' sexual self-determination and helpers' anxieties by preempting the possibility of any intimacy that helpers would then have to consider. It solves the problem by ensuring that it never arises.

Another way in which Swedes attempt to resolve this problem is through material and discussions that frame sexuality in relation to people with disabilities primarily as a threatening and dangerous activity. A plethora of publications in Sweden discuss sexuality and disability in terms of violence and abuse. They have titles like *Seldom Seen: Educational Material on Violence against Women with Disabilities* and *Violence against Women with Psychological Disabilities* (both published by the Ministry of Social Welfare), *When One Hits That Which Hurts: Violence against Women with Disabilities* (published by the National Council on Violence Against Women), *Violence against People with Disabilities* (published by the Swedish National Council for Crime Prevention), and *"Who Wants to Be Together with Me?": On Therapy, Sexual Abuse and Developmental Disability* (published by Save the Children, Sweden).[33] These documents all contain important information, such as discussion of nonverbal behaviors that might indicate that someone has been subjected to sexual trauma. If they circulated together with other publications that discussed sexuality as a source of pleasure and affirmation for people with disabilities (publications like the Danish *Guidelines about Sexuality—Regardless of Handicap*, for example), then interested helpers and caregivers would have access to a range of materials they could explore and learn from, to help them think about what their roles might be in relation to the erotic lives of people they help or care for.

But the emphasis in Sweden on sex as a source of danger to people with disabilities, particularly congenital disabilities, is not balanced by anything that acknowledges sex as a source of pleasure. This imbalance creates an atmosphere in which sex, almost by definition and certainly by default, is construed as being abusive. For that reason, it should therefore be hindered, prevented, or stopped.

An illustrative example of how this kind of framework is constructed is a film made for adults with intellectual disabilities by the Swedish National Association for Persons with Intellectual Disability (Förening för Barn, Unga och Vuxna med Utvecklingsstörning, FUB).

Titled *Say "Yes," Say "No": Who Gets to Hug Me? (Säga ja, säga nej: Vem ska få krama mig?)*, the thirty-minute film is about boundaries and intimacy.[34]

The film contains no moving images, only still photos and slowly paced narration in a soft-spoken female voice. It tells the story of Lena and Carina, two friends in their twenties with intellectual disabilities. Carina takes a bus to Lena's apartment, where the two young women have made plans to drink Coca-Cola and eat potato chips as they dress up for an evening dance (like the kind Lotta Löfgren-Mårtenson describes in her work). While Carina is waiting at the bus stop, a man—a complete stranger—walks up and sits down next to her. He suddenly puts his arm around her. "He smells of tobacco" the narrator says, "Carina thinks that is disgusting." In a series of still photographs, we see Carina throw the man's arm off her shoulder. The narrator says that Carina shouts at him, "I don't want you to put your arm around me! Don't touch me!" She then gets on the bus and goes to Lena's apartment. She tells Lena about the incident. The narrator says that Lena is proud to have a friend like Carina, who is so courageous that she can say "no" like that.

When Carina and Lena later get to the dance, they discover that another friend, Anna, is huddled in the restroom, crying. Anna reveals that her stepfather has forced her to sleep with him (*ligga med honom*). Lena calls her mother, who comes and comforts Anna and assures her that her stepfather will never touch her again.

The feature of this film that makes it characteristically Swedish is its resolute focus on sexuality as a source of aggression and abuse. The narrative about sexual harassment at a bus stop and rape by a stepfather makes it clear what "Say no" in the film title means. But it is never apparent what the "Say yes" might refer to.

At several points in the film the narrative is interrupted by interludes consisting of still close-up photographs of young women and men with intellectual disabilities. As these photos appear onscreen, we hear what presumably are the voices of the people depicted, talking about things like how important it is to say "no" ("I'm the kind of girl who has courage, who dares to say 'no'").

In one two-minute interlude, just before Carina and Lena find Anna crying in the restroom, the voices also talk about intimacy in more affirmative terms. What they say, however, is the following:

> Yeah, I have a friend who is a girl [*en flickkompis*] in Vetlanda whose name is Karin. And we have fun together. We hug [*Vi kramas*]; yeah, that happens sometimes. She has a cat named Carola. A black cat.
> —voiced over a photo of a smiling young man

We like each other. We hug and kiss [*Vi kramas och pussas*]. It feels a little tingly [*pirrigt*], like that.
　　—voiced over a photo of a young woman

She hugs me sometimes, my mother. Sometimes. It feels really good. It feels good when I am sad. I get so sad sometimes. So it's nice when some-one sits beside me and comforts me.
　　—voiced over a photo of another young woman

Yeah, lots of hugs, lots of hugs. Really good. You can horse around [*busa*] too [laughs]. Mama and me, we horse around all the time.
　　—voiced over a photo of a laughing young woman with Down syndrome

Intimacy, in these voice-overs, consists of hugs and smooches—the Swed-ish word *pussa* that the speakers use denotes not an erotic kiss, but rather the kind of affectionate peck one bestows on children, or grandmothers. This is perhaps what the filmmakers want to convey as affirmative intimate behavior—the kind of activity to which disabled adults might want to say "yes." But the use of the chaste word *pussa* juxtaposed against the sequence of comments about hugging opposite-sex friends and about hugging one's mother creates an impression that the intimacy desired by adults with intel-lectual disabilities has little to do with sex. In fact, in the film the word *sex* occurs only once, as does *intercourse* (*samlag*). This happens at the very end, when the narrator is summing up. "Everything went well for Anna," the nar-rator concludes. "The stepfather confessed to the police that he had forced Anna to have intercourse with him. He had committed a crime, and so he went to prison. Anna never saw him again. Every person has the right to decide whom they want to kiss and hug. If someone tries to kiss or hug you, or have sex with you, and you don't want to, you need to get help."

It is striking that neither of these two words, *sex* or *intercourse*, are elabo-rated or explained in a film about sexuality for young people with intellectual disabilities. The words occur without comment, as though their meaning must be self-evident to any viewer. But notice the context—the sole context—in which they occur: in the middle of a series of allusions to confession, force, "the police," someone who "committed a crime," "prison," someone never seen again, the idea that "you don't want to," and the need to get help. How anyone with an intellectual impairment (or anyone else) watching this film might come away from it with anything other than a profoundly anxious impression of sex is difficult to imagine.

Say "Yes," Say "No": Who Gets to Hug Me? was made in 1995, but little has changed in Sweden since then. In September 2012 the Skåne county provincial regional council and the Malmö city council in southern Sweden organized a conference called Sexuality—Possibilities Different Conditions (Sexualitet— möjligheter olika förutsättningar). The conference title was odd and rather inscrutable, even in Swedish, but the information provided by the organizers made it clear that the conference was about sexuality and disability.

In keeping with the enduring Swedish tendency to frame questions of disability and sexuality in medical terms, the conference took place at Malmö University Hospital. It was attended by 320 Swedish professionals who worked in some capacity with people with disabilities (mostly intellectual disabilities). The plenary lectures at the conference included two talks about Denmark—one by Jens, who presented the research we discuss in this book, and the other by a Danish official from the Ministry of Social Affairs, who talked about the work being done at the time to revise the *Guidelines about Sexuality—Regardless of Handicap*. Both presentations highlighted the facilitation of sexuality.

In stark contrast, *all* of the Swedish presentations focused on sexuality and disability as a problem. One plenary speaker talked about his work with young men with Down syndrome who have sexually assaulted others. Another talk was by a woman who worked in a private clinic specializing in sexual abuse, sexual trauma, and "sexualized behavioral problems" (*sexualiserade beteendeproblem*).[35] A third lecture, canceled at the last minute, was to have been by a Swedish social work researcher whose work focuses on trying to stop adults with intellectual disabilities from having sex in return for money or presents.[36] The issue of sexual pleasure was not completely absent from this conference—it was raised in the two presentations about Denmark. But the fact that it occurred *only* in the talks about Denmark highlighted it as something of a foreign concern, of limited interest to Swedish professionals, who are otherwise occupied—with issues of abuse, trauma, and prevention.

:: :: ::

Denmark also has its share of literature and information on disability and sexual abuse. The *Guidelines* document contains a section on "Problematic sexual behavior" that discusses how helpers should respond to behavior that is socially inappropriate or illegal. An NGO called Social Development Center (Socialt Udviklingscenter, SUS) has created a number of publications for helpers and for people with disabilities that discuss sexual harassment and sexual abuse. These include an easy-to-read booklet titled *Sexual Abuse—No Thanks!* and booklets titled *Good Advice on Seeing and Preventing Abuse* and *A Literature Review: Sexual Abuse of People with a Handicap.*[37] A detailed "toolbox" (*værktøjskasse*) developed by a state-funded project about sexuality in schools for people with disabilities (Projekt Seksualpolitik på specialskoler) provides interested schools and group homes explicit guidelines for devising policies relating to sexual harassment and abuse.[38] The Danish National Board of Social Services (Socialstyrelsen), has a website for social workers and other professionals titled "Prevent Sexual Abuse of People with Handicap" that provides a wide range of downloadable brochures and publications, as well as links and videos on the topic.[39]

The significant difference between Sweden and Denmark, then, is not that Danes who work with people with disabilities are not concerned with issues of sexual abuse. The difference is that Danes who work with people with disabilities produce and circulate materials on sexual danger and sexual abuse *even as they also* provide materials about sexual pleasure for interested helpers, concerned parents, and curious people with disabilities. So a booklet like *Sexual Abuse—No Thanks!* directed at people with intellectual disabilities contains illustrations on how to say "no" like the one in figure 4.3. But the same publication also contains images that provide affirmative, or at least relatively nuanced, images of sexuality, such as the one in figure 4.4.

Even in a context where the point is to help people with intellectual impairments say "no," sex is presented in figure 4.4 as a variety of activities—"many things"—to which a person might also conceivably say "yes." The activities being considered by the man and woman thinking about them are not depicted as intrinsically sinister. They are presented simply as examples of what sex may consist of. The text lets readers know that they may not like all kinds of sex and that sex is not something that anyone likes all the time. But the image does not patronize its intended audience. The range of sexual activities depicted as available to people with intellectual disabilities is no different from the range available to anyone else. And the decision that readers are invited to make is *whether* they want to have sex, not just, as it is in Swedish material, how they might most effectively say "no" to sex.

Danish sexual advisors and others encourage disabled adults to explore their sexuality partly *in order to prevent* sexual abuse from occurring. They are adamant that the most fertile ground for the sexual abuse is a culture that

HVORDAN SIGER DU NEJ?

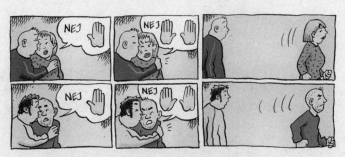

STOPPER DEN ANDEN IKKE, SKAL DU GÅ.

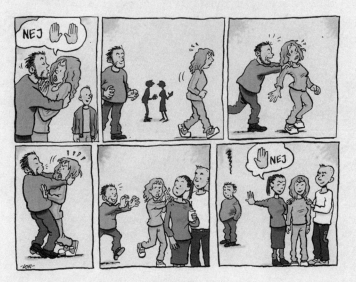

FØLGER DEN ANDEN EFTER DIG – SØG SAMMEN MED DINE VENNER
ELLER ANDRE DU KAN STOLE PÅ.

4.3 *How do you say no? If the other person doesn't stop, walk away. If the other person follows after you—go to your friends or others you can trust.* From the Danish booklet *Seksuelle overgreb—Nej tak!* (2010).

4.4 *Sex is many things. You should not do anything you don't like! It's not always that you are in the mood for sex. It's not good to feel pressured.* From the Danish booklet *Seksuelle overgreb—Nej tak!* (2010).

denies the sexuality of individuals with disabilities and refuses to talk about sex in affirmative terms. They insist that only by engaging positively with people's erotic interests can one provide them with knowledge and experience that will allow them to identify and understand abuse should it ever occur.

As an example of this, a sexual advisor named Alida told Don the story of Dorte and Ragnar, a couple whom she helped have sex. Dorte lives in a group home for adults with cerebral palsy. She has intense spasticity and no verbal language. She communicates by making a variety of sounds and by using the thumb of the one hand she can control to point at a tray on her wheelchair on which are drawn letters, numbers, and many commonly used words. When Dorte was in her late thirties she began a relationship with Ragnar, a man ten years older than her, who lives in another group home. Alida has worked in Dorte's group home for many years, and the two women know each other well. When Dorte and Ragnar became a couple, they asked to speak to Alida. "The two of them wanted to have intercourse," Alida said, "And I talked to them about how they could do it because they didn't know. Well, Ragnar said that he had had a few other girlfriends. When we talked about it he said that he had been to bed with a couple of other women, and the last one he was together with, they had had intercourse, and she was handicapped too. So my understanding was that he had it all down, and he was clear about what we were talking about. But I knew that for Dorte all this was completely new."

Alida said she was happy to assist. She told them that given the configuration of Dorte's body, and her spasticity, the way the couple would probably have to have intercourse was with Ragnar lying behind Dorte and entering her from behind. Alida helped the couple lie in that position, with their clothes on, so that they could decide whether or not it felt comfortable. But that didn't really work. "I could see that Dorte, she didn't really get what I was talking about," Alida said. "And Ragnar seemed uncertain too."

So Alida brought one of her colleagues into Dorte's room, "and we lay down on the floor, me and my colleague, and showed them what we meant. We lay together, spooning, and showed them what we meant. And I told them things like, 'Ragnar, he should lie like this, do you see?'

"So they said they would try that. So we left the room and Ragnar undressed and helped Dorte undress, and they tried it out."

Later on, Alida asked the couple how everything went. "I asked, 'Well, how did it go? Do you want to talk about it?'

"And Ragnar says, 'Yeah, it's all good. It's good, good.' Dorte, she nods."
It turned out, however, that all was not well. Alida continued:

OK, a few months go by and I feel like Dorte has changed. She seems, she seems almost like she's in a kind of depression. She gets like, she just sinks into her own thoughts. I see all the signs of sexual abuse. And suddenly a light goes on and I think, "Oh no, there's something really wrong here."

So I say to them, "I'd really like to have a talk. I'm curious to know how things are going." That was fine with them. And it turns out that Ragnar didn't actually know which opening he should put his penis in. That really caused Dorte a lot of pain, because he was putting his penis in her anus instead of her vagina. And Dorte doesn't know, because she's never had intercourse before. She doesn't like it, but she really wants to be "normal," so she just lets it happen. She doesn't tell him to stop. Boy, that was hard for me, because I felt it was my fault because I hadn't checked, really checked, that Ragnar knew what we were talking about. Because it turned out that he didn't.

So I talk to him and find out that yes, he has had sex before, but I seriously doubt that the experience was particularly enjoyable for the young woman he had it with. So we have a long talk about how sex is about both partners feeling pleasure, and how maybe they should do something else besides this, and that Dorte needs to be ready for it, needs to want it, and that he just can't stick it in and that's the end of it, you know?

And it all resulted in Dorte saying no to any more sex for a long time. Then at some point they tried again, and then Dorte decided she didn't want to anymore. So now they don't have sex.

Alida went on to say that Dorte's relationship with Ragnar has been bumpy. "He doesn't do it anymore," she said, "but at one time Ragnar had a temper, and Dorte was also a little afraid of him because he could get so angry [hidsig] if he felt pressured."

There was a period when the staff were tired of the fact that he was always here. He butted in and had opinions about how the staff did their jobs. Because he has language, he can speak, and he would sit at the table and tell the staff what to do. But he doesn't live here; he's a guest. And so sometimes they would say something to him.

When they did, he would go into Dorte's room and shout at her. So Dorte was a little afraid of him. After a while, Dorte opened up and said that she was afraid that Ragnar might hit her. I could tell that she wasn't telling me everything, and I told her, "Dorte, if there's anything more you want to tell me, you can talk to me. I'm not going to spread what you tell me to all the staff here." Because she was afraid to tell me because she thought that if the staff found out, then they'd make Ragnar even more unwelcome, and that would make it even worse for her when the two of them were alone.

So when she told me she was afraid. I asked her, "Would you like us, together, to have a talk with Ragnar about this?"

Yes, she wanted that.

So I made it clear to Ragnar that there was no way we could accept any violence here. No way. We have responsibility for the people who live here, and if we see that anyone is being subjected to something they haven't agreed to, we're going to intervene. I told him, there is no way I am going to ever accept any violence here, and if I discover it, I'm reporting it to the police, whether Dorte wants me to or not.

Alida recounted the story of Dorte and Ragnar to make the point that unless she had been trusted to be involved in the couple's erotic life, the discomfort and abuse that Dorte suffered in her relationship with her partner would have been difficult to detect and resolve. Alida realizes that the advice she initially provided resulted in something other than the happy effect she had anticipated. But the way to improve that situation, she makes clear, was to talk more about sex, not less. Alida has her own opinions about Dorte and Ragnar's relationship, but she has no illusions about how, at the end of the day, none of that matters very much. What matters, she told Don over the course of several conversations, is not treating Dorte like a child. Alida says that she hopes the fact that she has shown that it is possible to speak openly and affirmatively about sex has helped Dorte to learn to recognize the boundary between affection and abuse. And she says that she hopes that Dorte will feel secure enough to turn to her and to others for help, should she ever need it again.

This is the same approach that the staff in Pernille's group home finally settled on in relation to her relationship with her bus driver boyfriend. As we mentioned above, the staff in that case were all absolutely convinced that Pernille was being exploited—but there was nothing they could do about it. Pernille, an adult, asserted that she was satisfied in the relationship, and there was no evidence that her bus driver beau physically abused her. So all the staff could do was stay aware, talk to Pernille, and do their best to try to help her ensure that she was not being treated like a doormat.

The Boundary between Sex and Reproduction

While all of the tensions, anxieties, and problems we have been exploring in relation to sexuality and disability are important and pervasive, we come at last to the two issues in particular that loom above all others whenever the sexual lives of individuals with severe disabilities are considered as a topic for discussion. Those issues are gendered. When it comes to male sexuality, the one that occupies much public concern and debate is the purchase of sexual services. Is it acceptable that men with significant disabilities, who may be unable to find partners in the way many nondisabled people do, buy sex from prostitutes to satisfy their sexual needs? This inflamed question is part of a topic that we will discuss in detail in the next chapter.

As far as disabled women are concerned, the issue that occupies everyone involved with their sexuality is the risk of pregnancy. This subject generates much more discussion and anxiety in relation to women with intellectual disabilities than it does in the context of women with physical disabilities. This is so partly because some women with physical disabilities are incapable of becoming pregnant. This is partly so also because it is easier to simply ignore the sexuality of significantly physically disabled women. If a woman does not have verbal language and is unable to draw attention to her sexuality—for example, by obviously flirting or by masturbating in public— then any sexual desire she may feel can be disregarded by anyone who does not want to recognize it.

The final reason women with physical disabilities raise less concern in regard to pregnancy than do women with intellectual disabilities is because many women with physical disabilities are vocal, articulate, and demanding. They do not tolerate other people meddling in their reproductive choices, and they are willing to do battle to defend them.

Intellectual disabilities present another picture. One social worker who works in a group home for people with intellectual disabilities in Denmark identified pregnancy as everyone's "worst fear" (*største skræk*). What we might call "the pregnancy problem" is absolutely central to how many people think about the sexuality of women with disabilities, and it structures policies and practices that relate to their capacity to have an erotic life.

For decades the pregnancy problem in many parts of the world was dealt with mercilessly. Women with disabilities (and some men with disabilities) were sterilized without their consent and even against their will. The reason was eugenic, the desire of social engineers to prevent the spread of what they called "defects." Scandinavia has a particularly shameful past in this regard. Denmark had two laws regulating sterilization, the Sterilization and Castration Act of 1935, which regulated voluntary sterilizations and castrations, and the Feebleminded Act of 1934, which allowed for sterilizations and castrations without the consent of the persons concerned. More than 12,000 "voluntary" sterilizations and 6,839 forced sterilizations (of women, in 87 percent of the cases) were carried out in the country until the laws were abolished in 1968.

In Sweden, the first Sterilization Act was adopted in 1935 and amended in 1941 so that it was applicable to a wider range of people (not only hereditary insanity and feeblemindedness but also other "grave illnesses," such as epilepsy and syphilis, were included). Formally, Swedish law did not allow for forced sterilizations, but a majority of those sterilized were patients of asylums, and their discharge was often made conditional on their consent to sterilization. The number of people sterilized during the forty years the Sterilization Act was enforced was also three times higher in Sweden: 62,888 people were sterilized there, 93 percent of them women.[40] The law was only rescinded in 1975.

As an acknowledgment of this ignominious history and as a gesture of redress, in both countries today, surgical sterilization is difficult to obtain. No sterilizations are performed without the written consent of the person undergoing the procedure. In both countries, anyone over twenty-five who wants to be sterilized must meet with a doctor or a medical counselor to discuss the decision and sign a consent form stating that one has been informed about other methods of preventing pregnancy besides sterilization and about the consequences of sterilization. Individuals between the ages of eighteen and twenty-five must receive special permission from the National Board of Health and Welfare in Sweden (Socialstyrelsen), and, in Denmark, from one of the Councils on Abortion and Sterilizations (Samråd for Abort og Sterilisation) that operate in each of the country's five medical administrative units.

Despite the fact that the age of involuntary sterilization is past, disabled women's reproductive capability continues to be actively limited, partly by staff ensuring that they take some form of contraceptive. The preferred contraceptive is the matchstick-sized Implanon rod, which is injected just under the skin along the back of the upper arm and remains active for up to five years. Legally, no one can be forced to submit to contraception against her will. This means that women with intellectual disabilities have to agree to accept it. The process by which they come to do so will be looked at more closely below.

It should be clear by now that, in addition to contraception, the problem of potential pregnancy is also dealt with—especially in Sweden—by making it difficult or near impossible for disabled women to have sex. Women with physical disabilities who cannot manage to have intercourse without an assistant's help are likely to never have intercourse in Sweden because no assistants will help them. So someone in the same situation as David's girlfriend Lisa, whom we mentioned in the last chapter, would live without sex in Sweden. Women with intellectual disabilities often do not need any physical assistance to have sex. But, once again, Lotta Löfgren-Mårtenson documents how social workers and staff members police their activities so as to prevent them, as best they can, from ever being in a situation where sex is possible. Löfgren-Mårtenson's observation that people "often react with uncertainty" (osäkerhet) when young people with intellectual impairments express the desire for children is a vast understatement.[41]

In Denmark the situation is more complicated because sexual advisors and many others are committed to facilitating for women with disabilities the same sexual freedoms that nondisabled women have. But this comes with a risk—a sexually active heterosexual woman can become pregnant. If her partner does not use a condom she can, of course, also potentially contract a variety of sexually transmitted diseases, including HIV. But the greatest fear on everybody's mind is that she can become pregnant.

Susanne is a twenty-eight-year-old woman who lives in a group home in Denmark for people with intellectual disabilities. A pale, slight woman with auburn hair and a smooth, girlish face, Susanne is gentle, quiet, and focused. Everywhere she goes, Susanne carries around a life-sized infant doll she has named Niklas. The doll's body is soft and filled with material that makes it weigh about what a two-month-old child would weigh, but its limbs and its bald head with puffy blue eyes that never close—these are hard, beige plastic. Staff members in Susanne's group home have programmed the doll to cry and make sounds that its caregiver is supposed to respond to. Susanne is very attentive to these sounds. Whenever the doll cries, she comforts it, cradling it and putting a pacifier in its mouth. When it makes sounds that she interprets as hunger, she puts a bottle in its mouth. The doll has its own bed—not a bed for a doll, but an actual child's cradle. It also has a large baby stroller with an umbrella. It has a number of small outfits and shoes that Susanne has bought in baby stores. On one of the first occasions Don visited Susanne in her room, she held her iPhone above the cradle and filmed the doll for five minutes, looking at it adoringly the entire time.

When Don first got to know Susanne he was uncertain about whether she actually realized that the baby she was caring for was a doll. She does, after all, live in a group home for people with intellectual disabilities. Since she treated the doll with such attention and love, Don assumed that she probably thought it was real. But one day she told him that she would be going to Greece with her family for a summer holiday later in the season. "Who will look after Niklas when you go?" Don asked, in a tone he hoped conveyed empathy and concern.

"I'll just switch him off and leave him here," she answered, shooting him a look that suggested she reckoned he might be a bit slow.

Susanne had acquired her doll as part of a project about children that her group home had run in order to acknowledge and articulate the desires that some of the young female residents had expressed to become mothers. For the better part of a year, three of the group home's sexual advisors met for two hours a week once every three weeks with women who wanted to be included in the project. Eight young women participated in these meetings, which consisted of discussions about what it means to be a mother, what kinds of needs a child has, and what kinds of duties and responsibilities come with having a child. At every meeting, in addition to talking, the young women made posters. They drew on large sheets of paper and pasted pictures they cut out of magazines. The posters were a way for the sexual advisors to try to assess the individual women's understandings of things like an infant's needs. The group also discussed how a child develops and how mothers do not only just care for their child by feeding it and holding it; they also need to stimulate it in a variety of ways.

An important part of the project was a guest appearance by two women with intellectual impairments who had had different experiences in relation to children. One of the women had decided to have herself sterilized; the other had opted to become pregnant. Both of the stories they told were wrenching. The woman who had had herself sterilized said she did so because she felt pressured by her parents. Her message to the young women listening was that they shouldn't allow themselves to do something they did not feel was right for them.

The woman who had opted to have a child narrated the story of how her child was taken from her after it was born. This woman had contact with her daughter, but she had been judged incapable of raising her, and the child lived with foster parents. The message that this woman conveyed was that women with intellectual disabilities need to understand one thing: they can decide to become pregnant, but they cannot decide what will happen to their baby once it was born.

This message, and the rest of the activities and discussions that occurred during the "parenting project" (*forældreevne projekt*), put a chill on the maternal desires of most of the young women who participated. But even after much discussion about how county authorities necessarily become involved with the child of a woman with intellectual disabilities and, in most cases, take the child from its mother, a few participants still insisted that they wanted to become mothers.

This is how Susanne got her doll. Susanne was one of the young women in the group home who continued to insist that she would be a good mother. To help her change her mind, two of her group home's sexual advisors borrowed a friend's summer cottage and took Susanne away with them for a long weekend, together with a life-sized baby doll that could be programmed to fuss and cry.

Eva was one of the sexual advisors who went with Susanne on this retreat. She explained its purpose. "We wanted Susanne to make a well-considered decision about having a baby," she told Don.

> We bought a doll with money from the parenting project. It's a doll that you can program to do certain things. It has thirteen different programs, and we took the one that was a bit over the middle level of difficulty. You get this CD, and you install the program on your computer, and you activate the doll with a button. The person caring for the doll has an armband, and that registers how well that person cares for the doll. So when the doll cries and wants food, it only stops crying when you put a bottle in its mouth. It registers that its needs have been met.
>
> And so, me and Mette [the other sexual advisor] were there with Susanne for three days in this summer cottage we borrowed. The doll registered when it was held and when it was fed, but we were there to observe

the emotional contact—eye contact and closeness and how she managed to hold the child, that sort of thing. We made notes about that every hour.

Eva said that Susanne surprised her and her colleague. "We were impressed at how well Susanne managed," she said.

She managed the doll really well. Damn well, in fact. So we decided that we needed to make more demands on her. So we told her, "Okay, but remember that you're also going to have to make some food for the doll when the doll is asleep. You've got to wash the doll's clothes. You have to remember your own hygiene. You have to go out and shop and do all those other things that people do when they have a child."

And that she couldn't manage [*det magtede hun ikke*]. She couldn't manage. All her focus was on the doll, and nothing else. She didn't bathe, she didn't brush her teeth, she didn't have any energy left for anything else except caring for the doll.

During those three days, Eva said, Susanne began to understand that she would not be able to care for a child. "She came to the realization that she couldn't manage a baby because she couldn't manage to care for herself, too. We talked about that a lot with her, that if you're going to take care of a child you have to take care of yourself, otherwise it doesn't work. And she began to understand that during that weekend. She came to the conclusion, 'I don't want to get pregnant, I don't want to have my own child. I want this doll.'"

And so it ended. Susanne had wanted a child, and instead she got a doll. She was allowed to keep the programmable doll, and she had herself sterilized.

Eva is forthright in stating that this outcome, which amounts to what one researcher has called a "conversion of an intellectually disabled person's desire for offspring into a desire for infertility," was the one hoped for.[42] Eva is the sexual advisor who told Don that a pregnancy among the residents is a group home's "biggest fear." The reason for the fear is partly that a pregnancy would draw attention—from parents, the social welfare system, and possibly even journalists—to the policies and practices in the group home that facilitate the sexual lives of residents. While the social workers and sexual advisors who have developed and implement those policies are proud of them and can easily defend them, they realize that a pregnant intellectually disabled woman is an easy target for anyone who might want to discredit them. Social workers also worry about the child born to an intellectually disabled woman—how it would be raised and who would take care of it. This is also the concern of most parents of disabled women.[43]

Mostly, however, the fear Eva identifies concerns the woman who would become pregnant. Eva and the rest of the staff at the group home recognize that an intellectually disabled woman's desire to have children is understandable and natural. "They watch television and see movies, just like everybody else," the director of the group home told Don. "They see staff members who have been away on parental leave come back to work with photos of their babies. They see them smiling—they see how happy people get when they have a baby. And especially if they have a partner, those kinds of feelings become very strong. It's absolutely natural." It is the very fact that the desire for motherhood is so natural that the consequences of motherhood for women with disabilities are so painful for staff members to contemplate. The way they see it, they are being honest with residents who want children. Their job, they say, is not to sugarcoat reality. This is why they emphasize to the women they work with that the child welfare authorities are automatically brought in when a woman who lives in a group home becomes pregnant. It is why they stress that the chances are minimal that such a woman, who, they emphasize to the woman herself, is in the group home because she needs a substantial amount of help to get by in her day-to-day life, would be allowed to keep a child. The heartbreak of seeing a young woman bond with her baby only to have the baby taken away from her would be too much for anyone to bear.

To prevent this from ever happening, women in group homes are given a great deal of counseling and advice about contraception. Men are counseled, too, about condoms and about respecting a woman's "no" to sex. But the emphasis is on women taking precautions to prevent pregnancy. Most women willingly accept contraception—they either take the pill (if they have an intellectual disability, they are reminded and assisted by helpers to take it daily) or, more typically, they allow a nurse to inject an Implanon rod into their arm. Sometimes, as in the case of Susanne, they opt for surgical sterilization.

Those few women who resist taking contraception because they want to become pregnant are counseled until they accept it. The "parenting project" and the weekend away with Susanne are one way to inculcate in young women a "desire for infertility." Social workers like Eva also talk individually to women, explaining to any woman who resists contraception that many of the activities she enjoys doing—like going to a social club or spending all day watching DVDs of *Anna Phil*—will not be possible if she has a baby to take care of. "You have to be concrete," Eva told Don. "You have to say that these concrete things she will not be able to do if she gets pregnant."

Sometimes young women are taken to doctors, who add their voices to the chorus of staff members who are urging the woman to accept contraception. But the trump card is always the information that child welfare services will in all likelihood take a woman's baby away from her.

This combination of education, counseling, and subtle threats is remarkably successful in shaping the reproductive choices of women with disabilities. In the twenty years that the group home for adults with intellectual disabilities that Don lived in has existed, not a single woman has ever become pregnant. When Don talked with Susanne about wanting to have children, she kept repeating that she thinks she would have been an excellent mother. But the county, she said, the county would automatically take away (*tvangs-fjerne*) any baby she might have given birth to.

"They don't listen to the mother. They don't give you any chances. They just come and take your baby right after it's born."

Out of Bounds

In a provocative essay on how sex and disability is represented in culture, literature scholar Anna Mollow discusses the paradox involved in perceiving disability to be a sign of two seemingly contradictory states: asexual innocence, on the one hand, and sexual excess, on the other. She observes that

> cognitively disabled people are commonly depicted as childlike and asexual but are often feared as uncontrollable sexual predators. Similarly, websites for "amputee devotees" present disabled women in terms that evoke sexual excess (a photo of an amputee woman shopping or washing dishes is sufficient to provide "compelling sexual entertainment") and simultaneously emphasize lack ("A woman is not whole if she does not have something missing!" www.amputee-devotee.com announces).[44]

Mollow says that the conjoined structure of both absence and excess makes "disability" seem very much like sex; indeed, she proposes that sex *is* disability. "We desire what nearly shatters us," she says, referring to psychoanalytic understandings of sexuality as a force that disturbs and transgresses. "We desire what disables us."[45]

Mollow's point in linking disability and sex like this is to argue that disability, like sexuality, is a structuring feature of the human psyche. It is not so much a characteristic or quality that only some people possess as it is a fundamental trait that constitutes us all. And it isn't just that everybody is a mere car accident or burst blood vessel away from disability, as disability rights activists never tire of pointing out; it's that disability—the structure that comprises both absence and excess—is at the center of everyone's existence. For that reason, Mollow says, disability, like sexuality, is something that should be examined as a phenomenon that unsettles everyone's sense of themselves as independent and whole. "Rather than seeking to humanize the disabled (insisting that disabled people be treated 'as human beings')," she says that theories about disability should, instead, "ask how disability might threaten to undo, or disable, the category of the human."[46]

To "undo" a category or a concept is a prized plum for literary theorists, and Mollow's argument is in many ways typical of the cultural studies approach to disability that we were critical of in the introduction—the kind that enthusiastically and so effortlessly evaporates disabled people's actual lives into erudite theoretical ether.

But Mollow's exploration of the reasons why both disability and sex seem to be so unsettling also illustrates what is valuable and insightful in cultural studies approaches that examine representation. If both disability and sexuality, by their very natures, each separately disturbs decorum and transgresses boundaries, then it stands to reason that their combination in the sexuality of people with disabilities will constitute a particularly pungent challenge to a wide range of sensitivities, identities, divisions, and relations. Indeed, Mollow concludes by suggesting that one reason why our culture strives so relentlessly to desexualize people with disabilities is because they embody the inherent disabling essence of sex that we do not want to acknowledge or confront.

The boundaries that we have discussed in this chapter can thus be read as examples of flashpoints that ignite when cultural ideas about disability and sexuality, like the ones Mollow discusses, collide with lived realities. The erotic lives of people with disabilities are negotiated through talk about boundaries and through activities that both secure boundaries and transgress them—and sometimes refashion them. We saw that, in Sweden, the primary mode of engagement is to insist on the fixedness of boundaries and to constantly reinforce that fixedness. The unequivocal message conveyed to adults with disabilities is that sex is an activity that should not cross boundaries. It needs to be contained. If it must occur at all, it should not come to the attention of other people. It should happen in private, inside locked rooms, and with no assistance from any helper. The deeply transgressive relations that can develop between disabled children and their mothers are not discussed, and sex is discouraged by portraying it more as a dangerous threat than as a potential source of fulfillment and pleasure.

Danes are more boundless than this. Professionals, parents, and people with disabilities, too, acknowledge boundaries wherever sexuality is concerned. But they often are more willing than Swedes to negotiate those boundaries. Lone Hertz, Käthe Piilmann, and the mother who insisted that the staff of her son's group home make accommodations for his sexuality are examples of individuals who fully grasp boundaries, but who try to reconfigure them in ways that protect both their own integrity and the integrity of their disabled children. Residents of group homes who decorate their rooms with nude centerfolds mark the boundaries of their homes, and the staff who work there respect that. Feelings of violation incited by a physically disabled woman's pleasurable responses to being washed are aired in a frank discussion among staff and through sexual counseling with the woman, the outcome of which is satisfying to all. The attention-consuming boundary between having sex and having children is the focus of extensive conversations, activities, and interventions, which though debatable in terms of their ultimate goal of dissuading disabled women from wanting to get pregnant, at least take seriously the women's desire for children, engaging that desire honestly and with respect.

In all these cases, boundaries are recognized. They are regarded as essential dimensions of people's relationships and of a person's integrity and sense of self-respect. But they are fluid, not fixed. They are negotiable, not immutable.

This willingness to discuss boundaries and to explore ways of accommodating a variety of positions in relation to them is at the core of the differences between how sexuality and disability is engaged with in Denmark and Sweden. That core difference illuminates the most critical boundary of all: the one between the willingness to extend, and the refusal to get involved.

CHAPTER 5 :: paying for sexual services

Lone Hertz is in her midseventies now. A Julie Christie sort of beauty, with high cheekbones, flawless skin, and thick, flowing white hair, she remains well known in Denmark, not least because of her frequent interventions concerning disability. In 2009, for example, Hertz announced to the press that she had purchased sex for her son.

Hertz had arranged the prostitute's visits to her son, Tomas, many years previously, and she had written about doing so in *The Sisyphus Letters* (*Sisyfosbreve*), the book about her life with Tomas that was published seventeen years earlier, in 1992.[1] Her revelation in the memoir was mentioned in only two of the reviews that appeared, and in both cases it was offered as an example of the book's general tone, which was universally praised as "unsentimental," "heart wrenching," "harrowing," "moving," and "brutally honest."[2]

Lone Hertz decided to remind the public of her decision to purchase sexual services for her son because she was distressed that prominent politicians in Denmark had begun demanding that the purchase of sexual services be criminalized. Hertz opposed this antiprostitution rhetoric, partly on feminist principle that the state should not be in the business of telling women what they can and cannot do with their bodies. But mostly she opposed talk of criminalization because she realized that a law prohibiting the purchase of sexual services would seriously impact the disadvantaged group to which her disabled son belonged. "I think it is perfectly reasonable," she told the press, "that people with a handicap who can't get sexual release by themselves, for example through masturbation, might obtain peace of mind and body if others help."[3]

In her book she had expressed this thought at greater length, with eloquence and frustration. "I *insist*," she wrote, in direct address to her son,

> that it is a human right to achieve sexual release both physically and mentally. But everyone makes excuses, they don't want to acknowledge the problem. No matter what I say or do, Tomas, nothing happens. I feel suffocated by disinterest. An enervating form of resistance. It's nothing, not even oppositional. One boxes in a vacuum and one slowly loses one's energy. In the end, it's as if the problem never existed at all. The brainwashing is a success. But for God's sake, how many so-called normal people would like to never have sexual pleasure with anyone? To be locked in their own heads, always and forever? Alone with their thoughts and words? With their body and their needs? [emphasis in original][4]

Lone Hertz's revelation about her active role in her son's sex life, and her insistence that people with significant disabilities have the right to have a sex life, was reported positively in the Danish press. She was described as a "charismatic" actor and mother who "has devoted her life to caring for her brain damaged son."[5] One article featured a photo of Hertz holding her son Tomas close to her and kissing him lovingly on the cheek. Nobody editorialized or wrote in to suggest that Hertz was misguided or wrong to be concerned about her son's sexuality, and the tabloid newspaper in which the story first appeared, *Ekstra Bladet*, asked its readers what they thought of the actress's actions: 94 percent of the 9,367 readers who wrote in a response said they approved.[6]

Just across the Öresund sound from Denmark, in neighboring Sweden, a similarly well-known personality expressed similar thoughts about disabled people and sex. In this case, though, the outcome was anything but similar.

Sören Olsson is the coauthor of several beloved series of books for young people that all Swedes under about age thirty know well, not least because several of them have been made into movies and television series. Olsson is also the father of a teenage son who has Down syndrome and a serious heart problem. In an invited 2007 column in a magazine for the parents of children with disabilities called *Parent Power* (*Föräldrakraft*), Olsson wrote that he was unsure how he ought to handle his son's awakening sexuality. He recounted that he had recently asked his son why he seemed unhappy. His son replied that he "wanted a girlfriend. He wanted it to be exactly like it is in the films he's seen. They kiss each other and make out and they're naked together."

Olsson realized he didn't know what to do: "Obviously one would like to give one's son the possibility of exploring this exciting and arousing field [*detta spännade och kittlande område*]," he wrote. "But how do you help someone find love and closeness? The obstacles in the way feel frighteningly large."

Olsson goes on to tell how he mentioned this problem to a friend, who suggested that Olsson take his son to Denmark to buy sex. Olsson says he was appalled by the idea: "I left my friend feeling a combination of distaste and shame [*avsmak och skam*]." But then he began to think about it, and he began to lament that his son might never experience the kisses, the making out, and the lying naked with a female that he seemed to want so badly. "The boundaries that in the beginning seemed completely clear became more diffuse, and I realized that I could no longer give a definite answer," he wrote.

Olsson concluded his column by pointing out that he doesn't "advocate either for or against" his friend's suggestion about going to Denmark. But, he says, "if it serves no other purpose, then maybe this little column can incite a discussion about this subject?"[7]

The discussion that Sören Olsson invited took a turn he did not foresee. His column in *Parent Power* was picked up by Swedish Radio's news channel P1. The interview on P1 led to a phone call to Olsson from the tabloid newspaper *Aftonbladet* and subsequent publication of an article under the headline "My son wants to be with a naked girl."[8] On the basis of the *Aftonbladet* interview and the original column in *Parent Power*, another tabloid newspaper, *Expressen*, then published a story under a rubric which asked readers to decide, "Is it OK to buy sex for one's son?" (*Är det okej att köpa sex till sin son?*).[9]

The collective answer to the question posed by *Expressen* was not affirmative. Columnist Linna Johansson, in *Expressen*, declared that she was "seriously disturbed by this" (*blir upriktigt illa till mods av det här*).[10] Under the headline "Women are not sex aids" (*Kvinnor är inga sexhjälpmedel*), the free newspaper, *Metro Riks*, published a column by Hillevi Wahl, an author of children's books, in which she declared, "First of all, I don't understand why he sits there and talks about his son's sexuality in front of the whole Swedish nation. Isn't that an incredible violation of privacy and integrity [*oerhört integritetskränkande*]?" Wahl went on to remind Olsson that "it is not in fact a human right to be able to have sex with someone" (*det är faktiskt ingen mänsklig rättighet att få ha sex med någon*).[11]

In the newspaper *Helsingborgs Dagblad*, columnist Kristina Persson accused Olsson of wanting to take his son to a brothel in order to "gather material for the book on Bert's sexual escapades." (Bert is the title character of one of Olsson's most successful book series.) Persson concluded her column by vowing, "Never again a Bert book in my home."[12]

Insinuations and personal attacks like this led Olsson to refuse to discuss the matter any further. The news website Corren.se reported that Olsson declared that he "doesn't want to be part of this anymore. . . . He wanted to begin a discussion about a big and difficult topic, but the issue has been reduced to being about disability and prostitution."[13] Olsson confirmed this in an interview with us. He told us that he was shocked at how quickly and decisively the discussion he had hoped to incite "spun out of control" (*spårade ur*) and devolved into vicious personal attacks. He remembered that bloggers began to write about "what a horrible parent I was and what a horrible person I was and that I shouldn't even be allowed to have children."[14]

The contrast between what happened in Denmark when actress Lone Hertz revealed that she had purchased sexual services for her son and what happened in Sweden when author Sören Olsson merely raised the issue as a theoretical possibility for his son is paradigmatic of the dramatic differences that exist between the two countries when it comes to understandings of sexuality. That the contrast should be expressed with particular clarity in relation to prostitution is not surprising. Many people in both Sweden and Denmark regard attitudes and laws concerning prostitution as a kind of chasm that separates the two countries just as much as, if not more than, the waters of the Öresund sound.

The basic difference is this: in 1999 the Swedish parliament passed a law that prohibits the purchase of sexual services. The law was directly inspired by feminists like the American legal scholar Catharine MacKinnon, who insists that paying or receiving money for sex is necessarily and indisputably degrading, and that any kind of prostitution (the term "sex work" is vigorously rejected) is indistinguishable from sexual abuse; in fact, it is a form of sexual abuse.

The 1999 law left the selling of sex uncriminalized, because the law's advocates argued that anyone who sells sex, by definition, is a victim, and punishing victims is wrong. So while selling sex is legal in Sweden, purchasing it is a crime. Since 2011, when the 1999 law was made even tougher, the maximum penalty for purchasing sexual services is one year in prison.

In Denmark, too, 1999 was a significant year with regard to prostitution. The same year the Swedish parliament made the purchase of sexual services illegal, the Danish parliament decriminalized prostitution, with the argument that one did not help prostitutes by punishing them.

This contrast between the two countries echoes an earlier one, in the 1980s, which also had to do with sexuality. In the early years of the AIDS crisis Sweden adopted draconian measures to combat the epidemic. These included a nationwide ban on gay bathhouses and the forced incarceration of HIV-positive women and men (mostly drug-addicted sex workers and African immigrants) who doctors decided could not be trusted to inform their sexual partners of their positive serostatus. More than one hundred people with HIV have been incarcerated in this way. In 2005 the European Court of Human Rights held that Sweden had violated the right to liberty and security of an HIV-positive man who had been forcibly isolated in a hospital for one and a half years and continually threatened with detention for seven.[15]

In 1987, the same year the Swedish parliament passed those laws, the Danish parliament *abolished* the law on contagious diseases and instituted programs of cooperation with gay rights groups and with the owners of the gay bathhouses that existed in the country.

These kinds of contrasts between Denmark and Sweden vex the Swedish government and baffle Swedish journalists, who tend to explain them by invoking stereotypes of libertarian Danish sybarites who fail to grasp the severity of issues that Swedes respond to with well-reasoned and politically progressive prohibitions. Danes, for their part, dismiss the Swedes as being obsessed with prohibitions and believing them to be a remedy for whatever ails them.

Swedish laws regarding HIV have been softened slightly in recent years, partly as a result of bitter international criticism (since 2004, for example, gay bathhouses are no longer illegal—though there are none in the country). But Sweden aggressively markets its abolitionist prostitution law, especially in Scandinavia and the Baltic countries. Since the law was passed in 1999, various Swedish governments (alternating between a Social Democratic–led government and a coalition led by the Conservative Party, Moderaterna, a center-right party supportive of social welfare) have spent millions trying to influence other countries to adopt what has come to be known internationally as "the Swedish model."

In Denmark, a center-left coalition led by the Social Democrats won the parliamentary elections in 2011. The Social Democratic party convention in 2009 had committed the party to importing the Swedish law to Denmark. Once in government, however, the Social Democrats found that there was little support in their coalition to change existing law. Then, in late 2012, the Danish Council on Criminal Law (Straffelovrådet) issued a long-awaited, 900-page review of laws pertaining to sexuality in which it recommended *against* the criminalization of clients. Laws like the one in Sweden serve rhetorical purposes, the council concluded, but they impact negatively on precisely the people they are purported to help, namely, sex workers—who lose income and become increasingly stigmatized when such laws are passed. The Social Democratic prime minister, Helle Thorning-Schmidt, announced that the report's arguments persuaded her. Like the Danish legislators who had decriminalized prostitution fifteen years previously, Thorning-Schmidt said she no longer believed that criminalization was the best way to deal with the problems that can arise in connection with prostitution. In an about-face that angered many people in her party, she affirmed that her government would no longer attempt to introduce the Swedish law in Denmark.[16]

It should be clear by now that the purchase of sexual services is only a tiny fragment of the vast landscape that emerges when one begins examining the sexual lives and erotic desires of people with disabilities. Despite its relative insignificance to the lives of most people with disabilities, however, prostitution is an unavoidable subject, not least because it is guaranteed to arise—usually sooner rather than later—whenever sex and *congenital* disability is discussed. When the topic is acquired disability, talk tends to center on rehabilitation and on how the person who has become impaired can regain some of the sexual ability that he or she lost because of his or her accident or illness. But with congenital disability, like the kinds focused on in this book, discussion tends to turn quickly to prostitution, perhaps, at least in part, because many nondisabled people have a hard time imagining that severely impaired adults could ever hope to find anyone who would willingly have sex with them without getting paid to do it.

Congenital disability also sometimes figures in the arguments of people who want to legalize or regulate prostitution. The argument is one of charity:

state-run brothels, advocates say, would be a benevolence that would provide disabled people with access to experiences they otherwise might never have (this, recall, was Lars Ullerstam's argument in his book *The Erotic Minorities*). But any discussion that links the words *prostitution* and *disability* in the same sentence usually quickly turns to debate, and that debate rapidly comes to center on the to-be-or-not-to-be question of prostitution. Disability usually swiftly falls from view, except when commentators who regard sex work as inherently degrading point out that disability does not give anyone a license to abuse other people.

For those reasons, debates like the one unleashed by Sören Olsson's column in *Parent Power* magazine usually impede understanding more than they facilitate it. All the details and textures and fine nuances—the reasons why some people with disabilities purchase sexual services; the reasons why some sex workers accept disabled clients; the kinds of interactions that occur when disabled clients are visited by sex workers; the kinds of relationships that develop between sex workers and disabled clients; the kinds of help that disabled adults who want to purchase sexual services require or desire; differences and similarities between adults with physical impairments and those with intellectual impairments; between disabled women and disabled men; between those with verbal language and those without—all those dimensions of social life and erotic desire are elided in debates that focus exclusively and dogmatically on the issue of whether prostitution is right or wrong. In those debates, a world of relationships is overlooked. A universe of emotions, sensations, and perceptions is left unacknowledged and unexplored.

Disabled Women Who Pay for Sexual Services

I talked to my mother about how I had been feeling pretty bad about myself for a long time. You know, big mood swings. One day I'd cry over the stupidest things and the next day I'd be completely hysterical. I didn't have any control over my moods. I'm the kind of person who reflects about things a lot, but I didn't know what the problem was.

So I sat down and thought, "Okay, something is going on with me now that hasn't happened before. What is going on, and why?" You know? And I thought about how I was twenty-seven years old. And I had never had a partner or a sexual experience. Most people have their sexual debut long before they are twenty-seven. And so I thought, "Well, of course.

I'm having all these mood swings because my body and my psyche are mature enough for it, but I hadn't yet had it."

So I thought, "What can I do?" I've always been against, you know, going out on the town and coming back home with just anyone. I didn't want to do that. I need to feel secure and all that. So it was important to me to go onto the Internet and find someone who was a professional and who did it because he wanted to. And it was important for me to, like, pay for the service, so that I wouldn't be embarrassed that there were some things that I maybe wasn't able to do or that I needed to be taught how to do certain things.

Frigg Birt Müller is the sort of woman who comes to mind when most people imagine a Scandinavian beauty. Svelte body, straight hair so blonde it is almost white, bright smile, smooth pore-less skin that makes one think of a peach. Then there is her name. It's an unusual name in Scandinavia, but Frigg was the Nordic goddess of fecundity. Everything about Frigg the mortal signals the kind of natural grace for which Scandinavian women have become internationally renowned.

Don was sitting in Frigg's light, sparsely furnished, ground-level apartment on the outskirts of Copenhagen, interviewing her about her decision to go on national television and talk about the fact that she pays for sex.

We found out about Frigg the same way everyone else in Denmark did: in November 2011 she was featured on a television program called *Mormors Bordel*. *Grandmother's Brothel*, as that title can be translated into English, is a series of twenty-five-minute programs that address prostitution. The titular grandmother is a reference to the ages of the pair of women who host the show. One, sixty-three-year-old Suzanne Bjerrehus, is a former Miss Denmark who had minor roles in several Danish porn films in the 1970s. She married a wealthy businessman and became a talk show host. Her cohost, sixty-five-year-old Karen Thisted, is a journalist and former editor of the tabloid newspaper *Ekstra Bladet*. *Grandmother's Brothel* was produced as Denmark's parliamentary elections of 2011 were heating up, and debates about sex work had become increasingly common in both the mass media and political rhetoric. Several of the political parties on the Left, including the largest, the Social Democrats, had announced that they were in favor of adopting the Swedish law criminalizing the purchase of sexual services. The conceit of *Grandmother's Brothel* (which went on to air for a second season in 2012) is that Bjerrehus, the former Miss Denmark, is opposed to the Swedish law, whereas Thisted, her friend and antagonist, is in favor of it. But rather than just debate prostitution in a studio, the women "want to get out and see it," they say in the opening credits over shots of flying airplanes and Asian women in miniskirts. The various episodes include a visit to a German brothel, a trip to Gambia in order to try to understand female sex tourism, to Sweden to try to understand why the Swedes criminalized the purchase of sexual services, and, inevitably, to Pattaya in Thailand.

The third episode of the first season was about disability. But instead of simply chewing the well-masticated cud of portraying men with physical disabilities who buy sexual services from women, the producers of *Grandmother's Brothel* looked for, and found, a young disabled woman who bought sex from a male escort she saw online. That woman was Frigg.

Frigg told Don that the producers of *Grandmother's Brothel* found her because the young man she purchased sexual services from had already been interviewed by the grandmothers for another episode, on men who sell sex to women. This man told the producers that he knew a young woman who has cerebral palsy and sits in a wheelchair and who purchases sex. He said he would ask her if she would consider appearing on television to talk about it.

When her escort told her about the program and asked if she would consider appearing on it, Frigg was enthusiastic. "I thought that it was great to have the opportunity to push back a little against [*skubbe lidt*] people's prejudices," she told Don. She welcomed the chance to confront viewers' beliefs about the supposed asexual passivity of disabled people. Frigg also said it was important for her to do this with openness and confidence. When Don offered to give her a pseudonym in this book, she declined: "This is important to me," she said. "I think using my real name and showing that I am a real person makes this have more impact. If I don't use my real name, it seems like I'm embarrassed over this. And I'm not."

Another woman who is not embarrassed to talk about the fact that she purchases sexual services is Eva, a thirty-year-old woman with muscular dystrophy. Eva (a pseudonym, since she has not appeared publicly to talk about her sex life) does not buy sex from an escort—she uses a service called Handisex, a business run by a young woman and a young man in Copenhagen who studied sexology together and realized (partly through conversations with Eva) that the sexual options for people with disabilities were limited. Handisex offers disabled people who live in their own apartments or in group homes the kind of sexual assistance that Danish sexual advisors provide in the group homes in which they work. For between 350 and 800 Danish kroner (US$60–140) per hour, depending on the kind of service and its frequency, a person with a disability can hire twenty-five-year-old Michelle or forty-three-year-old Asgerbo to come to their home and give them advice about such things as choosing sex aids or how to find a partner. Michelle and Asgerbo also provide assistance with masturbation, and this is the service that Eva purchases, about once every two weeks.

Eva is unable to use her hands to reach her genitals or to manipulate the vibrator she uses to help her orgasm. So Michelle from Handisex does this. On the days Michelle comes to Eva's apartment, her assistant first undresses her and helps her into bed. The assistant then leaves, and Michelle comes into the bedroom.

"I have this thing that goes in, and that also has a part that sits on the clitoris," Eva told Don when he asked if she would explain how Michelle helps her.

> And she, like, puts it on, and in, and makes sure that it is placed right. And it has these different programs that I like to try out to see which one I want. Michelle goes through the different speeds and movements, and I tell her which one I want. Then she goes out and closes the bedroom door. Sometimes it isn't easy to get it to stay in place, and if it falls out I need to have help to put it back in. So I call for her and she comes in and does what I ask her to do, and then she goes out again. And afterward she washes it and puts it back where I keep it.

Eva is heterosexual, and Don asked her why she paid Michelle, and not Michelle's business partner Asgerbo, or some other man, to help her have sex. She replied that she has never had male assistants. She would feel very uncomfortable if a man washed her privates or helped her in the toilet, and she would never want a man who was not her lover to help her with a sex aid. Also, Eva said, she is opposed to prostitution, and paying a man help her have sex would seem too much like paying for sex. She uses Handisex because no prostitution is involved. "Michelle isn't doing anything with her body," Eva said. "I'm not abusing her, or using her. She's just giving me practical help, is the way I see it."

Frigg and Eva are examples of individuals who almost never figure in discussions of disability and sexuality, except as an absence: disabled women who pay for sexual services. The services that these two women pay for are certainly different: Frigg pays a male escort who has sex with her; Eva pays a female with whom she feels comfortable to help her use a mechanical sex aid. The two women also differ in their attitudes toward prostitution: Frigg is positive toward sex work; Eva is opposed to it. Across these differences, however, the two women have one thing in common: they both reach out to paid professionals to help them have an erotic life.

In so doing, Frigg and Eva are no different from the men with disabilities who are the usually ineluctable focus of any discussion about disability and paid sexual services. Like those men, Frigg and Eva have made a decision that their lives are more satisfying if they can have sex once in a while. And so they do, enlisting the services of individuals with knowledge and skills that allow them to experience sensations and pleasures that most nondisabled adults—especially most nondisabled adults in their twenties and thirties—take completely for granted.

The Myth of Sex Surrogates

In order to discuss disability and the purchase of sexual services sensibly it is first necessary to clear up a number of misunderstandings, myths, and falsehoods that frequently arise whenever the subject is broached. One of these concerns the topic we have just considered—the fiction that the only disabled adults who purchase sexual services are men.

Another legend that commonly circulates when sex and disability is discussed is the belief that there exists a cadre of women and a few men who, in English, are usually called "sex surrogates" or "sexual surrogates" and who, so the story goes, see it as their vocation to provide sexual services to disabled men. They are not prostitutes, because they have special training in healing or different forms of therapy. So the sex they provide is more than just common sex; it is therapeutic sex, it is healing erotic fulfillment. Whenever journalists report on sex surrogates, they usually imply hazily that there are scores of such professionals happily servicing disabled men, especially disabled men who happen to live in the Netherlands, Switzerland, Germany, Denmark, or California. Exactly how many of these surrogates there may be, or exactly how they work, is always left vague.

People who fit the commonly circulated description of sex surrogates do exist. The disabled author Mark O'Brien described one in a widely read autobiographical essay titled "The Sex Surrogate," which became the basis of the 2012 Hollywood film *The Sessions*. The essay describes how O'Brien, who contracted polio at age six and spent the rest of his life inside an iron lung, had his first sexual experiences, at age thirty-seven, with a paid sex surrogate named Cheryl.[17]

Another example of actually existing sex surrogates appears in the 2008 French film *L'Amour sans limites* (Love without limits).[18] That film contains brief interviews with two nondisabled people, a woman in her forties and a man in his fifties, who receive payment to have sex with disabled adults who go on weekend retreats at an organization called the Institute for the Self-Determination of Disabled People (Institut zur Selbst-Bestimmung Behinderter). This institute, located in the German state of Saxony, was also featured in a cover story about sex and disability that ran in the German weekly magazine *Der Speigel* in August 2012.[19] The 1996 book *The Sexual Politics of Disability* makes a passing reference to what it calls a "surrogate therapy service in the Netherlands," Stichting Alternative Relatiebemiddeling, that was featured on a BBC television program in the early 1990s.[20] In Los Angeles, an organization called the International Professional Surrogates Association provides training and certification to what they call "professional surrogate partners." These are trained professionals who engage in sexual practices with a client under the supervision of a therapist.

So while it is undeniable that there are some people who provide what used to be called "sex therapy" to disabled clients, the number of such people worldwide is miniscule—a recent congress of professional surrogates in Florida attracted twenty-five participants.[21] The practice is also contested. Many disability rights activists object to sex surrogacy because they bristle at the implication that the only people who will want to, or are able to, have sex with disabled people are professionals who have undergone special therapeutic training or New Age consciousness-raising.[22]

Another problem with the term is that it carries a suggestion that sex surrogates are somehow better than sex workers. Sex surrogates, the label seems to say, are more healing, more involved, more professional—they are, in a word, a bit classier than common prostitutes. The female "sexual companion" (*Sexualbegleiter*) interviewed in the French film just mentioned—a woman named Eva Zylka—makes this explicit. In describing her sexual activities with disabled men, Zylka says, "I don't just give my body, I give more. I give my heart, my soul, and I look after my partner's heart and soul. It's not only about the activity; it's not only about the technique. I see the total person. That can also happen in classic prostitution," she says, "but I dare say that it is rare."

Language of erotic uplift like this might help to make paying for sex more palatable to some people with disabilities or to caregivers of disabled people who are frightened or repelled by the idea of prostitution. But a claim to provide more empathy, care, and concern than is offered by women who work in "classic prostitution" should also perhaps be heard as a way of staking a class (and probably also a race) distinction. It is difficult not to hear talk like Eva Zylka's as a covert assertion that sex surrogates are more sophisticated, better educated, and more European (that is, whiter) than common prostitutes. Zylka's romanticized description of what she does is like the distinction that the British painter Stephen Gilbert made between erotica and pornography, where erotica is what you like and pornography is what other people like. It is a—perhaps unintentionally—stigmatizing language that does its best to elide the fact that regardless of how much heart and soul someone like Eva Zylka might claim to put into her job, she still receives remuneration, just like a sex worker does, for having sexual relations with paying clients.[23]

This kind of stigmatizing language is explicitly rejected by the woman who is arguably the world's most famous sex professional who works with disabled adults—a blonde woman in her midthirties with a ready, dazzling smile named Rachel Wotton. Wotton is one of the founders of Touching Base, a nonprofit organization in Sydney, Australia, that helps facilitate contacts between people with disabilities and sex workers. The organization runs workshops on the topic of disability for sex workers and on the topic of sex work for individuals with disabilities and those who care for them. It also provides information about how to contact sex workers who accept disabled clients. Already well known in Australia, Wotton became an international celebrity in 2011 when a documentary about her, *Scarlet Road*, was screened at the Sydney International Film Festival and later shown on television and at film festivals around the world.[24] *Scarlet Road* follows Wotton as she teaches at workshops, speaks at international conferences, and has erotic sessions with clients with disabilities. It documents her advocacy work for both sex workers and people with disabilities.

Wotton never refers to herself as a sex surrogate. Both the film and media interviews she did after the film was released make it clear that while she sees her work as a vocation, and while, as she told one interviewer, "It's my job to provide a really good service, and companionship, and being able to talk and be focused on the client, and be present," she does not see herself as any different from other sex workers.[25] On the contrary, Wotton is adamant that she is not a therapist or a healer—she is a professional working in the sex industry. Her advocacy work is focused on improving the public perception and the social conditions of both sex workers and people with disabilities. She sees these two groups as confronting similar prejudices, patronizing attitudes, and outright discrimination.

Sex Workers and Disabled Clients

Rachel Wotton's sense of affinity between sex workers and people with disabilities, and her special concern for and activism on behalf of adults with disabilities, are not particularly common among sex workers, in our experience. A Swedish sex worker we interviewed did share with Wotton a particular liking for disabled clients, partly because she had a certain soft spot for what she called "the invisible people"—"You know," she explained, "people who others just don't see: the kind of person who talks a little bit too much and too long to the checkout person in the supermarket, the ones who strike up conversations about the weather on buses, the kind who die and rot and nobody even notices until the smell gets really bad." Many disabled people, this woman said, are not really seen by others. But when you do actually see them and treat them with respect and empathy, "they come back. If you treat them well, they're the best regular clients you can get. They come back, they plan in advance, and they keep the times they've booked with you. The only time they cancel is when they don't have enough money. But then they tell you in advance, 'Sorry I can't come next Thursday because my housing allowance hasn't come when it was supposed to.'"

Most sex workers can acknowledge a point like this, in theory. In practice, though, most are wary of disabled clients. Some simply don't find bodies with impairments appealing; others dislike the thought that they might have to be more active with a disabled client than they would have to be otherwise, where they can just "lay there and be a little bit tender and sweet" (*ligge der og være lidt sød og rar*). Many others are afraid that they might inadvertently hurt a disabled client, or be hurt by him. This is not an unreasonable concern—sex workers, after all, are usually no more knowledgeable about disability than anyone else in the general public, and unless they happen to live in Sydney, Australia, it isn't as though there are any special courses available to instruct them about what is different, and what is the same, about people with physical and intellectual impairments and people who do not have such impairments.

Other sex workers are afraid they will say something or do something that is unintentionally offensive. One woman told Don, "I've always had difficulty with handicapped people—not because I feel any kind of repulsion [*væmmelse*] toward them, but because I'm afraid that I'm going to transgress their boundaries. How much can you look? How much can you ask?"

Despite these kinds of commonly felt anxieties, some sex workers do accept clients with disabilities. In Denmark, the ones who do so, for the most part, are mature—in their thirties or older, usually with several years of experience in sex work behind them. No one we spoke with specializes in disabled clients—sex workers couldn't, really, if they wanted to earn a decent living. One reason for this is that adults with disabilities are hardly a moneyed group. Most of them are not employed, and the monthly pension they receive from the Danish state amounts to about 10,000 Danish kroner after tax, which is the equivalent of just under US$2,000. The equivalent of about $1,200 of this pension goes to living costs, such as rent and food, if the person lives in a group home; more if he or she lives in an apartment where rent is determined by market prices. This leaves the equivalent of about $800 a month for savings and living costs, such as clothes, toiletries, entertainment, vacations, and so on. A budget like this, while generous by international standards, is hardly luxurious, and it limits how much any buyer of sexual services is able to avail himself or herself to them.

As the woman cited above points out, some people with disabilities can become regular clients. But in countries as small as Denmark or Sweden, a sex worker who tried to specialize in clients with disabilities would soon find herself having to look for supplementary employment to help pay the rent. There is also the issue of why a sex worker would want to specialize in this way. One woman we interviewed told us that she hated it when the topic of disability and prostitution came up in the mass media because, whenever it did, she said, she sensed a lurking subtext that prostitutes were somehow suddenly redeemed if they offered their gold-hearted services to disadvantaged souls who could benefit the most from their benevolence. "But I'm not fucking Mother Teresa," this woman said acidly. "I'm a businesswoman, and I do this; it's a job, to support myself. I am not a charitable institution."

This same woman, nevertheless, did accept disabled clients. And she began doing so the same way all the other sex workers we spoke to did—by chance.

Camille, another Danish sex worker, is a blowsy, expansive woman in her forties with red hennaed hair, heavily kohled eyes, and a loud, infectious laugh. She baked a cherry pie for her and Don to snack on when he interviewed her in her tastefully decorated, one-bedroom apartment, which she also uses as her workplace.

Camille told Don that she began sex work as a result of going to swingers clubs—clubs where men and women go to meet people for sex. She sought out the clubs because her husband of the time had no interest in sex and she couldn't accept living "like a nun." The swingers clubs were a revelation to her, she said. "I discovered that—wow [*hold da op*], I'm not just someone who likes sex; I'm someone who likes to have sex as something central in my life. It's like a carnival; there's always some new door you can open."

From having sex with many people for free to charging money to have sex with many people was a relatively small step for Camille. In the swingers clubs she had met some women who told her they worked as prostitutes. At first she was shocked. "I didn't know much about it, but I had always thought that prostitutes were victims. That they'd all been victims of incest, they were forced, they all had pimps, they were beaten, and that prostitution is self-destructive and exploitative of women [*kvindeundertrykkende*]."

But getting to know women who actually sold sex convinced Camille that her beliefs about prostitution were mistaken. By that time she had left her husband and had a new lover, but she continued to enjoy one-night stands with other men. And so in the end, she thought, "fuck it [*fuck det*]; why not take money for it? And my boyfriend was supportive," she said. "He was like, 'Go for it. I think it's wild [*pisse frækt*] that you have sex with other men.' And at the same time, he became more special, because other men are gonna pay for what he gets for free, you know?"

After Camille began charging for sex she soon discovered something that surprised her. "All those guys who had dated me, who thought I was a cheap tramp [*billig luder*] because I had sex with them for nothing, that all changed. When they pay for it, it's really uncommon that men treat you with no respect. And if they do, I just think, 'Fuck you, you've just handed over money for it, so I don't give a toss what you think.'"

Although Camille's path to prostitution through the epiphanies she experienced in the swingers clubs is different from the other sex workers we interviewed, she is similar to the others when it comes to her experience of clients with disabilities. She hasn't had very many—perhaps five in the four years she has been selling sex. And like most others, she didn't seek out or give any particular thought to men with disabilities. One evening, though, she got a call from a potential client who seemed concerned when she told him that her apartment was on the fourth floor and that there was no elevator.

And so he came, and I opened the door, and there he stood with a crutch. And I felt bad. I said, "I'm sorry you had to go up all those stairs."

He said, "That's alright."

And that's why he had seemed worried about the fourth floor. But he comes in and we agree on how long he's going to stay, and he gives me the money and I show him into the bedroom, where I work. I tell him to take his clothes off. And so he begins to take his clothes off, and he takes off his pants, and then he takes off a leg. Because he has a leg prosthesis. It was a strange experience because I wasn't at all prepared for it, and he just took it off like the most natural thing in the world. Pants off, then leg. And I'm like, "Hmm." And he had some kind of bandage that he also took off, while he made small talk. Which was surely the best way to do it.

And I'm looking at it, and trying to behave like it's the most common thing in the world. I asked him later how it happened—you can tell that I talk a lot and I always talk a lot to my clients—and I asked him how it happened and if he was born like that or what. He'd been in a boat accident.

Anyway, while we were having oral sex, and I'm laying between his legs, I was thinking, "This is really practical and really nice"—I'm thinking this while I'm laying between his legs and sucking him off. I'm thinking, "How practical that there's nothing there, there's lots of room." And I was about to say that to him, it flew into my head to tell him that, but I didn't. But I did think it was a fun experience [*en ret sjov oplevelse*].

In a kind of cosmic coincidence, the first disabled client that Sanne, a sinuous thirty-three-year-old who works in a brothel in central Copenhagen, ever had also wore a leg prosthesis. It probably was not the same man because, whereas Camille's client had no leg at all, Sanne's client was only missing his leg from below the knee. But Sanne's reaction to seeing the leg prosthesis was similar to Camille's. "I hadn't noticed anything different about him," she told Don, "and I left the room and came back and there he stood with a metal leg."

He'd left his sock on the metal foot, but he'd taken it off his real foot. I didn't know what to say. So I said to him, "Aren't you going to take your other sock off?"

He said, "I can't feel it so it doesn't make any difference to me."

And I said, "Um, okay." And I thought, "Shit, what am I going to do? Is he going to be able to do things in the normal way and lay in a normal way and do the things that other guys do?"

And so we got into bed and he took off his leg. And I thought, "Oh, that's why he didn't take off the sock."

Like Camille, Sanne was nervous and discombobulated at first. "What if I turn around and accidentally tilt him over? What if he falls?" she worried. But just like in the encounter between Camille and the one-legged client, everything went well in Sanne's first experience of sex with a disabled man. "He was just like any other man," she concluded. "I didn't even really notice that he didn't have a leg, because he was used to being in bed with only one leg. I was the one with no experience."

After barrier-breaking first experiences like these, some sex workers realize that men with disabilities are not a different species, nor are they dangerous, or fragile, or overly sensitive to curiosity about their disabilities. And so they relax at the prospect of accepting a disabled client from time to time, and they even come to like them. Jute—the sex worker who resented being seen as Mother Teresa—said she actually kind of likes clients who are what she called "socially handicapped"—that is, men with various degrees of Asperger's syndrome or autism, men who she said "have difficulty interacting with other people and conducting themselves properly [begå sig], and saying the right things." Jute had worked for many years as a nurse in psychiatric and mental wards, and she thinks her experience there has helped her understand people with social impairments and help them relax. Peter, a homosexual sex worker, said he gets something out of providing monthly sexual services to a significantly impaired man with cerebral palsy because he regarded it as his "small contribution" (mit lille bidrag) to making life better for the man. The male escort whom Frigg Müller regularly paid for sex said he enjoys making Frigg happy. "I can see her developing," he told the two grandmothers who interviewed him on Grandmother's Brothel. "I think that I am making her have more self-confidence and that she'll maybe get up the courage to have a sex life with someone else at some point. And that she won't just throw herself into a relationship with the first person who comes along, because now she knows a bit."

This is not to say that all sex workers are Samaritans. Sexual advisors in Denmark tell of women who charge disabled clients the equivalent of several hundred dollars for an hour and then rush away after ten minutes, as soon as the client has had an orgasm. One sex worker refused to remove her panties for a man with cerebral palsy—something that was only discovered when the sexual advisor who helped arrange the visit talked to the man afterward. (This sexual advisor called the brothel where the woman worked and complained, and the man was issued a full refund.)

Among people with disabilities, stories also circulate about how sex workers can cheat clients or humiliate them. Swedish author Johan Nordansjö's autobiographical novel *My Naked Self* (*Mitt nakna jag*) narrates an episode in which the main character—Max, a young man who, like the author, has cerebral palsy and sits in a wheelchair—arranges for a sex worker to come to his apartment. Max has mentioned his disability in an e-mail to the woman, and she has responded that everything will surely be all right (*Det går säkert bra*).

At the appointed time, Max goes down to his apartment building's entrance to meet her. The woman arrives, pauses before she gets out of the taxi, and then gets out and greets him. She asks him if he has change for a large note that she was about to pay the cab driver—the driver doesn't have change, she says. Max goes up to his apartment to get some change for her, and when he comes back down, the woman and the taxi are gone.[26]

Nordansjö describes this interaction from the point of view of Max, who is left humiliated by the woman's hurried departure. "Did I look so horribly handicapped that not even a sex worker would have sex with me?" Max asks himself. While his distress is certainly understandable, a narrative written from the female sex worker's point of view might highlight another perspective. Even though the woman had been told in an e-mail that Max had cerebral palsy and sat in a wheelchair, she may have been inexperienced, or she may not have been prepared for the severity of Max's disability.[27] Some sex workers might have responded to a surprise like this with aplomb, and they might have reacted with the cool that Camille or Sanne did when they realized they were about to have sex with a legless man. But other sex workers don't respond well, or always particularly rationally, to surprises like absent limbs or significant impairments.

Clients with Significant Physical Impairments

One kind of disabled person who raises particular challenges for both sex workers and everyone else who wants to facilitate such a person's access to an erotic life is an individual who is so significantly impaired that she or he has limited mobility and little or no verbal language. People like this require a great deal of assistance to even come into contact with a sex worker. In Denmark they can receive such assistance from a sexual advisor or some other person—it could even be their mother, as in the case of Lone Hertz's son Tomas—who understands their desires and agrees to help them.

The way this happens in practice is that, first of all, it gets determined that the person with a disability wants to visit or be visited by a sex worker. If the disabled individual has verbal language, that determination is not a problem—the person who wants to meet up with a prostitute simply says so, and he (it is usually a he) requests any help he might need to contact the sex worker he has set his eye on, such as help with sending an e-mail or a text message, or dialing a telephone number.

If the disabled individual who wants to have sex with a sex worker has no verbal language, the whole process is much more difficult and time-consuming. Once communication about this has been worked out, everything can be lightning-quick. Dirk, a social worker who has worked for twelve years in the group home for people with cerebral palsy where Don lived, told him that all that Flemming, one of the home's most significantly impaired residents, needs to do to alert him to his desire for sex is to say *isse*. "Flemming can't say *fisse* [cunt]," Dirk said, laughing, "but he can say *isse*." Whenever Dirk hears Flemming begin to hiss like a leaky radiator, he knows it is time to spring into action.

But getting to the point where a person like Flemming's desires are understood often takes time, patience, alertness, and empathy.

Take Rasmus, for example. A handsome, stocky forty-two-year-old man who wears designer glasses, Rasmus lives in a group home for people with cerebral palsy. He cannot control the movement in his arms or legs, and he has limited head movement. His language consists of a variety of one-syllable words and sounds that people who have known him for a long time can interpret but that are largely incomprehensible to most others. When those who are able to understand Rasmus's sounds interpret them, they ask him to elaborate by responding to yes/no questions to determine what he wants them to do or talk about.[28]

Rasmus, it turns out, is gay. For the past two and a half years he has been paying the equivalent of US$300 (1,700 Danish kroner) for a male escort to come to his group home once a month for an hour. This escort—a stout, soft-spoken, dark-haired man in his forties—is the only person with whom

Rasmus has ever had sex. Rasmus anticipates the escort's visits with excitement and delight, and the staff in his group home all know about them.

Don first heard about Rasmus's escort on a quiet evening in the group home when several people were sitting in the common room, distractedly watching a dating game show on television. During a commercial, Rasmus turned his head to Sara, one of the young female staff members, who was feeding a snack of coffee and cake to one of Rasmus's housemates. He looked at her and said, "Tish."

Sara saw that Rasmus was talking to her and asked, "What?"

"Tish," he repeated, "Tish."

"Tuesday?" (*Tirsdag*) Sara asked.

"Mm."

"What about Tuesday?"

"Pe," said Rasmus.

"Peter?" replied Sara. "Is Peter coming on Tuesday?"

Rasmus smiled broadly.

"Oh, that's great!" (*Nå, det var dejligt*) Sara said, with a big smile—to which Rasmus responded with an even bigger one.

At the time, Don did not know Peter was the name of Rasmus's escort. After he found out, he thought back to this interaction and reflected on how meaningful Sara's spontaneous affirmation and happy smile must have been to Rasmus, who seems to have mentioned Peter to her in order to share his own buoyant anticipation of Peter's impending visit.

But Don also wondered, given Rasmus's limited ability to communicate, how did he come to let others know about his sexual preference? And how did he manage to find and make contact with a male escort when he is unable to use his hands to type at a keyboard or make a telephone call?

It turns out that Rasmus's sexual identity was discovered by the staff at his group home not because he managed to make a little speech, but because they paid attention. Several years previously, the town where the group home is located had hosted a Sexpo—a weekend exposition where businesses that sell sex toys, lingerie, porn films, tattoos, New Age crystals, and other kinds of sexy or edgy merchandise rent a large exhibition hall to display and sell their products. When the Sexpo came to town, the staff at Rasmus's group home asked the residents if anyone wanted to go. Rasmus was one of the people who said yes.

While at the Sexpo, a couple of staff members observed that Rasmus did not seem terribly interested in the lingerie or the models showing their breasts or in the DVD tables full of heterosexual porn. Instead, he rolled off in the direction of the gay section.

Sometime after the Sexpo, the sexual advisor at the group home had a private conversation with Rasmus. She told him that several members of the staff had noticed that he'd seemed a bit more interested in men than in the women. Had this been correctly perceived? Yes, Rasmus answered. Did he want to talk about it? Yes, he said, he did. Those conversations led to one of the social workers (Jan, who is gay himself) taking charge of Rasmus's *éducation sentimentale*.

Jan helped Rasmus start searching the Internet, and together they identified gay porn sites that appealed to Rasmus (it turned out he was partial to "bears"—hairy, beefy men who like leather). After several months, Rasmus and Jan found an ad in the tabloid newspaper *Ekstra Bladet* for a male escort who ended his profile with the words "Offers visits to handicapped persons too" (*Tilbyder også handicapped besøg*).

The rest, as they say, is history.

How to Contact a Sex Worker

Rasmus's case illustrates the kind of trajectory that can occur when even people with significant physical impairments want to contact sex workers. If a person with a disability like Rasmus's is either contacting a sex worker for the first time or wants to contact a new one, this has to be worked out together with the person who has agreed to help him. One resource that a surprising number of people in Denmark use, even in this age of the Internet, is the tabloid newspaper *Ekstra Bladet*. Every day this paper publishes several pages of "Massage and Escort" ads that include short descriptions of the escort and of the services offered as well as a telephone number and perhaps a website or an e-mail address. Another section, "Clinics" (using the Danish euphemism *klinik*, from *massageklinik*), provides information about brothels. Readers paging through these ads sometimes find one that appeals to them. Otherwise there is the Internet. Ads on the Internet are often much more detailed than those in the newspaper, and it is sometimes possible to search a site for a word like *handicap*, thus making it easier to determine if particular escorts are willing to accept clients with disabilities.

Once the person with the disability has indicated a preference for a particular escort, the helper decides whether he or she is willing to contact that individual. A social worker in a group home for people with cerebral palsy told Don that the contact typically occurs like this:

> I call up and introduce myself, and then I say who I'm calling for. I explain that that person is a spastic [*er spastiker*], and that means such and such, like there can be some involuntary movements, he has no verbal language but he understands everything you say if you just speak clearly, that kind of thing. I say that the person I'm calling for is heterosexual, that he would like you to sit on top of him, or, in other cases, if he can, he wants to lie on top of you. Those kinds of details.

None of the sexual advisors we spoke to have any particular views on individual men's erotic tastes when it comes to sex workers, with one important exception: most refuse to contact anyone who is not Danish. The reason many of them give for this restriction concerns language. Sexual advisors say that the sex worker they speak to needs to understand Danish well, because the sexual advisors have to feel certain that the escort has understood what the person with the disability wants, what kinds of limitations that person has because of his impairment, and also what kinds of things relating to the disability are irrelevant to a sexual encounter.

But even more important than language is the sexual advisors' concern that they not facilitate the purchase of sexual services from someone who is not in the business willingly. Anne, a sexual advisor who has worked in the same group home for people with cerebral palsy since it was established twenty years ago, told Don that she once had a very unpleasant experience that caused her to rethink her theretofore boundless acceptance of whatever the resident who requested her help wanted. One of the residents in the group home became interested in Thai women (who, reports say, have become the largest group of migrant sex workers in Denmark).[29] He wanted to buy sexual services from one. Anne said she felt dubious about phoning up a Thai prostitute, but since this was expressly what the man she was helping wanted, she didn't feel it would be ethically defensible to impose her own concerns on him and overrule his choice.

Together they found an ad in *Ekstra Bladet* that the man liked, so Anne phoned the number in the ad. She explained who she was and that she was calling for a man with severe cerebral palsy, who had no verbal language, but who understood Danish well and who wanted her to come and have sex with him. Anne felt uneasy during this call, because the woman's Danish was broken. But an appointment was made, and the woman arrived at the agreed-upon time several days later. She went into the man's room and left after about an hour. Anne checked with the resident who had paid for the woman's services, and he was happy and satisfied. Everything had gone well, Anne said, except for one thing: she had noticed that in the group home's parking lot a man had been sitting in a car the whole time, smoking, waiting for the Thai woman. As soon as the woman emerged from her encounter she got in this car, and it drove off.

The different aspects of the interaction with the Thai escort, which already had Anne on edge because of the language problems and because of her uncertainty as to whether she could be sure the woman was selling sex because she really wanted to, coalesced into a kind of horror when she saw the car door shut and the mysterious man drive off into the night with the woman. Thinking about all the television shows and news reports she'd seen about sexual trafficking, Anne said that when she got home later that evening she felt terrible. She had no idea who the man was, but the suspicion that he might have been a pimp or a trafficker who made the woman sell sex against her will made Anne feel as though *she* had been violated. The boundaries for what she felt comfortable doing had been transgressed, and she was angry with the resident in the group home who had put her in a situation where she had transgressed them.

But most of all, she said, she was angry with herself for having "suppressed" (*undertrykte*) her own sense of what she was willing to do, and for not having made it clear to the man that she had her own principles, and that sometimes those were not negotiable. The next day she went into the man's room and told him how she felt and that she would not contact any non-Danish women for him ever again. If he wanted another Thai woman in the future he would have to ask someone else to help him, not her. She also told Don that several weeks after the incident one of the Danish television channels showed a documentary about prostitution in Thailand. Anne made a point of informing the man when it was going to be on, and she told him that maybe he ought to watch it.

Another social worker who works in a group home for people with cerebral palsy told Don something similar. When asked if there was anything he would refuse to do for a resident who wanted help to contact a sex worker, Dirk, the social worker who knew that Flemming's "isse" was shorthand for "I want you to help me find a prostitute," said,

If I call up a prostitute, I want one who understands Danish. It can't be someone from Thailand who came here illegally two months ago. It has to be someone who understands Danish. The only scruple [*skruppel*] that I have in relation to calling up prostitutes is that I don't want to call any foreigners [*udlændinge*]. I won't call Thai girls. If I find out that the prostitutes are from Eastern Europe, like Poland and over there, I say "no." But if I see that the women are sensible young Danish women who are well along the way and have chosen to do this because of—whatever their motive might be—it can be for school, to save money, that sort of thing, then it's perfectly fine [*fint nok*].

Sex workers with experience receiving calls from helpers like Dirk know they can ask questions and be explicit about what they will and will not do with a client. Peter, the male escort who visits Rasmus once a month, described the first time a social worker from Rasmus's group home phoned him. "He told me about Rasmus," Peter said, referring to Jan, the social worker who phoned,

and he told me about Rasmus's situation. Jan said that he was gay himself, and he talked a little about himself. It was clear from the conversation that he knew a lot about Rasmus's situation and had a high degree of empathy for him. He was able to tell me what Rasmus's physical condition was. He said that he was a spastic [*var spastiker*], and he told me that he was very hard to understand. He also communicated that he was very close to Rasmus. And they had a close understanding that meant that Jan had a lot of insight into Rasmus's life. And as I understood it, Rasmus had expressed to Jan that he liked men, which was a sign that they had a close relationship.

So I told Jan that he could go to Rasmus and tell him what I could offer, what I looked like, and he could show him the pictures on my website. ["Do they show your face?" Don asked Peter. "No," he answered, "they're dick pictures" (*pik billeder*).]

And he could also tell Rasmus what I expected from him, which was that he should be bathed and clean, that I am there for an hour, that I don't get involved in any kind of social interaction with the staff or anyone else at his group home, but that I have a high degree of empathy and that when I am with him I will try to listen and understand what he wants.

Once an encounter like this is arranged, the role of the helper is to get the person with the disability ready when the time for the meeting draws near. This always involves making sure the person is freshly bathed and that the room in which the encounter will take place is clean and inviting. In the group home for people with cerebral palsy that Don lived in, encounters with sex workers usually did not take place in the resident's room, because most residents have narrow adjustable hospital beds with bars on the sides to protect them from falling out at night. These beds cannot accommodate two people, so the room normally used for physical therapy was put to new use. That room has a wide, low-cushioned table big enough for two, which residents lie on to be massaged and manipulated by physical therapists.

Whenever the physical therapy room is put to use as a boudoir, it is always freshened up with linen and candles and perhaps a small vase of flowers. A radio is made available, in case anyone wants music. Soft drinks are provided. Don asked Peter to describe what happens when he comes to meet Rasmus once a month.

> Rasmus is always happy when I arrive. He makes this particular squeal [*hvin*] when he sees me. When I arrive, he is on the bed, with no clothes on except a towel over his privates. They've given him a bath, and he lies there on the bed, or he is sitting up, and there are clean towels, and he's got aftershave on. They are very diligent about his hygiene. So he's all ready.
>
> And my strategy is to spend the first minutes communicating with him at the same time that I touch him. I leave my clothes on for the first fifteen or twenty minutes or so because if I take them off, he immediately gets an erection and he wants action. That's the way Rasmus is. But when he has an orgasm, he gets incredibly tired. Really tired. He can actually fall asleep.
>
> And so I think, "Well he isn't going to get much pleasure out of my visit if it's all over in a couple of minutes." So I spend time communicating with him and touching him before I undress. You saw yourself how his hands are defective [*defekte*] because of his spasticity. He can touch me but only in a kind of awkward way.
>
> And so I'm there for an hour. So after about twenty minutes, more or less, I'm touching him and he gets an erection. At that point he is really keen to have an orgasm [*er meget opsat på at få en udløsning*]. And so we pause and drink some cola. The social workers have put some cola in the room, and we drink some—I help him drink by holding the glass and putting the straw in his mouth. All this is to prolong everything a bit.
>
> And so I massage him. I massage his back and arms and legs. I use oil, and it's clear that he really enjoys it. And so it goes until he has his

orgasm. I massage him, and I put a condom on him and suck him. I won't let him suck me because he's spastic. His jaw could suddenly lock.

When he's had his orgasm, I dry him off with a towel, give him some more cola, and we talk. To be honest, there are only about five words he says that I understand. The social workers where he lives give the impression that they understand more, which I'm sure they do because they know him better than me. But I try to stretch out the conversation so that it is about something the social workers have left me a note telling me is going on in Rasmus's life, like a holiday that he is planning on going on, that sort of thing.

Clients with Intellectual Impairments

Until now, we have been exemplifying encounters and relationships between disabled individuals and sex workers through stories involving people with physical impairments. But some people with intellectual impairments in Denmark also buy sexual services from sex workers. Some of these people require the assistance of helpers to make the contact or get to a klinik where the sex workers work. But an important difference between people whose disabilities are intellectual and those who have physical impairments is that individuals who are not physically impaired can move around. They do not necessarily need helpers to make the contacts they desire.

Camille, the talkative redhead who enjoyed the space afforded by the absence of one of her client's legs, has also had clients with intellectual disabilities. Three of them came to her at different times during a short period when she was working in a brothel in a southern German city. "I think there must have been some kind of sheltered workplace or something near the brothel," she told Don, "because they all reminded me of one another. They weren't mongoloids [*mongoler*], but they kind of looked alike; they had thin arms and were thin and had faces that looked kind of alike. The first one who came, his glasses sat crooked on his face and they were all greasy. And he spoke a little strangely. When I opened the door and saw him there," she said,

I had a feeling that he was . . . what can I call it? Backward [*tilbagestående*]. He's not 100 percent like us. That's a dumb thing to say, but you know what I mean. And I had some doubts because sometimes you get men under eighteen who come and want to have a go. In Germany there's a limit, the age limit for sex is fifteen, but I think that for prostitution it's eighteen. And

I wouldn't want to have sex for money with a seventeen-year-old kid. I'd feel like it was a taboo I'd broken. And I also want him to be at least eighteen so that he like knows what he is doing, you know?

And with this guy, I had doubts that it was defensible to take his money because I thought that he's kind of like a child, you know? But at the same time, I could see that he knew the kind of place he had come to. I talked to him and I asked him, "Are you sure you want to come to me? Do you want to pay me money?" That kind of thing.

And I could tell that he knew in advance that it was something that cost money and how much it cost. He had the money with him. And I thought, well, he's an adult, you know? So be it.

I was extra careful and I talked even more than I usually do. He talked like a child of seven or eight. He told me that he had been somewhere and won some money, and he talked about how he and his friend went places and that he's been to Italy and that they had good ice cream there. It was completely weird [*mærkeligt*] because he talked about children's things, and he was really happy.

"They were all really happy," Camille continued, "all three of the ones that came. And they wanted me to pet them [*de ville som regel at jeg kælede for dem*], and they pet me, like this"—Camille leaned toward Don and slapped him roughly on the shoulder and then stroked his arm clumsily, almost pulling on it. "Hard, like that. As though they didn't really know how to do it. And afterward I thought about it, and I think about it still today—can it be that they'd never been properly caressed?"

Another sex worker, who works in a klinik in Copenhagen, told Don something very similar about men with intellectual disabilities. "I had a young man, who came with a helper," she said.

At least that's what our appointment girl [*telefonpige*] said he [the helper] was. I didn't talk to him, and he only came the first time. He sat out in the waiting room, and we gave him a cup of coffee, and when the guy and I were done, the two of them left together.

The guy had Down syndrome [*Downs syndrom*]. You know, there's different kinds, and he was very Down syndrome. He was fun. He got off a lot. The only thing that made me feel kind of funny was that he seemed so young in the way he acted [*han virkede så ung af sind*]. He wasn't that young, but he was just like a teenager, even in the way he spoke. It made me feel a little funny, almost like a pedophile. But he was a fun guy [*en sjov fætter*]. He got off a lot—he would cum and still have an erection. He had good control over his body, and there was no doubt that he knew well what sex was.

But there was one thing, though, the whole thing about stroking and touching and being sensual, he didn't know how to do that. It's exactly like the Japanese. I've had a few Japanese clients, and they're the same way, I don't know why. They don't know how to touch you. They're extremely uptight about the body [*kropsforskrækkede*], I don't know why. Really uptight. And with them and with this guy I had to teach. I had to take his hands and say, "Do it like this," and I would run them up and down my body. It was all very controlled, very weird. Really weird. But kind of fun [*lidt skægt*].

The fact that the young man described by this sex worker came to the brothel with a helper illustrates the fact that even though people with intellectual disabilities are often much more mobile than people with mobility impairments—and, hence, can visit kliniks that may have steps or other barriers that would stop anyone in a wheelchair—they sometimes require assistance to identify sex workers who are willing to accept a client with a disability and to negotiate things like prices and services.

Søren, a sexual advisor who has worked for many years with people with intellectual and psychological disabilities, says that when he counsels men about sex he always tries, initially, to steer them away from prostitution. "Hey, couldn't you try masturbating by looking at some images of lovely ladies [*dejlige damer*] or get a girlfriend, or something like that?" he says he urges. Søren's concern is not moral; it is financial. He worries that men with a limited understanding of practicalities like financial planning and, perhaps in some cases, of the difference between a sex worker and a girlfriend, might easily end up erotically fulfilled but broke—especially if they decide that they are in love with the sex worker.

Prostitution in Denmark is not cheap. Going directly to a klinik is a great deal cheaper than having a sex worker come to you. But even in a klinik, prices vary according to the service the client wants. Many kliniks helpfully provide a menu of services and their costs. Here, for example, is the menu (translated from Danish, including the explanations in parentheses) handed to clients who go to a medium-sized brothel in Copenhagen. The explanations in parentheses explain exactly what the services include. The menu begins with the words "All prices are only guidelines [*vejledende*]. We also happily issue gift cards."

Swedish (with the hand)	500 kr. (= US$90)
Spanish (between the breasts)	500 kr.
Girl Masturbation (the girl plays with herself)	500 kr.
French (oral sex on you or on the girl)	500 kr.
Deluxe French (oral sex, the tongue explores balls and shaft)	600 kr. (= US$105)
Deluxe Danish (intercourse in various positions)	600 kr.
Mutual French (mutual oral sex)	700 kr. (= US$120)
Mutual Deluxe French (oral sex on you, the tongue explores balls and shaft, and oral sex on the girl)	800 kr. (= US$140)
French and Deluxe Danish (oral sex on you or the girl, and intercourse in different positions)	700 kr.
Deluxe French and Deluxe Danish (oral sex, the tongue explores balls and shaft, plus intercourse in different positions)	800 kr.

Many people with intellectual disabilities, even those who have literacy skills, would have trouble deciphering a text like this. This is one reason why a sexual advisor like Søren feels he needs to do some preparation before he accompanies an interested client to a klinik. Søren says he knows several kliniks in Copenhagen very well. He has visited them on many occasions and has spoken to the women who are in charge of booking appointments and also with women who sell sex on the premises. Like the sexual advisors who work with men with physical impairments, Søren feels it is important to determine to his own satisfaction that the women who work in the kliniks are Danes who speak the language and who seem to be there willingly. He also needs to make sure that the klinik accepts persons with intellectual disabilities (*udviklingshæmmede*), and he says he talks to women in the klinik about that. Kliniks of any size employ a woman— called an "appointment girl" (*telefonpige* in Danish)—who schedules appointments with the different sex workers who work there. This woman will know which sex workers accept clients with disabilities, and she will schedule an appointment when she knows one of those women will be working.

Before he arrives at a klinik with the person he is assisting, Søren will have spoken to the appointment girl and made it clear that the person for whom he is calling has an intellectual disability. On the agreed-upon day, Søren then accompanies the person he is helping to the klinik, explains anything that needs to be explained, such as the sex menu, and then behaves like the helper mentioned earlier. "I sit in the waiting room, and they usually offer me a cup of coffee," he told Don. "I sit there and wait, and afterward I ask if it was good or bad or what, and I ask what the person liked about the experience.

"I've had some amazing experiences in those situations," he added. One he felt was particularly notable concerned a young man with Asperger's syndrome. This man had difficulty understanding social boundaries, and one evening he approached a prostitute working the street and did or said something that she found offensive or abusive. A man who was looking out for the woman came to her assistance and punched the man with Asperger's, leaving him with a black eye. As a result of this incident, the man with Asperger's became obsessed with getting revenge. He happened to be an engineer, Søren said, and he wanted to make and then detonate small bombs in all the brothels in Copenhagen. Søren, who had been called in as a consultant by a psychologist at an autism center, told the man that he was impressed by how much thought he had put into his plan. But he suggested that maybe there was another way he could satisfy his desire for a proper response to the assault.

"And we talked and we reached the conclusion that what this guy actually wanted was to have sex," Søren said. He told the man that he would help him, but only if he agreed to behave himself and go to a proper brothel, not to a street prostitute. Søren also told the man that he needed to write a small report afterward indicating that he had behaved properly. "I told him I didn't want to know the details," Søren said, "but I wanted both him and the woman to write that he had behaved well." If the man refused, Søren would not work with him anymore.

The man agreed, Søren said, but he told him aggressively that he wanted a woman who would pee and defecate on him. An experienced and grizzled sexual advisor, Søren was unfazed. "I don't care what you do," he told the man, who, he suspected, was just trying to provoke him. "As long as there is no coercion or force involved, do what you want. But I want to see the report afterward.

"And so this is what happened. He comes out of the room at the klinik, and he gives me a piece of paper. And there I read that what he did is lay his head on the woman's stomach and have her stroke his forehead. That's all he wanted. That's all he needed. That's what he needed help in achieving."

Sex Workers' Attitudes toward Their Disabled Clients

Søren's story about the man with Asperger's syndrome who needed assistance to find some sort of peace in regard to sexual contact is an extreme but illustrative example of what people with disabilities can get out of going to professional sex workers who treat them with understanding and kindness while also acknowledging and fulfilling their erotic desires.

We hope it is clear by now that those sex workers who accept disabled clients often go to some length to treat them with respect and tenderness. Recall Peter's story about how he interacts with Rasmus when he sees him for an hour once a month. Instead of quickly giving him an orgasm and leaving after Rasmus subsequently falls asleep, Peter paces the session so that Rasmus gets both social contact and extended sensual pleasure from the encounter. The escort Frigg Müller hired to provide her with her first sexual experience also was very supportive and caring. Not only did he speak with her on the phone for half an hour before they agreed to meet ("to see if there was any chemistry," she said), he had also taken courses in sexuality and psychology, and he took time to tell her things she didn't know about her body and about sex. "He knew how he could do things so that it was the least painful to me. He explained everything that he was doing, and we had an agreement that I would squeeze his arm if we needed to stop, you know? He knew all those little tricks that I didn't even know existed." Frigg recounted the following incident that occurred the first time they had sex:

> I thought it was sweet [*rart*] that the first time I was with him, right afterward, I suddenly had to pee really badly, you know? It was like, I have to go *now*. And so I swept out into the bathroom here and I hurry up and sit down and when I get up from the toilet I see this huge blood clot [*den største blodpølse*] there in the toilet, you know? And so I call out to him and I say, "Hey, come here," you know? "Look at this. Am I bleeding to death or is this natural?" And he came in and looked at it and said, "Don't worry, you're not bleeding to death. It's completely natural, it's just your virginity [*mødommen*]."

"Now that," Frigg concluded, "is something I'll bet I couldn't have asked some guy I'd just gone out and picked up in a bar."

The female sex workers with whom we spoke are similarly concerned with their clients' well-being. Swedish Sandra said, "I think that the sex workers who accept disabled clients are the ones who are actually interested in meeting people. The ones who think that the fifty-three minutes out of the hour when you're not having sex—at least not penetrative sex—are the most interesting part of the job. And with disabled clients, it's guaranteed that you're going to have a different kind of meeting."

"How do you mean?" Don asked.

"Because you have to be a little more personal. 'Right, how are we going to get you into the bed?' You have situations where a client can work his hydraulic lift himself, but sometimes they need help, and that means that they have to let you in a bit closer inside their personal sphere [*den personliga sfären*]. And if you want them to call you again, then you have to treat them with trust and respect. And that makes for an interesting meeting."

Annette, a Danish sex worker in her midforties, says that whenever a disabled person's helper phones her, she is always careful to assist the helper in articulating exactly what the potential client wants so that she can pass him on to another sex worker if she knows someone who meets the man's specifications better than she does. So, she says,

> I always ask them, "Tell me specifically what it is that you want help with." When they hear that the person on the other end of the line is interested in whatever the problem can be, then everything can go pretty smoothly. But calling up to get a sex worker [*en pige*] is not something these helpers do every day, and you know you can hear, especially at the beginning, how they clear their throats and stammer and don't know what to say. So you have to like give them permission to say the things that they've talked about with the person they are helping.
>
> I can hear sometimes that I'm transgressing their boundaries, but I tell them they have to be specific so I'll know who to contact and what the needs are that the guy has, that he is going to pay for. All that so it can be the best, the best for the guy, so that everyone can go home happy. And so that they can notice afterward when they see the guy, "Yes! We nailed it!" [*Yes! Vi ramte plet!*]

Another Danish sex worker, Jute, said her concern for her clients expresses itself partly through a rumbling sense of guilt. She has two clients who are paraplegic and unable to achieve erections. The sexual sessions these men pay for consist mostly of conversation and the man licking her genitals. They can't come to her klinik because there are steps, so she travels to them and charges accordingly—6,000 kroner (US$1,000) for three to four hours. "I feel a little like I'm exploiting them," Jute said. "Well, not exploiting exactly, but it is a lot of money to have me come out just so they can talk to me and lick me. I'm not completely comfortable with that. But I'm working on it."

A fact often not appreciated when prostitution and disability is discussed is one we have already mentioned—that most sex workers who are asked do not accept disabled clients. Men with relatively minor disabilities like a missing leg can slip through the firewall and (pleasantly) surprise sex workers like Camille and Sanne. But individuals with visible impairments like Down syndrome or many forms of cerebral palsy, especially if they are in a wheelchair, are turned away by most women who work in the sex trade. Individuals with these kinds of impairments know this, either from experience or from being told by others, and so they usually carefully plan their encounters with sex workers, and some rely on the help and the expertise of sexual advisors like Søren or Dirk or any of the others we have mentioned in this chapter. When they find sex workers they like, they often establish a relationship with them that can last many years. One man we know with cerebral palsy has been going to the same female sex worker three times a year for the past fourteen years.

Why Do Adults with Disabilities Purchase Sexual Services?

A question we have left unexplored until the end is why people with disabilities go to sex workers at all. Most, of course, do not, just as most nondisabled people do not. But those who do occasionally pay for sexual services report that they find the experiences vital, enriching, and valuable.

Many of the people with congenital disabilities with whom we spoke had their first sexual experience with a sex worker, usually when they were in their late twenties or thirties, and usually after they had lived through years of angst thinking they would never have sex—because they thought they were unappealing or physically incapable of having sex, because they were never able to meet anyone who was interested in them, or because they simply did not know how. Frigg Müller is one example of a person like this, as is Rasmus.

Another is the Swedish author Johan Nordansjö, whose autobiographical novel *My Naked Self* we discussed earlier. As we noted, the novel's protagonist, Max, shares many characteristics with Nordansjö, including severe cerebral palsy. The novel tells the story of Max's search for love and sex. Like

Nordansjö, Max needs assistance for most activities, including eating, dressing, and going to the toilet, and his speech is difficult to understand. The book discusses the difficulties a physically disabled person faces in forming romantic relationships. For example, Max always attended a regular school, and he remembers how he felt left behind as his classmates began to pair up, leaving him single and abandoned. He mentions how jealous he is of his two younger nondisabled brothers, both of whom are married. He describes the difficulties he has making contact with potential partners: "When I go out what most girls see is just the wheelchair, the uncontrollable arm movements that prevent me from eating or dressing myself, and that I have a difficult time keeping my head still. They don't see the person Max."[30] Max regularly falls in love with his female personal assistants, who bathe him and care for him, and who inevitably leave him as soon as he reveals his feelings for them. At age thirty-two Max is still a virgin, and with no prospect of meeting anyone to love, he feels desperate.

Deciding that he has exhausted his possibilities for ever meeting anyone who will have sex with him in Sweden, Max, together with a female friend, Emma, travels to Phuket, where Emma helps Max buy sex from a Thai prostitute. This encounter is the book's climactic scene, and it is depicted at length, graphically and warmly. It is a turning point in Max's sense of independence and self-confidence. Three pages before the end of the book, Max sums up how the experience enriched his life: "The trip to Phuket also helped me build up better self-confidence. The most important thing that happened during the trip was buying sex. I had longed so much to be able to fuck [*Jag hade längtat så mycket efter att få knulla*], and to finally do it, that was tremendous. A big day for me. Now I have the courage to talk to strangers. I have the courage to buy sex. I have the courage to make passes at girls. I have the courage to wear whatever I want."[31]

Mark O'Brien's essay "The Sex Surrogate" describes a similar sense of elation, achievement, and invigorated self-confidence that the author feels resulted from his contact with a sex professional. He describes his life before his sessions with Cheryl, the sex surrogate:

> Even though I was in my thirties, I still felt embarrassed by my sexuality. It seemed utterly without purpose in my life, except to mortify me when I became aroused during bed baths. I would not talk to my attendants about the orgasms I had then, or about the profound shame I felt. I imagined that they, too, hated me for becoming so excited.

I wanted to be loved. I wanted to be held, caressed, and valued. But my self-hatred and fear were too intense. I doubted I deserved to be loved. My frustrated sexual feelings seemed to be just another curse inflicted on me by a cruel God.[32]

O'Brien writes that when his therapist first proposed the idea of a sex surrogate he had resisted it, partly because of the expense, but also because "my initial fear was that someone who was not my attendant, nurse, or doctor would be horrified at seeing my pale, thin body, with its bent spine, bent neck, washboard ribcage and hipbones protruding like outriggers."[33] His most powerful moment with Cheryl was when, at the end of their fourth and last session together, she put her hands down on the bed by his shoulders and kissed his chest. "This act of affection moved me deeply," he writes. "I hadn't expected it; it seemed like a gift from her heart. My chest is unmuscular, pale and hairless, the opposite of what a sexy man's chest is supposed to be. It has always felt like a very vulnerable part of me. Now it was being kissed by a caring, understanding woman, and I almost wept."[34] He finishes his essay by saying that he came to realize that seeing Cheryl had made him more confident about his sexuality. This helped him develop the courage to approach a woman with whom he later fell in love.

In addition to facilitating self-confidence, experiences with sex workers also help some people with disabilities understand that they are physically capable of having sex. Recall that one of Frigg's main reasons for deciding to have her sexual debut with a paid escort was because she wanted to see what she could and could not do without the risk of embarrassment. Frigg's uncertainty about her body and its capacities is not unusual among people with physical impairments. Inger, a Swedish woman of short stature, began a relationship with a nondisabled classmate when she was in her teens. But before Inger and her boyfriend attempted to have sex, she made an appointment with a gynecologist. "I thought my genitals, my vagina, was weird [konstig]," she said. "Because everything else about my body is weird, right, so why shouldn't that part be weird, too? I thought that there wasn't enough space for a dick. I'm so short, I thought that if he put his dick in me, it would come out my mouth. I had all kinds of horrible fantasies about how that was going to go." The gynecologist assured Inger that there would be no problem having sex, and she says that she felt incredibly happy (skitlycklig). "I remember that feeling of, shit, I'm normal! I'm a real woman. I got that assurance that 'Your genitals are completely okay.' It was like, 'Go and fuck all you want!'"

Many people with mobility impairments rarely see their bodies because they are always either sitting in a wheelchair or lying in a bed, and they may have difficulty moving their heads. If they have short arms, or no arms, or limited use of their hands, they cannot feel their body. Mark O'Brien says he was surprised when Cheryl the sex surrogate held up a large mirror and told him to look at himself. "I was surprised I looked so normal," he wrote, "that I wasn't the twisted and cadaverous figure I had always imagined myself to be. I hadn't seen my genitals since I was six years old."[35]

A sexual advisor who works in a group home for people with cerebral palsy in Denmark said that she always spends a lot of time helping the people she works with see their bodies. She encourages them to install full-length mirrors in their rooms and to use the mirror to look at themselves. In the morning, when she helps individuals out of bed, on the way to shower and dress, she pauses their wheelchairs in front of the mirrors and invites them to have a good long look at themselves. This is the same sexual advisor who made a point of writing in Helle's plan of action that to help her masturbate a mirror should be positioned at the end of her bed so that she could see her entire body as she pleasured herself.

Sometimes a person with a disability who pays for sexual services is physically incapable of having certain kinds of sex. Neither of Jute's two paraplegic clients, for example, can achieve an erection. She may feel a bit guilty charging them money just to talk to her and lick her, but Don interviewed one of those two men, who sees many sex workers besides Jute, and he said:

> I can't do like a normal, healthy person, have an ejaculation and think, "That was great," and get satisfaction from that. I can't do that. I get satisfaction up in my head, and I have, what should I say, for the most part I have another kind of experience when I go out. I don't get, what should I say, sexual satisfaction. It's hard to explain. I don't think people can really understand it because it is something completely different, you know? It's a tension, and, how shall I say it, one's pulse goes up. Like I go to a woman and she stands with her clothes on, and she might look good with her clothes on, but maybe she won't look so good with her clothes off. So there's a tension there. And it's a kind of orgasm [udløsning] when you see her without her clothes on.[36]

Don asked this man, Anders, how, if he can't get erect and doesn't ejaculate, he decides when a sex act is over. Anders answered that his partner decides this. His goal in paying for sex is to satisfy the woman he is with;

he gets pleasure from pleasing her. An experienced buyer of sexual services, Anders said he can tell the difference between faked engagement and the real thing. "Most women, when they have an orgasm," he told Don, "they become kind of tired or relaxed, or whatever you want to call it, and they won't have any more desire, and they'll want to have a pause. And so you just lie there together and cuddle and chat, and then you slide up out of that. It's like, what shall I say, it's like a curve that goes up again. And then comes the climax, and you then you just slip quietly down again."

Anders told Don that he keeps coming back to forty-seven-year-old Jute—he's been seeing her regularly for the past six years—partly because he knows he is not exploiting her ("Nobody exploits Jute," he said, impressed) but mostly because "she's very involved [*meget medlevende*]. She's involved in the act; she's not only play-acting. One sees her real person [*der er et menneske bagved*]."

Anders is a kind of buyer of sexual services who is rarely considered when men who purchase sex are condemned as insensitive exploiters of victimized women. While one doesn't have to be as convinced as he is that the female orgasms he witnesses really are genuine, it would be blinkered and unperceptive not to see that the kinds of encounters Anders describes are complex. Anders doesn't go to Jute and other sex workers for sexual satisfaction, he says. He doesn't get that. What he gets, instead, is something that is "hard to explain." That "something" seems to be the opportunity to engage with others in ways that extend his capacities. There is no sense in which Anders's encounters with sex workers are attempts by him to forget or to try to "overcome" his disability—to use the patronizing phrase so beloved on television dramas about how people with disabilities should inspire us all. On the contrary, his meetings with women like Jute afford Anders opportunities that allow him to explore and enhance his capabilities as a disabled man. They permit him to refine skills, sensations, and relations with others that he regards as life-enhancing.

Many, perhaps most, nondisabled people have opportunities throughout their lives that allow them to develop capacities like those together with sexual partners who don't charge by the hour. But for many people with disabilities, this is not always so easy. Jonas is a thirty-four-year-old blind man who lives in Copenhagen. He has no intellectual impairment and he is much more mobile than many of the other people we have discussed in this book. Even though a large city, for a blind person, is not an unqualified safe place (Jonas badly damaged his arm a few years ago when he fell into an excavation site in the sidewalk that sewage workers had neglected to fence off), Jonas moves around freely in Copenhagen and goes anywhere he wants. But he described how difficult it was even for someone like him to go out and try to meet people in clubs and other milieus where nondisabled people often find sexual partners.

"Just making a first contact can be incredibly difficult," he said, "because people are sitting at a table talking to one another, and you come up to their table and you can't look at them. Other people can see if they are signaling that you can sit down with them or whatever, but you can't. You can try to make contact and joke or whatever, but it's not very easy."

The same is true about establishing contact on the Internet. Jonas said that whenever it emerged during a chat that he was blind, the contact invariably was broken. "I've done it in a lot of different ways," he said.

> I've written in my profile that I am blind because, who knows, I thought that maybe there are people out there who think it would be really cool [*fedt*] to have sex with a blind person. But nothing happened. And I've also tried slipping it in when I'm chatting with people that I'm blind. But that's always that. I have a blind friend and we've been talking about maybe trying again—it's been five or six years since I was on a dating site—we were talking about doing an experiment and trying again, to see if the trend has changed. Because it's like people are afraid, afraid of saying something dumb or saying something wrong. They're like, "Oh, he's blind, he can't do a lot of things." And that prejudice makes them nervous.

Jonas's comments about his difficulty meeting sighted people to date lead us to an issue that inevitably arises when disability is discussed in relation to paying for sexual services. Isn't Jonas compelled to pay for sex because he is just too picky? Why can't someone like him, who has a disability, just be satisfied with trying to find a partner with a similar disability? Wouldn't that be easier? Why does he spend so much time trying to find a sighted person who might be attracted to him, especially when experience has taught him that this is difficult to the point of potentially being impossible?

The idea that people with disabilities should stick to their own group in their search for sexual and romantic partners is rarely voiced explicitly, since most people seem to perceive that it smacks of insensitivity or even bigotry. It is, after all, far from politically or socially acceptable to suggest to ethnic minorities that it might be a good idea for them to restrict their search for partners to people who share their cultural background or skin color, or to tell people from working-class backgrounds that if they really are serious about finding a partner then they ought to perhaps limit themselves to looking for others who belong to their own class. When it comes to disability, though, many disabled people say they sense bewilderment and impatience from nondisabled people when they insist that they are not interested in establishing a romantic or sexual relationship with another disabled person. Jonas, for example, told Don that he often gets asked why he doesn't try to find a girlfriend who is blind.

"Because I don't want a relationship with someone who is blind," he tells them. "I want to be out in the world, I want to experience things, and I don't do that if I'm just around blind people all the time."

Jonas's lack of interest in finding romantic partners who share his impairment seems to be fairly common among disabled people of many varieties. Frigg, for example, was disturbed when she heard about a group home for people with cerebral palsy that ran a speed-dating evening for disabled people. The event consisted of arranged meetings where potential partners sat across from one another at a table and had a five-minute conversation before they moved on to the next potential partner and repeated the process. The evening was festive and concluded with dancing and the opportunity to exchange contact information for later, longer dates. Frigg liked the idea of speed-dating, but she objected to the fact that the event was only for people with disabilities.

"Why is it only for handicapped people [handicappede]? I don't have anything more or less in common with handicapped people than I have with you," she told Don. "I'm against that kind of thing, when everything becomes so handicapped-this and handicapped-that."

A common reason many people give for not wanting to form a relationship with someone who shares their own disability is that it is limiting. This is Jonas's view—that couples where both partners are blind can easily become isolated from "the world." The limitations can also be purely physical. A woman in a wheelchair interviewed in the French film L'amour sans limites says that she would never want to have a relationship with someone else in a wheelchair. She would want someone who could help her and extend her own experience and engagement with the world. If she were together with someone who had the same mobility restrictions as herself, she says, she would have the same problems she has herself—only doubled.

Pernille, who we discussed in the last chapter, was similarly uninterested in having a disabled partner. Maria, another woman with cerebral palsy who lives in a group home, told Don that she has no interest in disabled men. She wants to have a child, she says, and "I want a man who is able to take care of a child in the way I can't. To help me with the practical things." Anna, who also lives in a group home for people with cerebral palsy, and who has no verbal language, gets her most fulfilling erotic pleasure from being the submissive bottom in sadomasochistic sex play. Anna would not want to be with someone who has the same kinds of mobility impairments as she has because then the kind of erotic activity she enjoys most would be physically impossible.

Many people with intellectual impairments are also not particularly interested in looking for partners among others with similar impairments. In the course of her research among young adults who attended dances arranged for people with intellectual disabilities, Lotta Löfgren-Mårtenson came to understand that a dream for many of them was to find a partner who had no intellectual impairment or, failing that, an intellectual impairment that was less pronounced than the one they had themselves.[37] Löfgren-Mårtenson interprets this desire as a way for individuals to secure their sense of their own value. That the strategy often fails—for example, when young people fall in love with staff members or doctors who do not reciprocate their feelings—doesn't detract from the fact that the goal of finding someone who is less impaired than they are provides many young people with a way of dealing with stigma and of pursuing a sense of dignity and worth.[38]

A well-known and relatively easy-to-discern hierarchy of desirability exists among people with disabilities.[39] At the top of the scale is someone who has no physical or intellectual impairments. This is the most desirable category of person to have as a partner. After that comes those who have congenital impairments, such as blindness or restricted growth, or acquired disabilities like lost legs or spinal cord injuries. These individuals have intact language faculties, they have been socialized and educated in nondisabled contexts, and they are articulate, usually mobile, and can make demands to improve conditions that dissatisfy them.

Lower on the scale are people with mobility impairments, such as cerebral palsy or muscular dystrophy—the more restricted their mobility and the less verbal language they have, the lower they fall. Intellectual impairments tend to rank relatively low on the desirability scale of people with disabilities, even among individuals who, themselves, have intellectual impairments, as Löfgren-Mårtenson's work shows. Here, too, the more significant the impairment and the more it affects mobility and verbal language, the less desirable the individual will generally be held to be. At the very bottom of the desirability scale are people like Rasmus, the gay man we discussed earlier, who has cerebral palsy that greatly restricts his mobility and his language, to the extent that nobody really knows whether he may or may not also have specific intellectual impairments as well.

Unsurprisingly, this hierarchy of desirability is linked to, and in important senses is determined by, popular culture and conventional norms of attractiveness. This means, of course, that it is no different from the scale of desirability that influences the erotic choices of nondisabled people. And that fact is what causes many people with disabilities to take offense when they sense that nondisabled people expect them to apply different, and lower, standards of desire than nondisabled people apply in their lives just because they have a disability.

A very real consequence of this hierarchy of desirability is that the lower you are on the scale, the harder it will be to find a partner. This does not mean that it is impossible for even significantly disabled individuals to find love and have sex. Recall, for example, Steen and Marianne, each of whom has serious impairments but who maintain a relationship—one that includes sex—with the active support of the staff at Steen's group home.

It is undeniable, however, that a disability makes finding an erotic or romantic partner more difficult. This simple fact, which ought to be obvious to anyone who gives it even a moment's thought, is surprisingly often not conceded when nondisabled people discuss sexuality and disability. When Johan Nordansjö's book *My Naked Self* came out in Sweden, for example, the author was featured in several newspaper articles because he let it be known that he was in favor of state-regulated brothels. In one article, the newspaper gave the last word to a woman named Louise Eek, who was well known in Sweden in the early 2000s as a vigorous opponent of prostitution. Eek informed Nordansjö that his ideas about prostitution revealed that he has a "stale and lamentable view of people" (*en unken och beklaglig människosyn*). When asked by the journalist how she thought that a disabled person like Nordansjö should try to deal with his intimate and sexual needs, Eek responded coldly: "I think that disabled people should try to find a partner the same way that everybody else does."[40]

This kind of remark, which is at best insensitive and at worst cynical, reveals a profound inability to engage empathetically with the lives of people who cannot "try to find a partner the same way that everybody else does"—because they sit in wheelchairs that cannot enter many public spaces; because they cannot see to read signals that someone like Louise Eek registers without even thinking; because they have intellectual impairments that limit their abilities to manage many kinds of social contact; because they have no verbal language or no functional limbs to type text messages or use a computer keyboard; because their spasticity and their general appearance are stigmatized in a society that reveres nondisabled bodies. While many of these people do manage to find erotic and romantic partners—Johan Nordansjö himself later got married and has two children—many do not. And for those people, paying for sexual services is the only way they can experience the exaltation, discovery, release, satisfaction, joy, affirmation—and sometimes also the humiliation and heartbreak—that can come from having an erotic life.

When all is said and done, it is important not to dramatize sex too much, or give the impression that it always has a profound existential significance for people with disabilities. Sex does become important for many people with impairments because it provides them with a sense of their bodies and of their capacities that they do not get from any other kind of relationship. But disabled people pay for sexual services also simply because a satisfying sexual experience makes them feel good. People with cerebral palsy often report that their spasms reduce after sex because their bodies relax. Others are like Anders, who likes going to prostitutes because the pleasure he believes he gives them gives him pleasure in return. Frigg, remember, sought out an escort because she found herself having mood swings that were startling to her and unpleasant.

Don asked Frigg if her moods had improved after she started seeing the escort. She laughed and said, "Just ask my mother and my family. They say that they can always tell that I become a lot more harmonious and happy afterward. And then time passes and when I start to get disgruntled and obstinate [*sur og tvær*] my mother will come and say to me, 'It looks like it's time again.' So, yeah."

Eva—the woman who pays Michelle from Handisex to come and assist her with her sex aid once every two weeks—once had a partner, a nondisabled man, when she was eighteen years old. That relationship lasted a year and a half. After it ended, Eva lived without sex for many years. She told Don that not having sex wasn't particularly distressing for her. But now that she is having it again, she said, she has come to realize something: "Having an orgasm once in a while makes it easier to get through the rest of the day."

CHAPTER 6 :: why the difference?

In its idealized form, [the Danish notion] *frisind* does not simply denote permissiveness, but enlightened tolerance in matters of personal beliefs and moral conduct,
combined with a social commitment to establish the conditions for individuals to
think and live as they prefer. —Danish sociologist Henning Bech

According to what we have called a "Swedish theory of love," authentic relationships
of love and friendship are only possible between individuals who do not depend on
each other or stand in unequal power relationships." —Swedish historians Henrik
Berggren and Lars Trägårdh

Karl Grunewald, fit, alert, and still active at ninety-two, is an institution in
Sweden. By the time of his retirement, in 1986, he had worked with and on behalf of people with intellectual disabilities for half a century. During his ten-
ure as head of the Bureau for Handicap Issues (Byrån för Handikappfrågor) at
the National Board of Health and Welfare, he developed unrivaled competence and undisputed authority. He has published several books on intellectual disability, one of which—*The Care Book* (*Omsorgsboken*)—appeared in
eight editions between 1973 and 2004 and is the standard Swedish reference

source on intellectual impairments. His five hundred–page tome on the history of intellectual disability was published in Sweden in 2009.[1] After he retired, Grunewald founded the quarterly journal *Intra*, which we mentioned in chapters 3 and 4. That journal continues to set the agenda for discussions about intellectual disability in Sweden.

Jens met this Swedish legend at his home outside Stockholm to talk about his work and life. With the obligatory coffee and little sweet cakes set in front of him on the table of Grunewald's neat kitchen, Jens brought up the 1966 Apollonia meeting on sex and intellectual disability that Grunewald had chaired. At the time, Grunewald proclaimed the meeting to be a groundbreaking moment in disability history. As we recounted in chapter 2, his opening remarks predicted that everyone would look back on that November day as the moment when sexuality was finally and firmly put on the agenda for everyone who worked with intellectual disability.

So Jens wondered, what happened next?

Grunewald took a sip of his coffee and hesitated. "Well, I don't know," he said with an apologetic chuckle.

> I was afraid you would ask that. I actually haven't got much to say about it. I can say that, well, in Denmark they were more . . . let's say liberated . . . and they discussed homosexuality and pornography and all those sorts of things. They were more European, while we here were more backward [*efterblivna*] and square [*tröga*]. And the Norwegians, they were religious, so they were completely in the backwater.

Perhaps the most interesting thing about this response is its immediate recourse to stereotype. Despite having spent his entire long life working with and advocating for people with intellectual disabilities, when it comes to sexuality, Grunewald's explanation for the differences that exist between Denmark and Sweden doesn't mention politics, activism, his own or anybody else's actions, or any other concrete historical or sociological factor that may have played a role in shaping the kinds of differences between the two countries that we have described throughout this book.

Instead, Grunewald's response invokes well-fondled Scandinavian stereotypes about national ethos: Danes are permissive and European—the Italians of Scandinavia. Norwegians are buttoned up—the Scandinavian Calvinists. And Swedes are square—the, well, Swedes of Scandinavia. Grunewald's remarks are self-deprecating, but this presumably is an expression more of politeness than a belief that Danes have gotten anything right. Although he answered Jens's question by seeming to laud the Danes and apologize for the Swedes, his insistence at the Apollonia conference that one should not "poke around in" disabled people's sex lives, and his chastisement, when reviewing the *Masturbation Techniques* films, that "other people's well-meaning advice and meddlesome guidance is often more harmful than it is beneficial" indicate that, in fact, his assessment of how Danes came to engage with the sexuality of people with disabilities is probably not especially favorable.

Karl Grunewald's explanation for why Denmark and Sweden have such vastly different policies and attitudes regarding sexuality and disability is a common one that arises whenever Swedes or Danes attempt to account for the differences between the two countries. Partly because both many professionals and many people with disabilities themselves have a limited grasp of the history of sexuality and disability, and partly because, as recent research by media scholars has documented, "media images of Denmark and Sweden reinforce rather than challenge national stereotypes," differences between the two countries tend to get accounted for by stereotypes.[2]

This is not entirely unreasonable: platitudes about "liberated" Danes and "square" Swedes do in fact have some explanatory power. But to understand why, it is important to color in the stereotypes and nuance them with content—to ground them in history, politics, and culture and to explain the precise nature of the differences that get summed up in glib comments about how Danes are permissive and Swedes are squares.

Drink, Drugs, and Sex

Ask any Swede or Dane what it is that differentiates their two countries, and they will likely offer an answer that mentions alcohol, drugs, and sex.

Swedes regard Danish policies toward alcohol as being irresponsibly lax—except when they are relaxing in Denmark themselves, on holiday, sipping a glass of wine during the day and remarking to their companions what a refreshingly Continental country Denmark appears to be. The reason for this kind of ambivalence (Danes are quick to label it hypocrisy) is that Swedes are used to tightly controlled alcohol policies managed by a state-owned monopoly.[3] The Swedish state has a monopoly on the sale of any beverage that contains over 3.5 percent alcohol through its chain of retail liquor stores called Systembolaget (literally, The System Company). Until fairly recently, those liquor stores were dour places indeed—one foreign visitor to Sweden described their atmosphere as "part funeral parlor and part back-street abortionist."[4]

Nowadays, many of these stores have been spruced up, and customers are actually allowed to handle the bottles and cans they want to purchase, rather than queuing up to order them from behind a counter. But it is not possible to purchase anything chilled in any of the stores (too encouraging), and visitors are greeted with informational brochures warning of the dangers of drinking and offering advice on how one ought to talk about alcohol with one's teenage children. Systembolaget does not sell alcohol to anyone who is visibly intoxicated or known to be an alcoholic, or to anyone the salesperson suspects may sell or give alcohol to a minor or to an alcoholic. Its profits are channeled directly into the state budget, which partly explains why alcohol is so heavily taxed. It is very expensive to buy in bars and restaurants, where a pint of beer normally costs more than US$10 and a bottle of the cheapest wine will often cost almost US$50. Although any Swede who has traveled abroad recognizes that Swedish alcohol policies are restrictive, people still overwhelmingly—in 2012, reportedly seven out of ten Swedes—support the monopoly.[5]

In Denmark there is no alcohol monopoly, and beer, wine, and spirits are available for purchase in supermarkets and in shops that import alcohol directly and keep their profits after having paid the sales tax to the state. In bars and restaurants, prices are approximately half of what one pays in Sweden. A 2011 report comparing health statistics in the Nordic countries asserted that Danes have the lowest life expectancy in Western Europe (79.5 years) and that one of the reasons is their high consumption of alcohol (11.1 liters per person, per year). This report provoked debate in Denmark. A common reaction was that people thought it was better to have a short and happy life than a long, sober, dreary life.[6]

Laws and social policies pertaining to narcotics display a similar divergence. Swedish policies and public attitudes toward drugs are restrictive and punitive. In 1978, and again in 2002, the national parliament declared that the goal of the country's laws and policies on drugs was a "drug-free society."[7] Criminologist Henrik Tham has summarized the Swedish policy as follows:

> In the 1980s, the use of waivers of prosecution for minimal possession became quite restricted, the consumption of drugs was criminalised, and a law providing for the coercive treatment of drug abusers was passed. The police also changed their policy, and resources for combating drugs increased sharply. The new resources were primarily directed towards street-level drugs with a nation-wide drive in the early 1980s resulting in

a doubling of the number of arrests. . . . The number of convictions and prison sentences in the 1980s was twice that of the late 1970s.

The increasingly coercive model was also marked by a sharp resistance to syringe exchanges and by opposition to the expansion of methadone programmes. . . . The importance of demonstrating that society strongly repudiated any use of drugs was emphasised over and over again in the political and public debate. Increasingly, the fight against the use of cannabis was given priority on the grounds, first, that it is more dangerous to health than was previously thought and, second, that it is the stepping stone to hard drugs.[8]

In contrast to Swedish zero-tolerance, Danish policies relating to narcotics are based on a philosophy of harm reduction. Danes make a distinction (emphatically rejected in Sweden) between "hard" drugs that are highly addictive and injectable (heroin, crystal meth) and "soft" drugs like cannabis. Police tolerate cannabis possession for private use, and since the beginning of the HIV epidemic in the 1980s, the country has well-established methadone programs. Syringes are available without a prescription in pharmacies, unlike in Sweden, where a prescription from a doctor is required to obtain them. The local government in Copenhagen, especially, is well known for its inventive practical solutions to help prevent the spread of hepatitis and HIV and the degradation of drug users. The city has a mobile "fix room" (*fixerum*)—an old ambulance rechristened a "fixelance"—that IV drug users can climb into to inject drugs in a safe and hygienic environment.[9]

Finally, pornography and prostitution are the other social arenas that are readily identifiable to any Swede or Dane as significant points of divergence between the two countries. This contrast is rather recent: both countries have similar long histories of Lutheran repression of sexuality, repression that was challenged and overcome by sexual liberation movements in the mid-1960s. As a direct result of those movements, pornography was decriminalized in Denmark 1969 and in Sweden three years later, in 1972. Laws pertaining to prostitution were similar until the end of the 1990s. Denmark's recondite laws, which criminalized the selling of sex as the sole source of one's income (but which allowed it as a secondary income), were actually harsher than Sweden's, where the selling of sex, since 1919, had not, in itself, been a criminal act.

Beginning in the mid-1970s, however, the liberalism of the sexual revolution began to be criticized in Sweden. Feminist activists identified pornography and prostitution as cornerstones of patriarchal oppression and vigorously opposed them both. In February 1975 activists interrupted a "lesbian live show" at a strip club in Stockholm, unfurling banners proclaiming "Lesbian Love Is Not Porn," and later that same year a group of women gathered on the only street in Gothenburg where sex workers worked. The women waited for men to drive by with their car windows rolled down, and in a singularly Swedish gesture of protest, they hurled rotten sour herring (*surströmming*) into the cars. In 1976 feminists mobilized en masse to protest against a government inquiry that recommended revising and modernizing the penal code in relation to sexual crimes. Among other reforms, the inquiry proposed lowering the penalties for some offenses, abolishing the crime of indecent behavior, and lowering the age of sexual consent from fifteen to fourteen years. What ignited the protests was a proposal that the courts be permitted to take "into consideration the behavior of the coerced person before the abusive act" and possibly use that behavior to arrive at lighter sentencing in cases of rape. This was something the feminist movement could not tolerate; for many it was blatant proof that women lived in a patriarchal, sexist society. They needed more protection, not less, against men's predatory violence.[10] The protests succeeded in having inquiry's entire report withdrawn, and signaled a decisive turning point for attitudes toward sexuality in Sweden, from something to be liberated to something to be regulated.

Danish feminists never targeted either pornography or prostitution as obstacles to women's liberation. Indeed, feminist historian Drude Dahlerup found it notable that

> compared to the new women's movement in other Western countries there were two topics that the Danish Redstockings [of the 1970s and 1980s] were singularly silent about: pornography and prostitution. . . . The explanation is probably to be found in the fact that Danish leftist politics was part of the general Danish self-image that one is "broadminded" [*frisindet*] and thus unwilling to be part of the moral condemnation of prostitution and pornography. Moreover, it was leftist activists, with [the left-wing journal] *Politisk Revy* at the fore, who had fought for the liberation of pornographic images.[11]

A result of these differing attitudes during the past forty years is that, whereas the Danish state has repeatedly declined to restrict pornography (except child pornography, which has been illegal since 1980[12]) and legislate consensual sexual encounters between adults, Sweden has had a series of governments that regularly threaten to ban pornography and has passed numerous ordinances restricting displays of nudity. In 1999 it became, as we discussed in the previous chapter, the first country in the world to prohibit the purchase of sexual services in a national law.

The general theme that emerges when examining the contrasting policies and laws pertaining to alcohol, narcotics, and sexuality is that Swedish authorities, in response to issues that become defined as social problems, have a consistent tendency to opt for zero-tolerance and absolutist restrictions. Danish policies lean much more readily toward harm-reduction models that allow for individual choice. Those differences are the ones that Swedes and Danes can easily agree exist, and they are undoubtedly what Karl Grunewald had in mind when he remarked that Danes are "more liberated" than Swedes.

What are the historical roots of these kinds of differences?

Differences in Political and Public Culture

An important historical distinction between Denmark and Sweden concerns the level of diversity and dissent that is tolerated in public debate and in processes of decision making. Denmark has a relatively confrontational political climate, while Sweden has a tendency—noted by virtually every foreign commentator ever to write about the country—to manufacture consensus.

These national differences have histories that extend as far back as the seventeenth century and have to do with the structures of political authority that developed in each country. Sweden, in distinction to many other European countries, has always had a weak aristocratic class, which, moreover, was few in number. Swedish royalty maintained its authority by forming alliances with the peasantry rather than with the aristocracy. Kings and their council (which consisted of a small group of men from the highest nobility) negotiated directly with the landowning farmers for their provisions of soldiers, weaponry, and horses. Unable to levy these contributions to the state by force, the central power had to negotiate, which it did by granting political concessions to the peasantry. Consequently, Swedish farmers enjoyed a comparatively high level of influence in politics. They were represented in parliament from the fifteenth century, and the landowners in each parish formed a council that decided on local matters and prepared petitions to the king.

These arrangements, coupled with the fact that Swedish aristocrats never managed to obtain the same kind of extensive privileges as their fellow noblemen on the European continent, paved the way for the formation of what historian Eva Österberg has called a "negotiation state"—a state where the peasants were granted a degree of political agency and could influence politics.[13]

The political culture that ensued from this was, first of all, a culture of consensus. The parish councils lacked mechanisms for majority decisions, which meant that all of their members had to agree on each decision.[14] Dissenting opinions were smoothed out, overt conflict was stifled, Sweden pursued its "middle way." The "negotiation state" also fostered a climate in which the country's peasants, knowing that their relationship with the state relied on a system of negotiations via the parliament and the parish councils, developed a sense of confidence that they could influence policies that affected their lives.

These two aspects of Swedish political culture—a forging of consensus and trust in the state—became the constitutive elements for political life that still characterize how individuals think about the government and their relationship to politics and social reform.

In contrast to this, Denmark has a long history of autocratic kings and a powerful class of aristocrats that wielded enormous power directly over the population. This came about in the seventeenth century, when Denmark lost a war—and subsequently a third of its territory—to Sweden. The loss enabled the Danish king to impose autocratic rule and rein in the power of the nobility. The aristocracy became a class of landowners. From their estates far from the capital city, the nobility no longer had any direct influence on the decisions of the crown. But they had great power over their tenants, including the right to levy taxes, impose heavy workloads, and mete out corporal punishment. The overall situation of the Danish rural population was grim. Peasants were kept in serfdom until 1788 and had no say in parliament before 1835.[15] The domination of the population by the aristocracy, and the state's indifference to the suffering caused by that domination, led to a deep animosity toward the ruling classes and, historians are agreed, to a lasting distrust of the state.[16] This skeptical attitude toward the state was coupled with a culture of confrontation, in which authorities were frequently ridiculed or challenged.

Danish "Broad-Mindedness"

Today, two concepts—one a widely used Danish one, the other a more technical, scholastic Swedish one—are particularly helpful in thinking about how Denmark's more confrontational and diverse public and political culture differs from Sweden's more consensus-oriented ethos. The Danish concept is *frisind*, or broad-mindedness. Danish sociologist Henning Bech explains that frisind literally means "free mind" or "free spirit." Like other idioms of national peculiarities—such as the German *Anständigkeit*, the French *gloire*, and the Swedish *folkhem*, it is not easily translated into other languages. In its idealized form, it does not simply denote permissiveness, but enlightened tolerance in matters of personal beliefs and moral conduct, combined with a social commitment to establish the conditions for individuals to think and live as they prefer.[17]

Although the word *frisind* only gained currency in the 1930s, its origins can be traced to the mid-nineteenth century, when Denmark had been fractured by military defeats and suffered from a subsequent crisis of national identity. Early in that century, in 1807, the British navy bombarded Copenhagen and seized the entire Danish fleet because of fears that the Danes were on the verge of aligning with Napoleon. When Denmark did eventually do just that, and then ended up on the losing side of the Napoleonic wars seven years later, the country was forced to cede Norway to Sweden. Fifty years later, a catastrophic war against Prussia and Austria led to the loss of nearly half the country's territory and of two hundred thousand Danish speakers who suddenly found themselves living in an engorged Prussia. It was during this time of national trauma and soul-searching that frisind emerged as an ideology of national renewal.

A major inspiration for this cultural sensibility was the writings of the single most influential Danish intellectual of modern times, Nikolaj Frederik Severin Grundtvig (1783–1872). Grundtvig—who several years ago was the subject of an anthology titled *Grundtvig: The Key to Everything Danish?* (note: not just *a* key, but *the* key)—was a religious and political reformer, educator, one of the authors of the Danish constitution of 1849, and a prolific writer of historical tomes, political studies, religious treatises, hymns, sermons, and pamphlets. Grundtvig left his firm imprint on most aspects of Danish culture, and he is read, cited, sung, and lauded on numerous occasions in Denmark today.

Grundtvig's intellectual inspiration was a specific blend of German romantic nationalism (Herder, Fichte, Schelling) and British liberalism (Locke, Smith, Mill). The core of his philosophy was faith in the people, not in the authority of the state. One of his best-known works is a treatise on verse in Norse mythology in which he sought the basis for the nation in the ancient traditions of the Danish yeomanry. This kind of national romanticism was in vogue in the 1800s all across Europe and Scandinavia. But unlike many of his contemporaries, who developed a conservative ideology that exalted the monarch as the embodiment of the nation, Grundtvig combined national romanticism with a critical stance toward established authority. The future of the nation lies in the wisdom of the people, he asserted, not in the institutions of the state or in authoritarian education.

One of Grundtvig's most significant reforms was the founding of Folkehøjskoler. These "folk high schools," still important today, focused less on formal education than on personal development, they gave no exams and awarded no degrees, and they taught through Socratic dialogue rather than rote memorization. Consistent with this ideology of dialogue, Grundtvig's political writings also persistently call for freedom of expression. One of the most popular quotes from his work is his assertion that there must be "freedom for Loki as well as for Thor." This is a reference to the Norse deities associated with trickery (Loki) and righteousness (Thor). It means that society must facilitate the space for debate, and for coexistence, between different extremes of opinion and values.

Even though Grundtvig was not exactly a proponent of democracy (he believed in the wisdom of the people but not so wholly that he wanted the people to be directly involved in ruling the state), his ideas, as one Danish historian has summarized, "became a strong support for liberal and democratic opinions among his contemporaries, and especially for a critical attitude to state, authorities, and academic learning, in favor of a general trust in the judgment of the people and for equality, freedom of thought, and tolerance."[18]

After Grundtvig's death in 1872, his followers split into a conservative nationalist wing inspired by his national romanticism and a liberal wing focused on his antiestablishment ideas and his belief that the essence of the nation resided in its people. The liberal wing influenced radical critics in the 1880s and continued between the two world wars in the form of the so-called cultural radical movement. Most cultural radicals were inspired by Marx and were members of the Danish Communist Party, but the way they framed their communist ideology was fundamentally inspired by Grundtvigian Danish liberalism. Many of them were critical of Stalin's increasingly authoritarian rule, for example, decades before other European leftists began voicing similar concerns. And throughout the 1970s, inspired just as much by Grundtvig as by Marx, many Danish Marxists engaged in relentless criticism of the state and in defense of equality and freedom.[19]

The conservative legacy of Grundtvig's thoughts fueled nationalist movements, such as the populist, anti-immigrant Danish People's Party (Dansk Folkeparti). But it has provided inspiration also for less strident political philosophies, such as that guiding the right-of-center Liberal Party (Venstre), which was the majority party in the coalition that governed Denmark between 2001 and 2011. A striking feature of political culture and public debate in Denmark is that people across the political spectrum can and do invoke Grundtvig to support their viewpoints. What all Danes who do so seem able to agree on is that Grundtvig's writings license a wariness of authority and impel a willingness to question received wisdom. Danes regard those qualities as defining national traits. They are encapsulated in *frisind*, a concept that is claimed and cherished by both the political right and left.[20]

Swedish Statist Individualism
Despite their enduring significance in Denmark, Grundtvig's writings never really made it across the Öresund sound, and in Sweden, both his philosophy and the concept of frisind are all but unknown. Furthermore, in contrast to Danish distrust of the state, which Grundtvig encouraged, Swedes are internationally renowned for their *embrace* of the state. Every book about Sweden written by foreigners for at least the past seventy years has remarked on Swedes' robust affection for their strong, controlling, centralized welfare state. Reactions to that attachment vary between surprise, alarm, and disgust, depending on the political sympathies of the commentator. Conservative British journalist Roland Huntford, for example, begins his book about Sweden, *The New Totalitarians* (1971), with a quote from Aldous Huxley in which Huxley observes that "a really efficient totalitarian state would be the one in which an all-powerful executive of political bosses and their army of managers control a population of slaves who do not have to be coerced, because they love their servitude." Huntford continues darkly: "Of all people," he writes, "it is the Swedes who have come closest to this state of affairs."[21]

The French philosopher Michel Foucault spent four desolate years in Uppsala in the 1950s as a guest lecturer in French language and literature. He once told a journalist that his experience living in Sweden directly inspired some of the arguments about modernization and social control that he developed in *Madness and Civilization*.[22] German author Hans Magnus Enzensberger, who spent time in Sweden in the early 1980s, characterized Swedish citizens' attitude toward their government as "gullible and trusting, as though its benign nature is beyond all doubt."[23] A perplexed Danish journalist recently made a similar observation and wondered "while citizens of countries as different as the United States, Germany and Italy, in different ways and for different historical and contemporary reasons, regard the state's central power as something that should be resisted or at least reduced to a minimum, Swedes don't seem to get enough of it. The state is their friend, not their enemy. Why?"[24]

Swedish historians Henrik Berggren and Lars Trägårdh have proposed an answer to that question. Examining popular and philosophical writings, social movements, political decisions, and public policy, Berggren and Trägårdh argue that since at least the early 1800s, but especially since the consolidation of the welfare state throughout the twentieth century, Swedish society has been characterized by a particular kind of contract or relationship between the individual and the state. That relationship is one in which the state provides the means for the individual to flourish, independent of any familial or social ties. The state, in other words, promotes and enables a specific form of individualism. But it is an individualism that is different from, for example, the "rugged individualism" so lauded in the United States. American rugged individualism is defined in opposition to the state—one of its main features is the romantic ideal of an individual's absolute freedom from the reach or control of the government. In Sweden, on the contrary, *individualism is defined as a form of independence that is facilitated by the state*. It is, the two historians say, a "statist individualism."

Berggren and Trägårdh's concept of statist individualism emerges out of and addresses a seeming paradox that has long occupied both Swedes who meditate on "Swedish mentality" and foreigners who write about Sweden. Swedes, these observers note, are strongly conformist, but at the same time, they are also ardently individualistic. In an essay that still resonates today, American writer Susan Sontag, who spent seven months living in Stockholm in the late 1960s, expressed exasperation at how Swedes cooperated with one another, but only through elaborate choreographies that seemed designed to ensure that nobody ever becomes even trivially indebted to anyone else. She describes how it was "almost unheard of for one person to pay the whole fare for a taxi ride two or three have shared and uncommon for one person to take another to dinner; checks are split pedantically when people eat out together." Sontag reserved special incredulity for the Swedish custom of "borrowing a cigarette." Even close friends never simply took a cigarette from one another, she reported. Any cigarette lifted from someone else's pack was declared to be a loan, and verbose assurances were always given to the cigarette pack's owner that the borrowed cigarette would be returned—which inevitably, to Sontag's continual consternation and dismay, it was.[25]

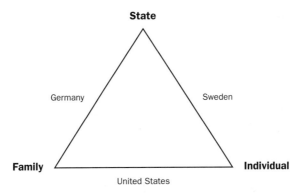

6.1 Power relations in modern welfare states. From Henrik Berggren and Lars Trägårdh, "Pippi Longstocking and the Autonomous Child and the Moral Logic of the Swedish Welfare State," in *Swedish Modernism: Architecture, Consumption and the Welfare State*, ed. Helena Mattson and Sven-Olov Wallerstein (London: Artifice Books on Architecture, 2010), 53.

Social conventions like the ones Sontag described are everyday manifestations of "statist individualism." They are expressions of profound discomfort with any kind of indebtedness to other people. This is a particular kind of sensibility, one that is possible only in the context of a society in which fundamental needs for security, welfare, and comfort are provided not primarily or necessarily by family, friends, and religious or social groups, but by something else. That something else is the state.

Berggren and Trägårdh explain statist individualism by contrasting the Swedish welfare state with the way the welfare state is organized and understood in the United States and Germany. The U.S. model of welfare, the historians say, frames the state in opposition to the individual and the family. The state may provide some support when an individual is unsuccessful in the job market or when he or she has no access to help from family or a charitable organization, such as a religious community. But the moral logic of the system is geared toward getting individuals to forge relationships with and dependencies on the market, the family, and non-state-funded organizations such as religious communities. In the German model, the state is seen as more responsible for social welfare than it is in the United States. But welfare is routed through the family and civic organizations, and these are supported by the government so that they can provide for the welfare of individuals.

Sweden differs from these other two models by aligning the individual with the state—*against* the family, the market, and religious organizations.

Berggren and Trägårdh explain that the goal of social welfare in Sweden is not to facilitate dependencies; it is to undo them. It is "to liberate the individual citizen from all forms of subordination and dependency within the family and civil society: the poor from charity, the workers from their employers, wives from husbands, children from parents—and vice versa when the parents become elderly."[26] The form this particular kind of contract between the state and the individual takes is one in which welfare benefits, such as child allowances (currently about US$160 per child per month, paid by the state until a child is sixteen) and access to health care, are universal, not determined by economic need. Spouses are taxed individually, student loans are given without a means test in relation to the incomes of parents, elderly people are guaranteed home care and, if necessary, a room in a nursing home. The Swedish Law on Support and Service to Certain Disabled People (LSS) discussed in chapter 2 is a further example: it applies to all citizens under sixty-five, regardless of income, and is paid directly to the individual with the disability, thereby facilitating a maximum of autonomy from parents, spouses, or anyone else.[27]

From the perspective of a person with a disability, the Swedish welfare state may appear positively utopian. Statist individualism's emphasis on individual autonomy and on the importance of providing the economic and material means directly to an individual so that she or he can maintain independence from the family, from charity, and from people in the community—all this may sound like independent-living philosophy on steroids. And in many ways, it is.

There is, however, a catch.

Statist individualism is grounded in a particular moral philosophy about how relationships between people should be managed. It arises out of, and continually reinforces, what Berggren and Trägårdh slyly call a "Swedish theory of love." What they mean by that phrase is this: the convictions that make statist individualism seem logical, sensible, and desirable entail a specific view of what a legitimate social relationship may involve. The "Swedish theory of love" is a set of understandings and conventionalized expectations about how people ought to relate to one another. Those understandings and expectations have deep historical roots, and Berggren and Trägårdh discuss how particular features of traditional Swedish peasant culture, such as the relatively late age of marriage and the consequently lower birthrate; the fact that newly married couples moved away from their parents to start their own households; the custom of sending children away from home to work in other (often newly started) households; the custom of *nattfrieri* (night courtship: an accepted form of courtship in which a young man and young woman slept together in the woman's bed at night without her parents' knowledge or approval)—all those factors shaped dominant Swedish understandings of the relationship between independence and dependency on others. They facilitated the building of the particular form that the welfare state took in Sweden, even as they, in turn, have been consolidated and reinforced by the welfare state.

As a normative ideal for how people ought to relate to one another, the "Swedish theory of love" authorizes some kinds of relationships and devalues and opposes others. Those it values are relationships between equally independent individuals: "Authentic relationships of love and friendship," Berggren and Trägårdh explain, "are only possible between individuals who do not depend on each other and/or stand in unequal power relationships."[28] The unstated but unavoidable corollary of this understanding of love and friendship is that relationships between individuals who depend on each other and/or who stand in unequal power relationships, whenever they exist, are regarded as undesirable, objectionable, and inauthentic.

That is the catch.

A moral philosophy of friendship and love that is able to accord authenticity and value only to relationships between people who do not depend on one another and who are in equal power relationships puts significantly disabled people like the ones we have discussed in this book in a difficult position. From the perspective of the "Swedish theory of love," any erotic relationships that significantly disabled people have or want to have will not only seem undesirable and unacceptable; in an important sense, such relationships will also be fundamentally incomprehensible. They make no sense.

Take Steen and Marianne—where he has cerebral palsy, is largely paralyzed, is deaf, and is mildly autistic, and she is deaf, nearly blind, and intellectually impaired, and both of them need elaborate assistance to be able to meet and sustain a relationship. Or take Rasmus and his escort, Peter. Or Pernille and her bus driver boyfriend, or any other nondisabled partner she may eventually find. Relationships like these can *never* be ones where dependency is lacking and power differentials do not exist. Therefore, in a framework defined by a "Swedish theory of love" these relationships can never be authentic. To recognize them as desirable and life-affirming would challenge the foundational assumptions of the theory, and to encourage them or offer them support or assistance would be to sanction relationships that contain features that this entire moral philosophy is dedicated to opposing.

Statist individualism and the "Swedish theory of love" that grounds it are in many ways progressive. The emphasis on individualism and the redistributive channels that have been put in place to ensure an individual's independence in relation to everything except the state have facilitated significant advances in gender equality, labor rights, and children's rights—advances for which Sweden is justly renowned and admired across the globe.

But by figuring dependency on other people primarily as a sign of subordination, and by regarding power differentials between individuals who care for each other as something objectionable and infringing, the "Swedish theory of love" also effectively excludes people with significant disabilities from its scope. The "Swedish theory of love" has trouble recognizing love desired or expressed by women and men with significant disabilities. Such love, from that viewpoint, can only really ever be *mis*recognized—as misguided, mistaken, impossible, or wrong.

Different Feminisms

In 2002 three Danish feminist scholars—Annette Borchorst, Ann-Dorthe Christensen, and Birte Siim—published an article arguing that feminist politics in Norway, Sweden, and Denmark operated very differently and were based on markedly different models of gender, power, and change.[29] Feminist politics in Norway, they wrote, can be characterized by a "discourse of difference." This is a view of gender grounded in perceived differences between women and men; one which holds that society will benefit as women's perspectives inhabit and influence politics, business, and culture. In Denmark, the authors argued, feminist politics could be summed up by what they called a "discourse of power-mobilization." This is a perspective that focuses on how participation in social movements empowers women. Feminism in Denmark tends to emphasize power from below, the authors wrote, and it highlights women as individual actors more than it concerns itself with overarching structural models.[30]

They characterized the Swedish model, in contrast to the other two, as a "discourse of oppression." Borchorst, Christensen, and Siim identified this Swedish perspective on gender as having three main features. First, they wrote, the Swedish model concerns itself primarily with political and economic structures rather than with individuals. Second, it embraces a statistical model of equality: gender equality is defined in quantitative terms of percentages and numbers—how many women serve on the boards of corporations, what percentage of the national parliament is female. Third, it is a top-down model, both in the sense that it holds that change is most effective if it is generated from above, through laws and social policies formulated by the state, and also in the sense that progressive change in Sweden for many years has been orchestrated by a vanguard of feminists who work in the government, or who cooperate with the government, by, for example, doing the research that informs the reports about gender and inequality the government uses to formulate gender-related policies and laws.

The three Danish feminists were not especially laudatory in their assessment of the Swedish model. While they acknowledged that women in Sweden had gained significant advances, they concluded that the Swedish insistence on seeing gender as oppression essentialized gender differences. One effect of this, they wrote, was to foster and maintain precisely the gendered and sexual inequalities they felt feminists ought to be committed to abolishing. The Swedish model also focused stubbornly on structure, the Danish researchers concluded. Its focus on numbers and percentages missed qualitative changes in women's influence. And its top-down directionality was not an effective way of thinking constructively about individuals and how they might more effectively be empowered in their lives.

The Swedish response to this assessment came from a professor of history named Yvonne Hirdman, whose work the Danish authors had used to illustrate the Swedish discourse of oppression. As if to remind readers of her status as one of the most influential Swedish feminists of the past thirty years, Hirdman was imperious. (In addition to authoring numerous books and articles, Hirdman also served on a landmark, agenda-setting government-appointed committee on power and gender equality.) She did not take issue with the Danish authors' assertion that Norwegian, Swedish, and Danish feminists worked with different models of gender and power. But effectively exemplifying their characterization of the Swedish model as one that emphasizes structure over agency, Hirdman criticized Danish feminists' emphasis on social agents, saying that focusing on agents leads one to romanticize them. She objected to the Danish authors' implicit conclusion that the Swedish model of gender equality was not the best, and she quibbled with the label "discourse of oppression" to characterize the model: Hirdman's own work did not use the word *oppression* (*undertrykkelse* in Danish; *förtryck* in Swedish); she wrote about "subordination" (*underordning*), she said.

Hirdman went on to suggest, condescendingly, that the Danish authors' inability to perceive the difference between those two concepts was partly because they have been influenced by postmodern theory and have a "normative, ideological attitude," and partly because of their "completely fascinating inability to read Swedish."[31]

Yvonne Hirdman's crabby response to a critical reading of Swedish feminism is a not-unusual reaction to any suggestion that the particular brand of feminism that has come to dominate Swedish politics and cultural life might not be the only way to think about gender, inequality, and sexuality. Feminism in Sweden today is a prototypical example of what political scientists call "state feminism" and what U.S. legal scholar Janet Halley has dubbed "governance feminism."[32] "State" or "governance" feminism is feminism "from above."[33] It is a form of advocacy for women that has been integrated into the state apparatus (laws, the courts, the legislatures) and whose politics and agenda also have significant influence on public policy and cultural debates (this breadth of influence beyond government institutions is why Halley, influenced by Foucault's more sweeping concept of "governmentality," prefers the term "governance feminism").

In Sweden from the mid-1970s, but especially since the 1990s, explicitly feminist interpretations of social relations and political life have played a central role in shaping national law and social policy. During the 1990s and the first decade of the 2000s, five of the eight political parties currently represented in the Swedish parliament made explicit declarations that they are "feminist." This includes the largest party, the Social Democrats, which in 1993 also instituted electoral gender quotas whereby women and men are placed alternatively on party lists. Several other parties followed suit, and from the mid-1990s onward, Sweden's national parliament had among the highest percentage of female representation in the world. Female representation culminated after the elections in 2006 with 48 percent and currently, after the 2014 elections, is 42 percent.

The increasing number of women in politics, many of the most vocal of whom explicitly have identified as feminists, put what those women purposely label as "women's issues" or "gender issues" high on the political agenda. A turning point in the relationship between feminism and the state was the publication, in 1990, of Maktutredningen, a government commissioned inquiry referred to in English as the Commission on Power. Yvonne Hirdman served as an expert, and in the commission's final report she formulated her theory of gender subordination, which had a decisive influence on several key politicians.[34]

The Commission on Power was followed by another commission, this one specifically devoted to investigating women's power in society. The Commission on Women's Power (Kvinnomaktutredningen) published fourteen reports, each several hundred pages long, written by sociologists, economists, and political scientists. Its final report summarized the commission's conclusions by stating that Sweden is not gender-equal and that women who are employed by the state in the public sector are exploited. Provocatively, and in the derisive tone that animates many discussions about gender in Sweden, the report also asserted that "men are like corks; they always float" and "it's better [for women] to change sex than to try to advance by getting better education."[35] Running parallel to the Commission on Women's Power, still another government commission, the Commission on Violence against Women (Kvinnovåldskommissionen), prepared its report, which resulted, among other things, in the criminalization of the purchase of sexual services.[36]

As with so many things between the two countries, feminism in Denmark is different. Already in the 1970s several of Denmark's political parties on the Left, including the Social Democratic Party, introduced gender quotas, and for a brief time they established women's caucuses within the parties. But in contrast to Sweden, in Denmark those same parties *abolished* the quotas and *disbanded* the caucuses in the 1990s, arguing that gender equity was not facilitated by segregation and enforced gender dichotomies.[37] In Denmark, unlike in Sweden (which has a strong tradition of maintaining separate women's leagues within political parties), the short-lived women's caucuses in the political parties never became a significant political force. Furthermore, feminists in Denmark, as the Danish feminists Borchorst, Christensen, and Siim pointed out in their overview of Scandinavian feminism, have never aimed to achieve the kind of top-down power that has so concerned Swedish feminists.

These differences have not significantly affected the number of women in politics, which is also high in Denmark. After the 2011 elections, the percentage of women in the Danish parliament was 31 percent—the third-highest in the European Union. In 2011, Denmark also appointed its first female prime minister (Social Democrat Helle Thorning Schmidt), a landmark that Sweden has yet to achieve.

In those countries where governance feminism exists, the specific agenda and goals it pursues vary. But as we mentioned in the previous chapter, the version of feminism that dominates across the political spectrum in Sweden is one inspired by the American legal scholar Catharine MacKinnon. Its cornerstone, as Borchorst, Christensen, and Siim point out in their summary of the Swedish model, is the conviction that men oppress women and that this oppression is a structuring feature of society.[38] This "gendered power regime," *könsmaktsordning*, as it is commonly referred to by Swedish politicians, journalists, and academics, is seen as a model of, and the basis for, all other forms of oppression.

The specifically MacKinnon-esque dimension of this view of gendered oppression is the firm belief that sexual violence and what some call the sexualization or the "pornografication" (*pornofieringen*) of the public sphere are the primary sources of men's power over women, as well as its ultimate expression. And like MacKinnon herself, over the past two decades Swedish governance feminism has increasingly moved in what sociologist Elizabeth Bernstein has labeled a "carceral" direction—it has become heavily invested in the legal apparatus of the state as a means of legislating acceptable expressions of sexuality and ostracizing and punishing acts and behaviors it regards as offensive to or oppressive of women.[39]

The 1999 national legislation criminalizing the purchase of sexual services is the most obvious example of this reliance on legislation to regulate sexuality, but the years since the 1990s have also seen a steady expansion of the scope of acts that qualify as sexual harassment, assault, and rape. The international arrest order issued by Swedish authorities in 2010 for Julian Assange—which includes the charge that upon waking up after a night of consensual sex, the Wikileaks founder "deliberately molested the injured party by acting in a manner designed to violate her sexual integrity i.e. lying next to her and pressing his naked, erect penis to her body"—is an instance when some of the more arcane facets of these increasingly sweeping punitive laws regulating sexuality have come to international attention.[40] The discussions among personal assistants about the kinds of activities that constitute sexual harassment by the men with disabilities who employ them that we mentioned in chapter 3 are intelligible in this context, as are the assertions we noted there about how male masturbation in hotel rooms creates a hostile work environment for the women who clean them.

A significant feature of Swedish feminism that differentiates it from feminism in Denmark is its hegemonic status with regard to questions pertaining to gender and sexuality. In Denmark, no single version of feminism dominates public discussion. Debates about issues like prostitution, gender quotas, or how women are represented in the media routinely attract a range of commentary from women (and men) who identify as feminist. In the spirit of frisind, there is no expectation or demand that everyone who calls herself or himself a feminist must share exactly the same views, and occasional attempts by some feminists to occupy the term and pass judgment on the orthodoxy of other feminists are sure to be challenged and ridiculed.[41]

Sweden lacks this kind of diversity. We mentioned above how this relative absence of conflicting opinions in the public realm has long been a feature of Sweden as a "negotiation state." It is also a feature of Swedish society that often is singled out for comment by observers. Susan Sontag was surprised over "the ubiquity" of left-liberal ideas that dominated the country when she was there. While she found much to be impressed by in a country where progressive ideologies were "establishment opinions," she was suspicious about the lack of substantive debate, and she wrote dyspeptically about how even politically radical Swedes seemed "largely paralyzed" when it came to finding anything to be critical of in their own country (their energies went into protesting U.S. involvement in Vietnam or supporting the liberation struggles in Angola and Mozambique).

More than thirty years after Sontag, Norwegian author Karl Ove Knausgård moved to Sweden and noted exactly the same thing. Knausgård was astounded by the level of conformity that characterized public discourse. In volume 2 of his best-selling autobiographical novel *My Struggle* (*Min kamp*, 2009), Knausgård wrote: "Just how conformist the country is, is impossible to describe. Also because the conformity appears as an absence; opinions diverging from the dominant ones do not in fact *exist* in public. It takes time for you to notice" (emphasis in original).[42] In an even more recent book, from 2011, Danish journalist Mikael Jalving wrote something similar, going so far as to argue that a structuring characteristic of Swedish society since at least the 1930s has been that "the three powers of the state—politicians, the media, and academics—work together. Not in a coordinated way—it isn't an evil plot or a conspiracy, but it is an unstated, shared, and comprehensive understanding of what counts as politics and morality, and what counts as polemic and stupid folk misunderstandings [*polemik og pøbel*]. . . . There is, in the new and modern Sweden, a pronounced degree of consensus about what is proper, and what is irrelevant or indecent to speak or write about."[43]

Instead of discussion and debate, Jalving says that Swedish public discourse is characterized by silence: an enforced unwillingness to advance or listen to any views that diverge from what the mainstream media, the political establishment, and the academic elite have decided to be the morally acceptable truth. Jalving sees this silence as one of the main chasms of difference between Denmark and Sweden—the subtitle of his book is *Travels in the Kingdom of Silence*. And the epigraph is a quote from a Danish academic who observed: "Danes believe that they can make problems go away by talking about them. Swedes believe they can make problems go away by not talking about them."[44]

The observations about consensus made by chroniclers as diverse as Sontag, Knausgård, and Jalving capture something generally true about how public discussion is structured in Sweden. But they have particular relevance to issues concerning gender and sexuality. Sweden exuberantly promotes itself around the world as a leader in gender equality, and Jalving's observation that there is, in Sweden, "a pronounced degree of consensus about what is proper, and what is irrelevant or indecent to speak or write about" is particularly apt whenever the topic is gender or sexuality.

A minor—but precisely, therefore, illustrative and telling—example of how this consensus is produced and enforced was what happened in February 2013 to Göran Jämting, a local politician in Åre, a small county of ten thousand residents known for its skiing resorts, located in a far northern corner of the country. Representing Sweden's center-right Conservative Party, Moderaterna, Jämting was a member of the local board of social welfare that grants alcohol licenses to restaurants and bars in Åre county. A newly opened strip club (which does not include nudity, because nudity in such establishments is illegal in Sweden) had applied for a license to serve alcohol, and the local newspaper interviewed several members of the board, asking about their views on the matter.[45] While everyone else interviewed expressed distaste for the club, Jämting told the reporter that he did not want to be judgmental. "I'm not terribly negative about prostitution either," he said, fatefully. "It's a bilateral agreement between a seller and a buyer. Who is actually exploited during an act of intercourse?"

This remark by a local politician in a local newspaper in a tiny rural county nearly seven hundred kilometers from Stockholm made national headlines. "Moderat politician in Åre is in favor of prostitution," announced the tabloid *Expressen*, the newspaper with the highest circulation in the country, in a variation of the headline that ran in all the other newspapers as well ("Moderat politician: Buying sex is OK" and "M-politician: Buying sex is completely OK" are other examples).[46] The particularly Swedish dimension of this incident—apart from the fact that it was treated as news at all—is that at no point in any of the reporting was it even implied that a view like Jämting's was possibly debatable. On the contrary, the only responses or comments reported were expressions of outrage. The Social Democratic vice chairperson of the board on which Jämting served was described as "shocked." She told radio and newspapers, "I think it's a disgrace that an elected official on the board of social welfare expresses himself like that" and "If he was in my political party, he wouldn't be nominated to serve on the board of social welfare, or anything else, with those views."[47]

Jämting's own political party unequivocally condemned his remarks and had what was reported to be a "crisis meeting" two days after the news broke. By the end of that meeting Jämting had composed a press release and resigned from the social welfare board. The press release read, "I am deeply repentant [*djupt ångerfull*] over my comments. I expressed myself wrongly and am ashamed of what I said."[48] Because he resigned, Göran Jämting never appeared at the board meeting that decided whether the strip club would be given an alcohol license. He was replaced by a female party member, and the decision was "no."[49]

:: :: ::

Gender oppression is a structuring feature of society, Swedish governance feminism insists, and sexuality is a primary means through which such oppression is maintained. Göran Jämting's remarks indicated that he was one individual who might not happen to always agree with that view. The result was public shaming and a forced resignation. Jämting's fate illustrates two things: "the ubiquity" in Sweden of a certain perspective on issues relating to sexuality, and the potentially serious consequences that face anyone who questions that perspective.

An understanding of sexuality that inevitably links it to oppression means that any discussion about sex (even sex between same-sex partners) will be colored by, and sooner or later segue into, a consideration of who might be being oppressed by whom. This concern, occurring as it does in Sweden against the backdrop of the "Swedish theory of love" that only accords legitimacy to relationships between individuals who do not depend on each other or stand in unequal power relationships, has the consequence of casting doubt on the authenticity of many kinds of relationships: any intimate relationship that exhibits a stark degree of difference between partners in terms of income, class, ethnicity, or age is likely to be regarded with suspicion.

But the combination of Swedish governance feminism's absorption with oppression and the "Swedish theory of love's" anxiety about dependency has especially toxic consequences for people with significant disabilities. It facilitates and encourages the discussions, films, and educational materials about abuse that we have shown are the sole feature of sexuality and disability that Swedish professionals enthusiastically pursue. But it makes it difficult to even imagine sexuality from a more affirmative perspective.

As we mentioned in chapter 3, one of the fears that Swedish professionals we interviewed frequently articulated was anxiety that individuals with disabilities who expressed an interest in sex might not really understand what sex actually entails, or else that the professional who was approached for advice or help might not accurately interpret the desires of the person with the disability. Women and men who work with disabled adults in Sweden told us that a question they pondered when they thought about whether they would ever consider assisting a disabled person to have sex was, "How can I be absolutely, 100 percent certain that I truly understand what that person really wants?" The unfailing answer to that question was always: "I can't." And neglecting to consider how anyone, anywhere, can be "absolutely, 100 percent certain" that they have ever truly understood what *anyone* really wants (including themselves, if one believes, like Freud, that people have an unconscious), the personal assistants, counselors, and other professionals who shared that concern drew the inexorable conclusion that because they can't read minds, any assistance they might provide in helping a disabled person have sex might be an oppression or an abuse. Better, therefore, to do nothing at all. Then, at least, one hasn't done anything wrong.

Different Agents

In addition to having different political and public cultures, and different kinds of feminism that play different roles in public life, Denmark and Sweden also have different people with different goals, who perform different concrete actions. The American political scientist John Kingdon has proposed a simple model of how social change can occur at the level of policy. It involves two factors: (1) a group of agents or "policy entrepreneurs" who have been working consistently for a long time to prepare for reform, and who have channels to power, and (2) a window of opportunity that makes it possible for the change to happen. That window can be a shift in popular attitudes toward some specific issue; it can be a change in economic conditions, the result of a political or mass media campaign, and so on. The important thing is that the policy entrepreneurs are there when the window is opened and can quickly offer solutions to some perceived problem.[50]

In both Denmark and Sweden, two windows of opportunity for reform opened in the second half of the twentieth century. The first one was flung wide open during the 1960s and 1970s when an entire generation of young people challenged the moral codes of their parents. Between 1969 and 1978, both Denmark and Sweden legalized pornography, made abortion a woman's own choice, and reduced the age-of-consent laws for homosexuals so that they were equal to those of heterosexuals. The social, cultural, and political groundwork was laid for the sweeping advances that have since come to benefit women and gay men and lesbians.

During that period, minority groups in many Western countries began demanding recognition and claiming rights, and people with disabilities were one of these groups. But while disability activists and their allies did eventually achieve significant victories, especially from the 1970s onward, engagement with the sexuality of people with disabilities was not among those victories, at least not in Sweden. In Denmark, as we have seen, the "normalization principle" included sexuality, and disability activists made sex a recurring topic of discussion and debate. In Sweden, sexuality and disability sometimes popped up in outré contexts like the book *The Erotic Minorities* or the film *More from the Language of Love*, but it was not a topic of mainstream consideration, and disability activists avoided it.

The second window of opportunity opened in the middle of the 1980s, when the issue of disability and sexuality reached the national parliaments of both countries. Initiatives that acknowledged that adults with disabilities were not asexual children proposed concrete measures to help disabled adults gain access to a sexual life. But the proposals and their results were completely different. The Danish Left Socialists' proposal—to improve sexual counseling and investigate how sexual assistance and training might be formalized—eventually led to the formulation and adoption of the *Guidelines about Sexuality—Regardless of Handicap*. In Sweden, the Communist Party's proposal to subsidize sex aids was buried in an unpublished inquiry by an isolated social worker, and the issue of sex and disability effectively dropped off the radar.

If those were the windows of opportunity that allowed the possibility of recognition of the sexuality of women and men with disabilities, who were the "policy entrepreneurs" who acted? In Denmark, unquestionably the most influential person in social politics at the time was Niels Erik Bank-Mikkelsen. As we discussed in chapter 2, Bank-Mikkelsen was the foremost representative of a new generation of social workers who defined and implemented the policy of "normalization." Far from having the conservative connotations that it has today, in the 1960s ideas about "normalization" were radical. The goal was to make it possible for people with disabilities to have a life "as close to normal as possible."[51] This meant living in society among other people and not locked away in institutions. And for Bank-Mikkelsen, "normalization" also expressly included the possibility of having a normal sex life; that is, of experiencing and fulfilling erotic desire.

To facilitate this, it was not enough to introduce gender-mixed institutions, create secluded spaces, and respect every individual's right to privacy. It was also necessary to provide sexual education and, in some cases, to actively engage with the sexuality of individuals with impairments. Bank-Mikkelsen's professional background was important in this context: he was a legal expert as well as a social worker. This dual competence enabled him to see that people with disabilities could never actively be assisted with sex unless the legal ramifications of such assistance were perfectly clear to everybody. Bank-Mikkelsen was also a former member of the Danish resistance who had spent time in a German concentration camp. This courageous defiance contributed considerably to his personal prestige. And, in addition, he was charismatic. Karl Grunewald remembered Bank-Mikkelsen as "a unifying person. People liked him because he never put on airs. He wasn't pompous, he talked in understatements."[52]

Bank-Mikkelsen's personal magnetism, his respected status, his conviction that sex was part of the "normal life" to which people with disability were entitled, and his position on the Danish National Board of Social Services made him a key actor in the process of sexual reform.

Two other agents whose work and advocacy were pivotal for both the adoption of *Guidelines about Sexuality—Regardless of Handicap* and the development of the certification program for sexual advisors were Jørgen Buttenschøn and Karsten Løt. In chapter 2 we recounted how Buttenschøn was originally a schoolteacher who got a job in a school for people with intellectual disabilities and perceived a need for an awareness of issues relating to sexuality. Buttenschøn was subsequently recruited by Bank-Mikkelsen to the Board of Social Services, and he became a significant reformer in getting

Danish professionals and politicians to act on issues surrounding the facilitation of sexuality for people with disabilities.

Buttenschøn's friend and colleague Karsten Løt came to share the responsibility for developing and teaching the courses for the sexual advisor certification program. Like Buttenschøn, Løt also was originally a teacher for young people with intellectual disabilities. He developed a range of pedagogical materials still used today and has been responsible for the courses for more than twenty years.

The socialist activists who formed *Handi-Kamp* were also crucial. Young people like Lone Barsøe spoke publicly about sexuality, both as a personal experience and as a political issue. *Handi-Kamp*'s cabaret group, the Crutch Ensemble, performed sketches and songs that insisted that sex was an important part of disabled people's lives and that anomalous bodies had their own beauty and allure: disabled men "use their time and energy on petting, closeness and tenderness," the activists wrote. It is sexy, they said, to be slack.

In Sweden, the most influential person among those who worked for and with people with intellectual disabilities is Karl Grunewald. Because he was part of a relatively small network of reformers that included his Danish and Norwegian colleagues in the 1960s and 1970s, Grunewald was well aware of what was going on in Denmark with regard to sexuality. Yet he never shared the Danes' interest in, or concern about, sexuality. Perhaps this is at least partly because, unlike Bank-Mikkelsen, Grunewald was a medical expert, trained as a child psychiatrist. This background appears to have inclined him to regard sexuality as a personal issue and sexual problems as primarily medical problems.

A certain unwillingness to perceive expressions of sexuality may also have played a role: when Jens interviewed him in 2012, Grunewald made the startling and hugely inaccurate claim that masturbation had long ago ceased to be an issue in group homes where people with intellectual disabilities lived. "That problem disappeared very quickly in the 1970s," he said, "because at that time we began organizing activities so that everybody would always have something to do."

Still, Grunewald helped revolutionize the way people with intellectual impairments were treated in Swedish welfare institutions. He was instrumental in abolishing the large institutions and creating smaller residential units, which have provided intellectually impaired adults with immensely better possibilities to develop and flourish. In his vision of a better life for people with intellectual disabilities, Grunewald did not completely foreclose the possibility of an erotic life: in his 1973 *The Care Book* (*Omsorgsboken*), he and his coauthor acknowledged that "the possibility to look for a life partner is just as important for the developmentally challenged as for other people."[53] Such a possibility, however, was to be facilitated by modifying the physical surroundings to provide more privacy, not by actively engaging anyone in discussion or assistance.

This was the philosophy that guided the reformist efforts of every one of the Swedes we discussed in chapter 2. Journalist Gunnel Enby—not exactly a reformer, but her book *We Must Be Allowed to Love* was one of few voices during the entire 1970s–1990s that advocated for a disabled person's right to have a sexual life—shared Grunewald's conviction that what people with disabilities needed was, as she put it, "one's own room, a key and the right to be alone with one's visitors."

Inger Nordqvist, the single most active individual in the country's history to advocate for the sexual entitlements of people with disabilities, also agreed. Unlike Grunewald—but similar to Enby—Nordqvist limited the scope of her interest to people who had physical disabilities, and who could benefit from rehabilitation. She held lectures, organized conferences, and published booklets on how it was possible to create a more sex-friendly environment for people with disabilities—by influencing attitudes, spreading knowledge of rehabilitation methods, and by promoting the development and use of sexual aids.

But all this was with a specific kind of person in mind: someone who either was capable of satisfying themselves in a decorous manner, because they were not intellectually impaired and because they had enough mobility to use a sexual aid if they could obtain one, or someone who already had a partner, or could conceivably find a partner who would take charge of private matters and see to it that their disabled lover obtained some sort of satisfaction, somehow—possibly with a sexual aid prescribed by a trained specialist who had carried out a diagnostic investigation.

This same imagined agent is the focus of the other important advocate of disabled people's sexuality, Spinalis rehabilitation clinic founder Claes Hultling—the man who compared a paraplegic man's sight of his own sperm under a microscope with a bank-shattering win in the lottery.

In considering all these potential agents of change who have acted over the years in the interests of people with disabilities, the single feature that perhaps most starkly differentiates them is the more expansive scope of engagement that characterizes the Danes. Swedes, for all the reasons we have discussed in this chapter, seem to have trouble engaging with the lives of individuals who are not articulate, mobile, and relatively independent. Individuals who require assistance to perform basic activities like eating, bathing, and experiencing sex, who may not have verbal language, who do not have partners, and whose sexual life will not sort itself out if they are handed a key to their door and a mechanical sex aid—those people almost never figure in Swedish discussions of sex and disability. On the very few occasions they do appear, such as in Inger Nordqvist's depiction of the "individual vibrator adaptation for woman who can only move her head," the kind of engagement they are offered is nothing if not disturbing.

Danes, on the other hand, are less inclined to ignore or neglect such people. On the contrary, as we showed in chapter 2, individuals who need the intervention of others to be able to understand and experience sex were precisely the ones who were the focus of the efforts of professionals like Jørgen Buttenschøn and the staff of the Mose Allé school, and they were the people whose perspectives and needs came to be accorded a central place in the *Guidelines about Sexuality—Regardless of Handicap* document.

This willingness to engage with significantly impaired adults in order to extend their capabilities in the realm of sexuality may partly be a consequence of less anxiety-ridden cultural attitudes around pleasure that exist in Denmark more generally, and perhaps also because of a seemingly deep-grounded sensibility that there must be "freedom for Loki as well as for Thor"—differences deserve engagement and debate, not repression and silence.

Whatever the reasons for the Danes' greater willingness to engage with the sexuality of people with significant disabilities may be, the practical result has been what amounts to a radical extension (or perhaps just a radical reaffirmation) of the old feminist slogan "The personal is the political." The power of that adage has always been its insistence that there is an interconnection between the private sphere and the public realm. The Danes we have discussed in this book have understood that that interconnection is not just there—in some cases, it needs to be facilitated. And they have also perceived something more: that the relationship between the personal and the political is not just a relationship between an independent agent and an abstract sociopolitical structure. It is a relationship between people, between individuals who care. It is a relationship between women and men who are willing to take a risk and extend themselves to engage with others—others whom they will never fully understand, but whom they nevertheless are able to recognize and acknowledge as fellow adults deserving of attention and dignity.

Why Do Swedes Not Know More about
What Goes On in Denmark?

As our research on sex and disability progressed and we learned more and more about the differences that exist between Denmark and Sweden in terms of policies, attitudes, and practices relating to sexuality and disability, we grew increasingly puzzled by a completely unanticipated discovery. Despite the two countries being separated by only a few kilometers of water, and despite sharing a language that, while not exactly mutually intelligible in spoken form, is certainly mutually accessible in its written forms, nobody in Sweden seemed to know much about what went on right across the Öresund bridge. That Danes with disabilities and the people who work with them did not look to Sweden for guidance in this area is something we came to view as understandable since, as we have seen, Sweden's way of handling the sexuality of women and men with significant disabilities is either to deny that it exists or else to see it as a problem that needs solving.

Denial and repression like that inevitably produce dissatisfaction and resistance, however, and a recurring feature of our discussions with Swedes were expressions of the conviction that the present state of affairs of not even really knowing how to talk about sex and disability could not continue; something needed to change. Whenever we asked people who voiced this frustration whether they had ever considered glancing over at Denmark for some idea of how the change they pondered might look, and how it might be achieved, the answers we received were dismissals. Swedes firmly believe that the Danes' sole solution to the issue of sex and disability is to provide disabled men with access to prostitutes. Many repeat, with enthusiastic disgust, the myth that the Danish state provides welfare subsidies for men with disabilities to pay for sex. Only a handful of the Swedish professionals and people with disabilities—and this includes scholars and activists who have written entire books on the topic of sex and disability—had ever heard of the Danish *Guidelines about Sexuality—Regardless of Handicap*. And even those who had heard of the *Guidelines* had only the vaguest of ideas what they might actually be about. No one knew about the Danish plans of action (*handleplan*) that get worked out between people with disabilities and the helpers who assist them, and to the extent they had even heard the term *seksualvejleder* (sexual advisor), Swedish professionals and people with disabilities assumed it was a Danish euphemism for a sexual surrogate or a prostitute.

The compact uniformity of Swedish ignorance about Denmark is a manifestation of the culture of consensus that we discussed above. But as the example of local politician Göran Jämting illustrated, the Swedish culture of consensus is not just an immutable natural fact. It is manufactured, in large part by mass media that highlights perceived broaches to dominant opinions primarily in order to stigmatize them and reinforce the received wisdom of the status quo.

This approach by the Swedish mass media is a principal reason why Swedes are either ignorant of or have nothing but misconceptions about sexuality and disability in Denmark. Some of this has to do with the fact that Swedish television and the Swedish press only rarely pays attention to Denmark. Generally speaking, Swedes' knowledge of their neighboring country is as meager as Americans' knowledge about Canada. Swedes living in the south of the country can tune into Danish TV1 without paying a cable subscription, and some of them travel over the Öresund bridge occasionally to spend time in Copenhagen or other nearby Danish towns. Those individuals may know something about Denmark's politics and culture. But the overwhelming majority of Swedes would have no idea who the current Danish prime minister is, which political parties make up the government, which social or cultural issues are the subject of Danish public debate, or much of anything else about the country.

As we discussed earlier, it *is* common knowledge in Sweden that Denmark has less restrictive laws regarding alcohol and that Danes have what Swedes usually refer to as a more liberal (*liberal*) attitude toward things like narcotics and pornography. But *liberal*, in this context, is a pejorative label that means something more like *libertarian*. It contrasts with what Swedes who use the word regard as their own more socially responsible stances. Swedes also know—partly because of the worldwide furor that erupted when the Danish newspaper *Jyllands-Posten* published cartoons mocking the prophet Mohammed in 2005—that Danish policies regarding immigration have become increasingly restrictive during the past fifteen years.[54]

This general lack of knowledge about Denmark, combined with a widespread belief that Danes are socially irresponsible hedonists who are fond of their drink and have recently turned into racists, primes Swedes to feel a kind of smug dissociation in relation to their southern neighbor. Swedish mass media stoke this condescending sensibility by reporting on Denmark usually only to highlight those aspects of the country that reaffirm well-established stereotypes.[55]

As far as sex and disability in Denmark is concerned, reports about that in Sweden are not exactly common—in the mainstream media during the past twelve years there have been three: two television shows and one long feature newspaper article. All three accounts report on the situation in Denmark only to dismiss or reject it. The newspaper feature, published in the largest daily, *Dagens Nyheter*, and titled "Sexköp med bidrag" ("Subventions to buy sex")—that myth again—repeats in scandalized tones how "far" things have gone in Denmark: "In Denmark it is legal to buy sex and authorities [*myndigheter*] *go so far* as to help handicapped men contact prostitutes," it informs readers. "A handicapped man in Århus *has gone so far* that he demands that his county subsidize his purchases of sex" (emphasis added in both quotes).[56]

One of the two television shows (a documentary about sex and disability) is more nuanced, but throughout its segment on Denmark it undermines all the information it provides by consistently giving the last word to people in Sweden who know nothing about Denmark. An informative interview with a Danish sexual advisor about sexual assistance in a group home for people with cerebral palsy, for example, concludes by cutting to a forty-year-old married disabled Swedish woman in Stockholm who has neither seen the interview nor exhibited any knowledge at all about Denmark. Yet she is given the opportunity to scoff: "Take all that stuff that the Danes have come up with [*hittat på*]," she says. "To be satisfied by a prostitute. It's so crazy [*korkat*] that I can't believe it's true. Typical Danes, I'd say. And how would that work? Is Stina-Berta gonna come at 10 AM next Saturday to masturbate me? Never in a million years! [*Aldrig i livet!*]"[57]

The content and tenor of Swedish reporting about Denmark appear in their most condensed form in an episode of a half-hour program called *The Cerebral Palsy* [CP] *Show* (CP-*magasinet*). The CP Show aired in eight episodes on Swedish TV2 in spring 2004. The program was regarded as a watershed in the representation of disability. It featured young people with disabilities as reporters and program hosts; it was confrontational and irreverent toward the politicians, social workers, and religious leaders who were interviewed; it was fast moving and often funny. When it aired, the CP *Show* was universally praised as being savvy and edgy.[58] It was awarded the Stora Journalistpriset, Sweden's equivalent of a Pulitzer Prize, in the category "Innovator of the Year."

The show's episode about disability and sex in Denmark deserves to be examined in some detail, partly because it illustrates the way Denmark is portrayed in even the most progressive contexts in Sweden, and also because the program received a great deal of publicity and attention, which means it is the source of many Swedish people's knowledge about the topic in Denmark. In that light, it is significant that every claim made in the show is either misleading or wrong. The program hosts are condemnatory to the point of being rude, and the interviews are edited so as to portray the people being interviewed in the worst possible light.

The episode opens with a shot of the two program hosts at the seaside, under a bridge. One of the hosts is Jonas Franksson, a man in his late twenties who has mild cerebral palsy—he has no speech impairment or involuntary spasms. He uses a wheelchair most of the time, but he can stand and walk. Franksson's cohost is Olle Palmlöf, a nondisabled journalist in his early thirties. In the opening scene, Jonas is sitting in a wheelchair while Olle stands behind the chair and pops a wheelie with it. The following conversation occurs as Olle bends down and addresses his cohost:

"Jonas, if you have CP, can you get turned on?" [*kan man bli kåt när man har cp?*]
   "Yeah."
   "But it must be terrible to be so CP that one can't fuck [*knulla*]."
   "I can fuck."
   "*You* can fuck. But you're like a super-crip CP [*lyx-cp*]. Surely there have to be some people who have CP so badly [*som är såpass cp-skadade*] or that have the kind of disabilities so that they live their whole lives and then die as unhappy virgins."
   Jonas looks down and answers in a heavy voice, "Yeah" [*Jo*].
   Olle turns directly to the camera and says, "As you've probably already noticed, today the *CP Show* is about sex and love."
   Jonas continues, "And a large part of this show will take place over there in Denmark [*därborta i Danmark*]"—he points out across the water—"among johns and prostitutes who have specialized themselves to only service disabled clients" [*bland torskar och prostituerade som har specialiserat sig på funktionshindrade kunder*].

The easy, off-color banter and friendly chiding between these two hosts sets the tone that characterizes this program and is one of the reasons why the *CP Show* was regarded as a breakthrough in media representations of disability. Here, though, already in the opening few seconds of the broad-cast, the hosts have done two things that characterize Swedish reporting on sex and disability in Denmark. The first is that they have framed the issue as being exclusively about prostitution. The second is that they have already made claims that are not true. Contrary to the host's confident assertion, there are no prostitutes in Denmark who have "specialized themselves to only service disabled clients." Anyone who had had even the slightest inter-est in discovering the actual situation in Denmark would have easily been able to discover that this assertion is false. As we shall see, though, the facts about sexuality and disability in Denmark are almost entirely irrelevant. Jonas and Olle go to Denmark not to discover anything about it. They go to condemn it.

The first person Jonas and Olle interview in Denmark, appropriately enough, is Jørgen Buttenschøn. Viewers are informed of Buttenschøn's iden-tity because his name appears on the screen. But he is identified onscreen as "Sex Political Chief Ideologist" (*Sexualpolitisk Chefsideolog*)—words that have the same alarming connotations in Swedish as they do in English. They imply both that the policies Buttenschøn discusses have been devised by leftist zealots, and that Buttenschøn is the fanatic brain behind their sinister triumph in Denmark.

At the time of the CP *Show* interview in 2004, Buttenschøn was in his late sixties, a dignified bearded man dapperly dressed for the occasion in a vest and tie. He is shown explaining to the hosts that when it comes to sexuality and disability, the focus in Denmark is on the person with a disability. If that person wants help with sex, he says, then it is the duty of the helper to provide it.

Left unelaborated, a statement like that could easily be interpreted to mean that the helper must provide sexual services to the person she or he as-sists. As we have seen throughout this book, that is *not* how sexual assistance in Denmark works, and as one of the main drafters of the Danish *Guidelines* document, Buttenschøn would have been well aware that the *Guidelines* ex-plicitly prohibit helpers from having sex with the people they assist.

The CP *Show*, however, does not attempt to clarify this. Indeed, as the program continues it becomes clear that the lack of follow-up questions or of explanation about this point is an intentional strategy. The show goes to some length to convince viewers that the job of sexual advisors is to act as sex surrogates or prostitutes for disabled men. For example, a later sequence featuring a sexual advisor named Kirsten Klitte Sørensen is introduced as follows: "This is Kirsten Klitte Sørensen. She is a sexual advisor [*sexualvägle-dare*]. It's her job to provide practical help for disabled people to satisfy their sexual needs."

This introduction cuts to a mid-close-up shot of a rustically dressed woman in her thirties sitting on a couch and saying: "Some people want to learn how to masturbate, some want to be put into contact with a prostitute. It's those kinds of things."

The host asks her, "You say 'learn how to masturbate.' What does that mean?"

"Learn how to masturbate?"

"Yeah."

"If you can't achieve an ejaculation, then you can't satisfy yourself. And if you don't know how it is done, one can help them with that."

"They want *you* to help," says one of the hosts, off-camera.

"I can certainly help them," the sexual advisor replies. As she says this, the host says, "Give them a hand" (*hjälper till*).

"I can help them. We help—I've never done it" (*Det hjælper vi—Det har jeg ikke gjørt nogen gang*).

The last part of Sørensen's comments, where she says, "We help—I've never done it," is not translated into the Swedish subtitles that appear onscreen during the interviews with the Danes who are featured on the program. The interview is also edited at exactly that moment. There is a momentary blackout, and when the interview resumes, Sørensen is sitting in a slightly different position. The interview continues with the following question, asked by the off-camera host:

"Do you guide it up and down?" (*För du den upp och ner, eller?*)

Looking distracted and slightly confused, as though the question doesn't quite make sense, Sørensen says, "Yeah."

"How is it?"

"What?"

"How is it? How do you feel?"

Sørensen shakes her head as though clearing it, or as though she suddenly understands what the host is asking her. And she answers, "I don't think about it so much. I don't spend a lot of time thinking about it. Sometimes I wonder what the person I help thinks about it. But it's sometimes hard—I've not done it. Because the people I help a lot have intellectual disabilities [*er udviklingshæmmede*] and are . . . I don't think they think about it a lot."

"So you mean that it isn't sexual for you."

"No, I don't think about it like that. I am indifferent [*Det er jeg ligeglad med*]. No, I don't spend a lot of time thinking about it."

"And your husband doesn't get . . ."

"My husband?!" Sørensen laughs out loud in surprise, as though a question about her husband was the last thing she was expecting.

"He doesn't get upset?" the host continues, "Jealous?"

Sørensen laughs, and says, "He just celebrated our twenty-fifth anniversary with me. No, he doesn't care."

This conversation, like the earlier one with Jørgen Buttenschøn, does not define the meaning of the key word, *help*. Buttenschøn was not asked to elaborate on the parameters of the help he mentions, which invites viewers to interpret his remarks as meaning that a person who is paid to provide assistance to disabled men is also obliged to service them sexually, if that is what they want. The interview with Kirsten Klitte Sørensen cements this impression because the producers seem to have edited out the part of the conversation in which information about the actual help she provides presumably was supplied. In her explanation about what "learning to masturbate" entails in practice, it is not clear that Sørensen means anything more than providing information about masturbation to the men she assists. The CP Show, though, implies that she actually masturbates men.[59] The *host* defines the help Sørensen provides as "giv[ing] them a hand" and "guiding it up and down."

A few minutes after the interview with Sørensen, the program returns again to Jørgen Buttenschøn. One of the hosts asks him, in an impatient, belligerent tone, "How far can one take this? What's the limit? What if a man with a disability is a pedophile and wants children? What if that is his individual need? How do you feel about that?"

Buttenschøn responds calmly that the laws of the country apply equally to everybody, even to people with disabilities. Pedophilia is not a possibility.

"But sadomasochism, would that be OK?" the host presses, in a voice that implies it shouldn't be.

"Yes," Buttenschøn replies. When you remove those few sexual acts that are actually illegal, he says, "there are still a thousand ways to be sexual."

At this point the interview is edited. After a brief blackout, we return to a close-up of Buttenschøn speaking again. Now, though, the context of his comments is missing.

"Some people like urine sex, for example," he is saying, "others like sadomasochism. And it gets worse. Some like to smear each other in shit."

"Here in Århus!" cries one of the hosts, shocked.

"Yes," says Buttenschøn, "in Stockholm, too," he assures the Swedish hosts. "It's hard to understand if you don't like it yourself, but yes, there are people with those kinds of sexual preferences. And it's always the staff's obligation to help people with disabilities in what they want."

"So that would be approved. To be smeared with shit, for example, because it isn't illegal."

"Yes."

"And you think that a person like that if he's in a wheelchair should get help with that?"

Buttenschøn responds by explaining that in his more than thirty years as an expert involved with the sexuality of people with disabilities he has met a total of two men who had that particular preference. In each case, the issue was solved simply, by allowing each man ample time in his own bathroom, where he could indulge in his desires, and by making it clear that he would have to clean up after himself so that nobody who came into the bathroom afterward would know what had happened.

The interview with Buttenschøn ends here, but he appears one more time, toward the end of the program. His last appearance is simply a shot of him getting up from the sofa he was sitting on during the interview. As he stands, one sees that the fly of his trousers is undone. The CP Show's producers not only chose to include this shot; incredibly, the camera zooms in on Buttenschøn's unbuttoned crotch and holds the shot for a full four seconds.

One other Dane is interviewed on the CP Show: Tor Martin Møller, a thirty-six-year-old man with cerebral palsy who is an important and well-known disability rights activist in Denmark. Møller is also a certified sexual advisor—the only one in the country who is seriously disabled himself. None of his accomplishments or qualifications are mentioned on the CP Show, however. Instead, the Swedish interviewers present Møller as a *torsk*—a punter, a john. That is the sole dimension of his existence that interests them. And lest Møller be unaware of the scorn that Swedes like the hosts of the CP Show attach to that social category, they inform him early on in the interview that, "In Sweden, it isn't just illegal to buy sex. Men who buy sex don't have a particularly high status. There's a derogatory word—people say that one is a torsk. People look down on men who buy sex."

"OK," Møller replies, looking like he wonders when his interviewers will get on with it and start interviewing him.

When they do, the interview with Møller travels the predictable trajectory of typical Swedish interviews or discussions on the topic. Instead of inviting him to talk about, for example, the relationship he has developed with the woman he had been paying for sex three times a year for the past eight years (by 2011, when we interviewed Møller, the relationship was in its fourteenth year), or about any other dimension of his erotic life, the interview proceeds like a cross-examination. And it leads to and concludes with the inevitable question, always formulated as an accusation, in a way that ensures that any response offered will be damning: "Don't you ever feel that you are exploiting [*utnyttjar*] the prostitute? That you are exploiting her body so that you can have sex?"

Toward the end of the program the host, Jonas, provides a summary of his perception of sex and disability in Denmark. The scene in which this summary is delivered takes place in a taxi being driven down a highway at night. Jonas is in the back seat, sleeping against the shoulder of his cohost, Olle, who also is asleep. We see the two of them slouched in the taxi, and we hear Jonas's voice, saying in voice-over:

> I am the Swedish morality's Don Quixote doing battle with the Danish sensibility's windmills [*de danska sinnennas väderkvarnar*]. Olle is my Sancho Panza. And I want to say to all Danish CPs that this is very wrong. That Tor is a tacky punter [*simpel torsk*], that Kirsten is gross [*läskig*], and Buttenschøn is fixated [*fixerad*].

At that, Jonas suddenly awakens with a start and looks at the camera for a second before the scene cuts.

There are several ways one might interpret this little monologue. If the show had been less derisive toward the Danes who appeared in it, one could interpret the reference to Don Quixote battling windmills as a critique of *Sweden*—the message being that Swedish anxieties about the Danish approach to sexuality and disability are grounded in nothing more than misguided delusions. Given the condemnatory tone of the final comments, and of the program as a whole, however, that reading seems an unlikely one. Instead, the reference to Don Quixote and Sancho Panza seems designed to invoke the moral righteousness of those two literary figures, inviting Swedish viewers to identify with that. And having the insults delivered in voice-over was perhaps a way to allow the hosts of the program to openly denigrate the Danish experts and people with disabilities who agreed to be interviewed, such as Tor Martin Møller, by making it seem as though the invective was not fully conscious and, therefore, the speaker not fully accountable. Or maybe the producers wanted to suggest that Swedes are so morally upstanding that even when they are unconscious they are guided by politically correct perceptions of sexuality that instinctively reject "the Danish sensibility's windmills."

Swedish superego vs. Danish id.

However one wishes to interpret it, host Jonas Franksson's speech is exceptional in its condemnatory tone. At no point in any of the CP Show's eight episodes are such harsh words used to talk about anybody, including politicians and bureaucrats who are portrayed as having made obstructive or foolish decisions that adversely affect people with disabilities. This recourse to derision indicates just how bound up with affect issues concerning sexuality are in Sweden, even in contexts that present themselves as informative and progressive. The fact that the CP Show went to Denmark and returned with a program that contains nothing but misperceptions, self-congratulation, and lies is symptomatic of—and can help explain—why those Swedes who think they know anything about Denmark in fact know nothing except falsehoods and urban myths.

Change Can Happen

Forty years have passed since the sexual lives of people with disabilities first began to be discussed with any kind of empathy. They have been eventful decades. In Denmark, they have seen the development of policies and practices that ensure that women and men with significant disabilities there have some of the best possibilities in the world to be able to discover sexuality, explore it, and affirm it as a vital part of their lives. In Sweden, nothing much of any far-reaching positive consequence has happened—but the efforts of advocates like Inger Nordqvist and Claes Hultling, and of people like sexologist Margareta Nordeman, who made the *Masturbation Techniques* films in the 1990s, and social work researcher Lotta Löfgren-Mårtenson, have at least ensured that the issue keeps coming up and remains possible to discuss in a respectful way.

Recent years have seen some potential shifts in the situation in both countries. In Sweden, the topic of sexuality and disability has been raised in a way not seen since the 1970s and 1980s. And in Denmark, the political Left, influenced by the Swedish feminist discourse of oppression, has begun to enact reforms that could lead to the erosion of much that has been accomplished in the country since the 1980s and of everything that makes Denmark unique in this realm.

The past few years have seen an increase in attention paid to sex and disability in Sweden. In 2005 a popular cultural magazine called *Arena* published an article titled "Horny Cripples" ("Kåta krymplingar"). The author—a disability studies scholar from Uppsala University—criticized Sweden for the way the welfare state ignored the sexuality of people with disabilities. "Do you need a suppository inserted into your anus or a catheter put into your urinary tract? No problem," the article began. "Do you want to have sex? Forget it."[60]

That same year, *Ottar*, the colorful quarterly magazine of the Swedish Association for Sexuality Education (RFSU), published a themed issue on sex and disability. The conclusion was that the topic remains one cloaked in silence, prejudice, and fear.[61] In 2010 an entrepreneur named Glenn Hanzen, who has a disabled son, started a company in the south of Sweden called Spicy Mate, which sold "quality" sex aids online. Hanzen attended trade fairs and meetings of local disability organizations, emphasizing the need to talk more openly about sex and disability while also promoting his company (which folded in early 2012). In 2011 a government-financed organization called the Association of Mobility Impaired Youth (Förbundet Unga Rörelsehindrade) published a report by disabled activist Veronica Svensk titled "Secrets Known by Many ("Hemligheter kända av många").[62] Over the course of three years Svensk had arranged seminars on the topic of sex for members of the association, and she had conducted a number of interviews with those members. Her report concludes that sex and disability is a taboo topic in Sweden. Her proposed solution to this situation is to encourage people to talk about it more.

In 2007 the Swedish trade union journal *Municipal Worker* (*Kommunalarbetaren*) published a series of articles on sexuality and disability. The articles were an update of a special issue titled "Sex in Health Care" ("Sex i vården") by the same author, Ann-Christin Sjölander, that had appeared in the journal almost ten years earlier. Those original articles were sharply critical of how sex and disability was resolutely ignored in Sweden. Sjölander had gone to Denmark and was impressed by what she found there. She hoped that informing Swedish professionals about the programs and policies that were in place in Denmark would encourage them to learn more about them and to adopt some version of them in Sweden.[63]

Needless to say, that did not happen. In her 2007 follow-up, Sjölander observed with disappointment that "not much has happened" in Sweden during the years since the first series of articles appeared.[64] Swedish health care workers still found the topic uncomfortable and taboo, and people with disabilities found it all but impossible to request information or help. A survey of forty municipalities (*kommuner*) across the country revealed that only one had a written policy document that mentioned sex and disability. That is the policy we mentioned in chapter 4—the one that reads "Staff cannot forbid adults with disabilities from watching porn films. However, they can discuss porn with that person and tell them how things work 'in real life,' and they can suggest some other ('softer') film and perhaps limit the amount of time they can watch such films."[65]

This same policy document encourages staff "to discuss with the service user [*brukaren*] the consequences that particular kinds of behavior can have. For example: What can happen if one dresses provocatively? What can happen if one is unfaithful to one's partner?"

The barely disguised and rather old-fashioned moral attitudes expressed in those guidelines, and the explicit instruction that staff are entitled to enforce limits on the amount of time an adult might watch pornography, is as far as Sweden has come, in 2013, on this issue.

In the entire country we have found only one other policy document on sexuality and disability. This is from a private firm located outside Stockholm that hires personal assistants for people with disabilities. That company's policy on sexuality is less patronizing than the one we just cited, but it is not appreciably more progressive. It instructs employees: "Sexuality is important for most people and can importantly influence how we feel. People who are dependent on other people's help for a good life have the right to help and stimulation even in this realm [*hjälp och stimulans även inom detta område*]. To receive help to discover one's own body and to receive assistance with sexual activities should be on equal footing with other basic needs."

Despite this affirmation, though, the one-page document contains not a single word of practical advice about how such "help to discover one's own body or receive assistance with sexual activities" might actually proceed in practice. What it does contain instead is several paragraphs on prohibitions: staff may not "engage actively" in sexual acts. They may not have sex with the people they help. They must not initiate sexual activity. They need to set up boundaries and make sure they are respected. They need to act immediately if they have any suspicions about sexual abuse.

Sweden today has come full circle, back to the point in the 1960s and 1970s when the sexuality of people with disabilities was first openly acknowledged as a problem. Because that sexuality is still portrayed primarily as a problem, however, discussion is stuck in a remedial register: how do we get it to stop or help make it disappear from view? Despite a revival of interest in the topic, and despite the advent of reforms like the Swedish Law on Support and Service to Certain Disabled People (LSS), which gives disabled individuals far more control over their own lives than they had forty years ago, it could well be that the situation for people with significant disabilities, in terms of sexuality, is in some ways worse today than it was in the 1960s and 1970s. Then, in the heady days of sexual liberation, a window existed to at least talk about sex in an affirmative way. As we have shown, that window closed in Sweden quite rapidly.

But the fact that it opened at all means that reform was at least a theoretical possibility. Had Karl Grunewald been more like Niels Erik Bank-Mikkelsen, or Inger Nordqvist been Jørgen Buttenschøn, or had Swedish disability activists followed their Danish counterparts and insisted that sex was part of their lives and was worth discussing and fighting for—then the situation in Sweden would possibly be very different from what it is today.

Today it is hard to perceive a sex-positive attitude in Sweden. The ascent to dominance of a MacKinnonesque view of sexuality as a primary tool of oppression makes it difficult to think creatively about more affirmative dimensions of sex. When sex itself is a suspicious act, vulnerable people will need to be protected from it. And when even important disability rights platforms like the *CP Show* portray the sexual lives of people with significant disabilities as repellent (what exactly did the hosts think they were representing or advocating, one wonders, when they decided to disguise the nature of the assistance that sexual advisors provide, and make so much of their interview with Jørgen Buttenschøn be about pedophilia, sadomasochism, and shit?), then the chances of empathetic engagement with disabled people, and of developing progressive policies in regard to their sexuality, seem slim.

:: :: ::

For all its progressive laurels, Denmark, too, may be moving down a similar path of restriction and prohibition. That trajectory began in earnest in 2005, when a fifty-nine-year-old man named Torben Vegener Hansen brought legal proceedings against Århus county, where he lives. Hansen, who has cerebral palsy, sued because he wanted Århus county to compensate him for the extra costs he has to pay to have a female escort come to his home to provide him with sexual services. Hansen's claim was about equal access: the Danish Social Services law stipulates that local authorities must compensate disabled people for extra costs incurred because of their disability. Hansen argued that if he were not disabled, he would be able to go to a sex worker himself and, hence, pay a more modest sum. That he needs a house call raises the price (from the equivalent of about $115 to $250 an hour, he said), and that difference, he argued, ought to be paid by the state.

Hansen's case garnered international attention and was relayed around the world. The BBC reported the story, and Hansen was the "handicapped man who has gone so far that he demands that his county subsidize his purchases of sex" in the Swedish newspaper feature discussed earlier. In January 2006 Hansen lost his appeal. The National Social Appeals Board ruled that the additional costs he sought were not covered by article 84 of the Social Services law, which is concerned primarily with medicine, transport, and food and dietary preparations.

Hansen's case prompted debate in Denmark. Upset that the case could even arise, the Social Democratic spokesperson on gender equality, Kirsten Brosbøl, announced that under no circumstances should public funding be given to any man to purchase sex. She blamed the *Guidelines about Sexuality— Regardless of Handicap* for encouraging Hansen, and she denounced the document for making it a duty for, she claimed, all helpers to facilitate contacts between disabled adults and prostitutes.[66] In parliament, Brosbøl demanded to know whether the minister of social affairs and equality intended to revise the *Guidelines*. The answer was no, but the minister said she did not want to endorse prostitution either. However, she saw the issue of prostitution and disability as a question of equality. If prostitution was legal in Denmark, she said, then people with disabilities ought to have access to it in the same way the rest of the population did.[67]

The Social Democrats were an opposition party in 2005, so they did not have the votes in the national parliament to revise or scrap the *Guidelines* document. But together with the Socialist People's Party (Socialistisk Folkeparti), they did have a majority of seats in the city council of Copenhagen. And so in March 2006 the Copenhagen city council passed a "code of conduct" ordinance (Københavner kodeks) that forbade municipal staff from arranging contacts between persons with disabilities and sex workers. Any city employee who disobeyed the code could be dismissed for refusal to abide by employment regulations. "We have made this decision because we are of the opinion that prostitution is fundamentally harmful," the Social Democratic magistrate in charge of the city's social affairs announced at a press conference.[68]

In parliament, the minister of social affairs, who had said she was against prostitution, did not oppose the city council's ordinance. Local governments had the right to overrule the *Guidelines* document, she said. This was a fateful moment for the *Guidelines*. The principles that had been codified in the late 1980s were, in effect, declared to be no longer binding for local authorities.

The status of the *Guidelines* document has continued to be eroded since then. The spotlight focused on the document as a result of Torben Hansen's court case, and the Copenhagen city council's code of conduct made the government nervous, so it directed the National Board of Social Services (Socialstyrelsen) to revise the *Guidelines*, paying particular attention to the passages referring to prostitution. The revised document was published in March 2012. It contains a number of important changes.

First, the new document is no longer called *Guidelines*. It has been downgraded to *Handbook* (*Håndbog*), which means that it no longer has any official status as a policy document. The new *Handbook* is more extensive than the document it replaced—compared to the previous 2001 edition of the *Guidelines*, it provides a greater number of practical examples of situations that helpers may have to confront in their interactions with people with disabilities. It describes how role-playing and discussion groups can be organized, and it gives concrete advice about how to talk about sexuality among the staff.

But it has excised two of the most distinctive and important features of the *Guidelines*. The passage treating sexuality as a positive entitlement—that individuals "*shall have the possibility* to experience their own sexuality and have sexual relationships with other people"—is gone. It has been changed to a literal translation of the UN document it cites: "People with disabilities *must not be denied* the possibility to experience their own sexuality, have sexual relationships with others and be parents" (emphasis added).[69] And the crucial instruction that a helper who does not know how, or does not want, to assist a person with a disability with the help they request nonetheless has "the duty to see to it that another helper or a qualified expert is referred to that person"—this has been removed from the new version. Facilitating contact with sex workers is still mentioned, but it is now expressed like this: "In some cases, staff members may experience that a resident expresses a wish for help to contact a prostitute. Staff members do not have an obligation to arrange such a contact."[70]

A weighty feature of the earlier versions of the *Guidelines* document were statements by the Ministry of Justice and the attorney general that appeared at the end of the document and declared that the kinds of assistance prescribed by the *Guidelines* was not abuse. As we discussed in chapter 2, such assurance was important because it made it clear that there could be no legal substance to threats, like those issued by chief physician Gunnar Wad in the 1960s, to prosecute anyone who engaged with the sexuality of disabled adults. In the new *Handbook*, both statements have been excised. Instead, a note of uncertainty has been introduced, in clear reference to the city of Copenhagen's ban on staff contacting sex workers on behalf of individuals with disabilities. The new *Handbook* says "the municipality [may] specify, within the parameters of the law, a latitude for the staff to work with sexuality."[71]

The new *Handbook* has largely defanged the old *Guidelines* document. However, at least so far, its appearance has made little practical difference for sexual advisors and other concerned helpers who work with people with disabilities. In Copenhagen, all that happened after the 2006 code of conduct was adopted was that staff members asked by a person with a disability to help contact a sex worker started phoning colleagues in other municipalities and asking them to make the contact instead. (Sexual advisors and others do say, though, that the code has made people with intellectual disabilities more vulnerable, because they can no longer take a helper with them to a brothel if they visit one).[72] The advent of the *Handbook* was not a major point of discussion at the annual meeting of the Sexual Advisors' Union (Seksualvejlederforeningen) in April 2012. Most members were just relieved to see that prostitution is still even mentioned in the new text. They had feared the worst, and the organization's leaders had lobbied the National Board of Social Services and provided it with detailed feedback on successive drafts of the revised guidelines.

In their day-to-day work, sexual advisors and other helpers continue doing what they have always done, and those people with disabilities who know their rights continue to insist on them. They are all aware, however, that the climate in Denmark has become volatile. They know that all the gains that have been achieved over the past forty years are fragile. They are the result of hard-fought battles, and those battles may have to be fought all over again.

CHAPTER 7 :: disability and sexuality—who cares?

The encounter with dependency is, I believe, rarely welcome to those fed on an ideological diet of freedom, self-sufficiency, and equality. —Eva Feder Kittay

The priority for a progressive disability politics is to engage with impairment, not to ignore it. —Tom Shakespeare

So now we have described and accounted for the differences in two Scandinavian welfare states that share many features when it comes to different kinds of support for people with disabilities, but that diverge dramatically when it comes to the question of those people's erotic feelings and sexual lives. Denmark, we have shown, has a history of acknowledgment and engagement with the sexuality of people with disabilities. Social workers and others directly involved with disabled people have developed policies grounded in the conviction that sexuality is a fundamental dimension of human existence and that significantly disabled people can be just as desirous as most nondisabled people of developing an erotic life. Since the late 1960s Danes have worked out practices that encourage and facilitate disabled peoples' capacities to experience, explore, and enjoy sexuality. Those practices are not perfect—the concerted efforts to convince young women with intellectual disabilities to remain on contraception or to opt for surgical sterilization, for example, are nothing if not disputable. But even those more debatable interventions involve a tremendous amount of discussion, engagement with, and acknowledgment of disabled women's feelings and desires.

As we noted in the previous chapter, some of the Danish policies and practices we have described have recently come under threat. But they remain robust, for the time being at least, because they exist in a society where state-sanctioned guidelines explain to helpers how they can engage with the sexuality of disabled people without actually engaging in sexual relations with them; where there is a corps of social workers whose professional training provides them with expertise on the subject of sexuality and disability; where disabled people and individuals who assist them speak out on sexuality in the mass media, usually to public acclaim; and where a diversity of voices debate the role the state should play in regulating the sexual lives of its citizens.

Denmark's neighbor, Sweden, is very different. Whenever disability and sexuality is discussed there, the focus since the 1970s has almost inevitably been on rehabilitation, privacy, or abuse. Sex is insistently imagined to be a threatening and potentially dangerous experience from which disabled individuals, in the view of many people who work with and care for them, are better off being protected. Sex is portrayed more as an individual characteristic than as an interactional activity that develops and enriches social relationships. And rather than make adjustments in the environment to help disabled individuals discover and explore their sexuality—for example, by mandating that helpers assist with masturbation, as Danish sexual advisors do, or assist partners achieve intimacy by helping arrange them in positions they cannot manage on their own—Swedish engagement with sexuality and disability has always emphasized regimenting the individual disabled body to conform to the nondisabled environment by using mechanical sex aids that can be positioned and controlled without anyone's help, by making sex invisible through instructions to lock doors and clean up after oneself, and by defining sex as a resolutely "private" matter that has no business appearing in the "public" domain. The old medical model of disability, which mandated that disabled individuals should expect no accommodation but should just adjust to their environment, is firmly rooted in Swedish understandings of disabled people's sexuality and in the practices people engage in when faced with it.

It should be abundantly clear at this point that the differences we have documented between Denmark and Sweden are not trivial. On the contrary, we hope we have demonstrated convincingly that the differences between the two countries impact mightily on the quality of disabled people's lives and on their capacity to develop and flourish. If you have a significant disability in Sweden and you do not happen to have a romantic partner who is able to assist you, then the chances are very great that you will live out your life with no access to any form of sexual activity. Even if you discover that you obtain erotic pleasure from an activity not usually perceived as sexual— like being lifted out of a wheelchair to be bathed, for example—that activity can be halted if someone notices that it turns you on.

Across the Öresund sound in Denmark, conversely, even significant disability does not condemn one to a monastic life of enforced celibacy. There, a person wanting assistance to understand and develop his or her capacity for erotic fulfillment has a fair to good chance of receiving it, in a way that respects an individual's integrity and facilitates the development of different kinds of intimate social relationships.

In this final chapter we want to offer an assessment of the differences we have described. To be able to do this, we have had to set aside much of the professional training we received in our respective academic disciplines. Anthropologists and historians do not normally compare social and cultural phenomena in order to evaluate them. The concern is usually to explain rather than pass judgment and to invoke, if not sympathy, then at least understanding for the people being studied. And indeed, we hope that our presentation of the situation in Denmark and Sweden has provided insight into the lives of a wide range of women and men with impairments as well as the individuals who work with, care for, and assist them.

But to simply highlight difference separated by a slash of sea and end the story there with a winsome relativistic wave goodbye would be to leave out what we, through the course of our work, came to perceive as the most important point of comparing these two Scandinavian countries. That point is this: the kind of engagement with the sexuality of significantly disabled people that occurs in Denmark is ethically superior to that which is permitted to occur in Sweden. It is, we are convinced, better. It is more respectful, more humane. It is more just.

Examining the reasons behind this assessment will lead us to a more general discussion about impairment, ethical engagement, and social justice.

In addition to all the other divergences we have documented, one further striking difference between Denmark and Sweden that we alluded to in the previous chapter is the fact that *none* of the people with whom we spoke in Sweden—none of the people with impairments, none of the parents, none of the educators, none of the individuals who work with people with disabilities, none of the experts with years or even decades of experience talking and writing about sexuality and disability—*no one* thought that the situation in Sweden regarding sexuality for people with disabilities was satisfactory. But nobody seems to know what needs to be done to make the situation better. To the extent that the situation in Denmark is considered at all in Sweden, it is rejected as a model because of the Danish stance on prostitution and also because Swedes, as we showed in the previous chapter, are systematically misinformed about what actually goes on in Denmark with regard to sexuality and disability. Few people we spoke to had any concrete suggestions for progressive action other than some version of the shopworn mantra, "We need more knowledge" or "We have to talk about it more."

In stark contrast to this, in Denmark *everyone* to whom we spoke was relatively satisfied. Many people thought that engagement with the sexual lives of people with significant impairments could be better, and there is increasing unease that the situation might deteriorate if the kind of feminist rhetoric about oppression that has become hegemonic in Sweden gains any more traction in Denmark. But everyone was agreed that the general situation as it currently stands is good or at least potentially good. Certainly no one suggested that Denmark should look to Sweden for any guidance on this front.

This means that in offering our assessment of the policies and practices of these two countries we are not only expressing our own views about what constitutes ethically sound engagement and social justice. We are also articulating an evaluation that seems to be shared, albeit in an often diffuse and sometimes frustrated form, by many of the people we encountered during the course of this research, on both sides of the Öresund sound.

Putting Oneself in the Shoes of Another

Throughout this book we have seen that for many Swedes who work with, care for, and even advocate on behalf of people with disabilities, the topic of sex seems best not dealt with at all ("Don't wake the sleeping bear"). Whenever sex is considered, it is not as a right, an entitlement, or a source of fulfillment or delight. On the contrary, sex in relation to people with a disability is almost inevitably portrayed as a problem and a threat. At best, the problem is managed—through unrelenting surveillance or by detailed instructions about locking doors and making sure that stains stay off sheets. At worst, it is handled by pinching an aroused disabled man's penis with two fingers and felling it with the "penis-killer grip."

Even when Swedish commentators attempt to extend their own perspectives to imagine what life must be like for a person with cerebral palsy or Down syndrome, they usually get no further than themselves. They achieve only what philosopher Iris Marion Young has termed "symmetrical reciprocity"—that is, they put themselves, with their background, knowledge, experience, *and privilege* into what they suppose is the position of another, and they imagine that such a substitution adequately captures the perspective of that other or those others. This is the kind of narcissistic substitution that results in comments like the antiprostitution activist Louise Eek's declaration that disabled people who want to meet others "should go out and do so like everyone else does." Another example is a Swedish blogger who devoted an entry in July 2012 to the topic "Is sex a right?" Moved to address the issue by an article about a personal assistant who complained to her supervisors that the disabled person she assisted smoked, watched porn films, and sometimes wanted help putting on a condom, this twenty-eight-year-old woman wrote:

> I began to think about if it had been me. If I were to have something happen that left me unable to have sex or masturbate on my own. I have to admit that I am a pretty sexual person. I like sex, and masturbation, I like sex toys, I like . . . well, gosh [*jösses*], I like a lot, quite simply. If I were to lose the ability to feel pleasure, lose the ability to give myself an orgasm, for example, that would be a pretty big loss. But I have a really difficult time imagining that I could ever have someone who works for me help me with this. That if anything would feel really humiliating, in fact.[1]

This sort of well-meaning but ultimately only self-serving displacement by an individual who has sexual relations but who in a flight of fancy pauses to imagine for a moment what life might be like if she could not, is a prototypical example of symmetrical reciprocity. A misguided exchange like this constitutes one of the moral standpoints that allows nondisabled commentators (or disabled commentators who happen to have partners or be married, like the Swedish woman in the previous chapter who scoffed at the "crazy" things the Danes had "come up with" to assist disabled people have sex) to lecture people with disabilities about how sex is not, in fact, something that one should not be able to live without. "Sex isn't a need, like eating or sleeping," is a comment one hears frequently when the topic gets discussed in Swedish contexts. Therefore, for individuals with disabilities to request other people's help in an effort to achieve sexual release is an outrage.

The belief that one can put oneself in another's situation and imagine the world from his or her point of view is one of the reasons why sexually active individuals feel they are entitled to chastise disabled people who dare to suggest that sex might be a human right.

Iris Young highlighted the dynamics of "symmetrical reciprocity" in order to draw attention to the way fantasies of identification and similarity—of being able to put oneself in the place of another—efface difference and disguise relations of power. She points out that while trying to imagine the perspective of another is helpful in carrying one beyond one's own immediate standpoint, it is a mistake to think that we can ever capture or occupy the standpoint of the other person. "When people obey the injunction to put themselves in the position of others," she writes, "they too often put *themselves*, with their own particular experiences and privileges, in the positions they see the others being in." Hence, "when privileged people put themselves in the position of those who are less privileged, the assumptions derived from their privilege often allow them unknowingly to misrepresent the other's situation."[2]

Young goes on to describe how this kind of misrepresentation doesn't facilitate communication or understanding—instead, it actually impedes it:

> If you think you already know how the other people feel and judge because you have imaginatively represented their perspective to yourself, then you may not listen to their expression of their perspective very openly. If you think you can look at things from their point of view, then you may avoid the sometimes arduous and painful process in which they confront you with your prejudices, fantasies and understandings about them, which you have because of your point of view.[3]

Instead of "symmetrical reciprocity," Young encourages us to approach others with an awareness of what she calls "asymmetrical reciprocity." We can never fully understand another person. We can never completely share his or her perceptions, history, views, position, and standpoint. We can never actually put ourselves in the place of another. Therefore, in order to learn from others we need to show humility. We need to engage with others in a spirit that recognizes that their perspective is both necessarily different from, and may actually challenge, ours. This is an ethical relation, says Young. It is one "structured not by a willingness to reverse positions with others, but by respectful distancing from and approach toward them."[4]

The Limits of Ability

One might respond to this understanding of ethics by saying that it is a fine perspective to have in relation to people who can talk or express themselves clearly through some other medium, such as sign language or mediated communication. Young seems to restrict herself to this scenario; at least that is one way of reading her closing remarks that "dialogue participants are able to take account of the perspective of others because they have heard those perspectives expressed."[5] But what about "dialogue participants" who have difficulty expressing their perspectives? What should the ethical relation be with them?

This question has proven a difficult one to consider from perspectives on ethics that emphasize agency, empowerment, and ability. The disability rights movement, for example, is less helpful on the topic of sexuality than one might hope, not just because it has been hesitant to address it, but also because—as significantly disabled people like Cheryl Wade have pointed out—in its struggle to challenge the long-standing equation of "disabled" with "helpless," the movement has tended to emphasize what Wade calls the "new disability mythology of the 'able-disabled.'" In other words, the disability rights movement promotes the idea that, given equal access and sufficient support, individuals with disabilities can do anything nondisabled people can do. This is a profound advance that has resulted in significant legislative, social, and economic gains for people with disabilities.

But a problem with a strategy that spends "all its precious energy on bus access while millions of us don't get out of bed," as Wade puts it, is that it turns severely disabled people like her into a kind of disavowed abject. It inadvertently transforms them into a kind of figure that haunts the disability movement and perturbs it by stubbornly embodying all the qualities—vulnerability, dependency, passivity—that the movement so desperately wants to transcend.

As we discussed in the introduction, the same kind of emphasis on the "able-disabled" also characterizes a disproportionate bulk of the scholarship in disability studies and crip theory. Writing in those fields also tends to focus on people with disabilities who are articulate, who are often artistically or athletically gifted, and who tend to be politically aware and active. Most of the people surveyed in *The Sexual Politics of Disability*, for example, were active in the disability rights movement. Literary theorist Tobin Siebers, in his book *Disability Theory*, writes that "there are signs that people with disabilities are claiming a sexual culture based on different conceptions of the erotic body, new sexual temporalities, and a variety of gender and sexed identities."[6] Robert McRuer exemplifies what he calls a crip critique with Bob Flanagan, an author and performance artist with cystic fibrosis who gained fame in the 1990s through public displays of masochism, and by hammering a nail through his penis.[7]

That provocative, talented, eloquent, and politically committed individuals with disabilities are challenging stereotypes, making demands, and staking claims is significant and transformative. Nevertheless, one might wonder: where exactly does this kind of focus on vanguard verbal articulateness, performance virtuosity, and activist "claiming" leave disabled people who can do none of those things? People like Steen and his girlfriend Marianne? People like Rasmus, who had to rely on the attentiveness of a few alert staff members to begin to explore his sexuality? People like Helle, who, in her twenties, had never even seen her own entire body before a sexual advisor suggested that they place a mirror at the foot of her bed? How might we engage the individual desires and particular lives of people like them without waiting for them to stage a protest, create a performance piece, or claim a sexual culture?

Here is where we confront the limits of approaches to disability and sexuality (and to disability more generally) that too exclusively foreground agency, empowerment, and ability. To frame the issue of disabled people's sexuality in terms of "agency" and "independence" is clearly crucial. But to do so without simultaneously acknowledging *and documenting* the fact that certain physical and intellectual impairments also entail dependency can lead to an emphasis on independence and privacy at the expense of a careful consideration of engagement and responsibility. This is clearly what has happened in Sweden, where a deeply rooted ethos of "statist individualism," together with the conviction that sexuality is private, has resulted in a situation that goes beyond an encouragement—it has led to an enforced insistence that people manage their sexual lives by themselves, regardless of their ability to do so.

The Challenge of Inability

Part of the problem in thinking clearly about the issue of sexuality and disability is that the concept of "disability," in its everyday, activist, and scholarly senses, downplays the idea of *inability*. The British social model goes the furthest here when it defines disability solely in terms of barriers and oppression. In this view, a person is disabled not by his or her body, but by society. *Impairments*—the word used in this framework to designate the physical or intellectual limitations that restrict an individual's ability to engage with the world on his or her own and to flourish without the assistance of others—are acknowledged, but they are regarded as private impediments that need have little or no relevance in a good society that accommodates physical and intellectual variation.

This backgrounding of people's limitations has been criticized in recent, alternative definitions of disability, all of which have been formulated partly in response to the social model. But even in many of these alternative definitions, physical and intellectual limitations are recognized only to subsequently be sidelined. The idea that disability is best defined as an identity, for example, largely sidesteps the issue of impairment, except to mention that the body ought to be theorized more.[8]

An alternative like Tom Shakespeare's "interactional approach" to disability attends explicitly to impairments, which he defines as predicaments that make life harder, and that affect people in different ways according to their severity. The suggestion that impairments be thought of as predicaments is an important advance. Like Simone de Beauvoir's oft-cited observation that the body "is a situation"—that is, it exists as both a biological entity and a social and historical specificity—Shakespeare's notion of impairment as predicament highlights both the embodied nature of impairments and the social world in which they accrue meaning and become the target of discrimination or accommodation.

If there is a problem in thinking about impairments as predicaments it is that predicaments are typically viewed as troublesome situations to be overcome. Shakespeare himself notes: "The *Concise Oxford Dictionary* defines predicament as 'an unpleasant, trying or dangerous situation.' Although still negative, this does not have the inescapable emphasis of 'tragedy.' The notion of 'trying' perhaps captures the difficulties which many impairments present. They make life harder, although this hardship can be overcome."[9]

The swift move in a formulation like this—from acknowledging a predicament/impairment to overcoming it—resonates with disability rights activism and is of course crucial to consider when strategizing politics and formulating policy. But notice that what is glossed over or even lost in a formulation like this is a sustained engagement with the nature of the predicament itself. Shakespeare recognizes that intellectual and physical impairments imply limitations: "To call something a predicament is to understand it as a difficulty, and as a challenge, and as something which we might want to minimize but which we cannot ultimately avoid."[10] But he doesn't linger on the nature of that difficulty or explore what it is, exactly, that makes it so challenging or what that challenge might mean for theory, policy, and action.

In chapter 4 we cited a text by the writer and performer Cheryl Marie Wade that described how significantly impaired people like herself "must have our asses cleaned after we shit and pee." That passage is from a three-page polemic first published in *The Disability Rag* magazine in 1991. It is also one of the most-quoted passages in disability studies literature. Surely a reason why it keeps reappearing in book after book on disability studies is because it portrays the experience of significant impairment so nakedly. It rejects euphemism, stamps on squeamishness, and demands that readers actually picture—in full-blown Rabelaisian detail—shameful, lowly, messy bodily functions from the point of view of a disabled person who requires assistance to perform them successfully. "It isn't 'using the toilet,'" Wade chastises readers, "it's having someone's hands in your private hairs so you can live in the world."[11]

Why is this kind of unflinching, indecorous language so arresting? Perhaps because Wade's text is one of the few instances in the literature on disability where readers are bluntly confronted with inability—not so much as a predicament to be overcome, as an ontological position that will always be lived and never be transcended.

If we pause for a moment in Cheryl Wade's private hairs, it becomes possible to ask why the inability she describes is so discomforting. And if we consider that, we can ask the follow-up question of whether inability should be considered only in terms of a privation or a lack. Is it possible to think about the inability that Wade insists on not so much as a lamentable condition that afflicts her (and could afflict us) but, instead, as something, rather, that is *productive*, and that fundamentally concerns us all?

Such a view of inability has become popular in recent years, in the form of assertions that vulnerability and precariousness constitute a kind of ontological foundation of human subjectivity. Sociologist Bryan Turner makes this a central point in his book about how human rights need to be grounded in recognition of common, universal vulnerability. Anthropologist Sarah Jain, in her work on cancer, suggests that we are all "living in prognosis"—in the sense that our lives are lived in relation to bio-power governmentality that enmeshes us in statistics, risk assessments, and indices of mortality, fertility, and productivity. Using similar language, queer studies scholar Jasbir Puar writes that we are all "living with debility," that is, we all exist subject to economic relations and political forces that disempower and exploit us.[12]

These kinds of reminders about the fundamentally sociopolitical, interdependent, and fragile nature of human life are valuable, and it is no wonder that vulnerability is being stressed now, partly as a form of progressive resistance to neo-liberal ideologies and policies that insist we are all independent individuals equally empowered to make choices in the global marketplace, and partly because that same global marketplace is increasingly making sure that more and more people are becoming impoverished, uprooted, unsupported, and vulnerable. A serious problem with assertions that we are all vulnerable, however, is that they very quickly tend to lose track of the fact that we are not, in fact, all *equally* vulnerable. We are not all equally captured in prognosis or equally impacted by regimes of debility, and scholarship that concerns itself more with abstract theorizing about the self and its relation to discourse and regimes of power than with the actual lives of specific individuals risks blurring or eliding differences that ought to be documented and understood in their specificities.

In order to think more imaginatively about vulnerability and inability, it seems important to consider the meaning of inability in terms other than just as a common human ontology. One thinker who has attempted this—interestingly, by sidestepping the human—is the philosopher Jacques Derrida. In an article he wrote near the end of his life, Derrida cites Jeremy Bentham's famous discussion about the ethical treatment of animals. Breaking with all philosophical and theological thought on the issue that had preceded him for thousands of years, Bentham proposed, in 1780, that the relevant issue to consider when thinking about the ethically sound treatment of animals was not whether they could reason or speak, or make rational choices. The crucial, decisive issue that should govern our interaction with animals, Bentham proposed, was "Can they suffer?"

Derrida considers this a question that leads us to a direct engagement with inability. Asking if animals can suffer, he says, "amounts to asking " 'can they *not be able?*'" And *that*, in turn, compels one to think about inability as something other than privation. "What is this nonpower at the heart of power?" Derrida asks. "What is its quality or modality? How should one account for it? What right should be accorded it? To what extent does it concern us? Being able to suffer is no longer a power, it is a possibility without power, a possibility of the impossible" (emphasis in original).[13]

With questions like these, Derrida compels us to consider inability as something other than a wretched condition from which individuals might be rescued and empowered to overcome. This is the brilliance of his framing of the discussion of vulnerability and what he calls "nonpower" around animals, who, after all, will never be empowered to speak, organize protests, or collectively disrupt the influence that human beings hold over their lives. By focusing on animals, Derrida makes it clear that he is not asking us to think of vulnerability in the way Tom Shakespeare suggests, as a predicament that can be overcome. His point is different. Vulnerability, Derrida insists, is best considered in terms of a relationship. But not just any kind of relationship. Vulnerability constitutes "a duty, a responsibility, and obligation, it is also a necessity, a constraint that, like it or not, directly or indirectly, everyone is held to."[14]

Now given the long and oppressive history of likening people with impairments to animals—a history kept distressingly alive by none other than the leading proponents of Jeremy Bentham's school of utilitarian philosophy, such as philosopher Peter Singer, who is notoriously fond of comparing severely disabled people to rabbits, or dogs—it is both dangerous and potentially deeply offensive to suggest that discussions about animals have any relevance at all to discussions about disability.

However, we think that Derrida's insistence that inability entails responsibility is a powerfully phrased insight. It engages vulnerability not as an ontological foundation or a sociopolitical position we all share. Instead, it regards inability as a characteristic or a quality that is differentially distributed in the world. Some beings are more not-able than others. And that fact, "like it or not," obligates us all.

Why Care?

The question one might legitimately ask at this point is: why? Why should vulnerability obligate? And to the extent that it does, how does one evaluate the terms of the obligation? On what grounds might one judge that one particular way of engaging with and meeting our obligation to vulnerable others is better or more just than some alternative way?

The first question, in many ways, is the more difficult one. Scholars like Bryan Turner say that vulnerability obligates because we all share it. "Human beings experience pain and humiliation because they are vulnerable," he writes. "While humans may not share a common culture, they are bound together by the risks and perturbations that arise from their vulnerability."[15] As legal scholar Barbara Hudson has noted, this kind of appeal to a shared vulnerability is a version of the classical liberal argument about ethics that bases engagement with others on the recognition of similarity. It holds that I should treat others in the way I would wish to be treated "because my actions will affect others the same way they would affect me, and I can empathize because of the characteristics we have in common."[16]

One problem with this framework is that it compels by appealing to the kind of symmetrical reciprocity—of imagining myself in the shoes of another—that Iris Young has criticized so trenchantly. But another problem with an argument like Turner's, as Hudson points out, is that it overlooks philosopher Richard Rorty's observation that most people simply do not think of themselves as "a human being." They think of themselves as being a certain kind of person, usually defined in explicit opposition to other sorts of people—an able-bodied person defined in contrast to people with disabilities, for example.[17] In cases like that, an appeal to a common vulnerability might elicit sympathy, but it is just as likely to elicit an embarrassed turning away, and disavowal.

Like Turner, the philosopher Emmanuel Levinas also addresses ethical obligation by observing that human beings are vulnerable. But Levinas's perspective is arguably the more useful in the context of thinking about disability. Rather than suggest that we are obligated to others because they are similar to us (since they too share a common vulnerability), Levinas argues that we are obligated to others because they are *different* from us, and from this position of difference they make demands that enmesh us in a relationship—whether we like it or not.

People are different because each individual has a specific history, a specific place in social networks, a specific singularity. This singularity emerges through relations with others, whose existence, whose address, and whose behavior toward me are what determine a place for me and, thus, in a fundamental sense, are what make me *me*. This relationship of susceptibility to others binds me to other people—since my existence as a subject depends on them. It also obligates me to them, both as an object of other people's actions and as an agent in relation to others. Levinas insists that the obligation is an ethical one in that it is a response to others and also entails a response toward others.

Social life consists of encounters with other people who remind us, through their presence in the world, that we are not completely free and independent agents who can do whatever we want. These encounters make demands on us. The demands may sometimes be punitive and oppressive, but before they are anything else, Levinas maintains, they are first and foremost appeals for acknowledgment. These appeals emerge out of the inescapable vulnerability that each person has in relation to another, and they testify to that vulnerability: they both rouse it and remind one of it.

Therefore, the fundamental modality of the calls that other people address to us is one that expresses passivity. They are appeals from the position of susceptibility, appeals to provide support, offer kindness, accept accountability, share the world. And because they are formulated from a position of passivity—from the position that Derrida labels "nonpower"—they are calls that do not imply reciprocity. They ask us to act without any expectation of reward or even gratitude.

Levinas says we can ignore these solicitations from others. We can evade them and act irresponsibly in relation to them. What we cannot do is avoid them altogether.[18] Attempting to do so—for example, by asking a question like "Why should I care about people with disabilities?"—does not dispense with or annul a relationship so much as it affirms one. The fact that the question can be asked at all acknowledges that however one answers it, one *already* has a relation to people with disabilities. And it avows that the relationship entails responsibility—in the dual senses of both the "ability to respond" and the "impossibility of indifference."

Philosophical arguments for ethical obligation like those developed by Levinas are important because they offer a vantage point from which we can contemplate respectful engagement with others without requiring symmetrical reciprocity or without appealing to a common, shared humanity—which, of course, is precisely the characteristic of some significantly impaired people that utilitarian philosophers like Peter Singer dispute. Levinas insists that we are responsible for others not because they are similar to us or because we necessarily understand them or because we can hope or expect to get something back from them (a returned favor, gratitude, love). Instead, he says, we are responsible for them because they are living beings who exist in our world and who *therefore* deserve to be accorded dignity and the opportunity to flourish.

Of course a problem with philosophical writing like this is that its often intensely erudite nature can render it unpersuasive for many people because it is difficult to comprehend, because its premises or stakes are unclear, or simply because it is hard to see how the arguments elaborated by the philosophers might actually be applied in practice to help facilitate more respectful engagement. None of this is helped by the unwillingness of many of the most important philosophers to offer any normative guidelines for ethically sound engagement. Levinas, for example, declined to entertain questions about general rules or procedures that might derive from his writings on ethics. Derrida, on at least one occasion that was noted by a fellow scholar, elaborated his thoughts on ethical engagement with animals while dining on a steak tartare.[19]

For those reasons, another way of answering the question of why we should care for vulnerable others is to phrase it in terms of politics and social justice. This is the path taken by those feminist philosophers, sociologists, and political scientists who write about what they call the ethics of care. Like Levinas, these scholars emphasize what philosopher Eva Kittay labels the "inescapable fact of human dependency": that we are all dependent and are, at various points in our lives, the recipients of care.[20]

But unlike Levinas, authors who address the ethics of care directly link relations of dependency to the social arrangements and redistributive channels that structure our world. All writers on the ethics of care develop extensive critiques of the fact that the overwhelming majority of people who care for others are women, who are either unpaid or vastly underpaid, and whose caring labor is taken for granted, not recognized, or under- or de-valued.

Reflecting on the reasons for this glaring inequality—which include ideologies of independence and the resulting denigration and denial of dependency; the private/public divide; stereotypes about women's supposedly natural and compelling caring instincts; and the gendered structure of the labor market—these authors discuss an ethics of care as a political project. Political philosopher Joan Tronto views an ethics of care as a "political vision" that enhances democratic citizenship.[21] Sociologist Fiona Williams argues for a "political ethics of care" that would balance the "ethic of paid work" that prevails in contemporary welfare states like the United Kingdom.[22] Political philosopher Selma Sevenhuijsen suggests that an ethics of care is "a form of political ethics" that can transform how we think about collective responsibility and justice.[23]

Framing the engagement with vulnerability as an issue of social justice has a great deal of traction in the social democratic welfare states that are the subject of this book. In both Sweden and Denmark it is regarded as beyond question that a just society has an obligation to provide care for its most vulnerable members. Furthermore, at least since the 1960s and 1970s, it is generally agreed that a decent society should go much further than merely provide basic care; it should also facilitate independence and the ability to thrive of those who are most vulnerable. This is the reason behind the significant reforms that have been enacted in both countries since the 1970s—the dismantling of the large institutions for the handicapped and the introduction of direct-payment schemes to people with disabilities so that they can hire personal assistants they choose themselves.

So, given that from many perspectives, and certainly in comparison with the majority of countries in the world, both Denmark and Sweden rank highly as just societies in relation to people with disabilities, on what grounds do we base our contention that the kind of engagement we observed in Denmark is better, and more just?

Capabilities and Justice

We can begin to answer this question by noting that social justice is not a relative concept. An account of justice that argued that the discrimination of women is just in a patriarchal society or that inequalities between different racial groups are just in a society where racial hierarchy is considered a reflection of nature or ordained by God would be unacceptable to most political philosophers as well as to most activists who campaign for social justice. Social justice is a normative concept. Its role, as philosopher Martha Nussbaum has observed, "is typically critical: we work out an account of what is just, and we then use it to find reality deficient in various ways."[24] This means that to evaluate the material we have presented in this book we need to present an account of justice that provides a set of principles that can help us assess the policies and actions we have described.

With that in mind, we can turn to Martha Nussbaum and the "capabilities approach" to social justice that she has been developing during the past twenty-five years. First articulated as a way of thinking about women and development in India, and related to a similar approach in economics developed by Amartya Sen, Nussbaum's view argues that justice is about ensuring fundamental human entitlements that allow people to live with dignity and develop their capability to exist and flourish in the world.[25] Her approach to social justice seeks to complement a tradition of theories of justice that employ the idea of a social contract.

Contractarian theories of justice ask us to understand and assess justice from the perspective of persons who are free, equal, rational, and independent and who agree to leave an anarchic and hostile state of nature in order to establish principles of government. The government that these contractors institute necessarily curtails their independence and autonomy, since it involves cooperation and an awareness of and respect for the perspectives and needs of other people. But in return, it provides mutual advantage in terms of security and institutions for distributing resources and services.

The postulation of a state of nature is a thought experiment; its significance is that it asks us to consider what principles of justice might offer an optimal compromise between individual liberty and social cooperation. Social contract theories developed by philosophers such as Thomas Hobbes (1588–1679), John Locke (1632–1704), Jean-Jacques Rousseau (1712–1778), and Immanuel Kant (1724–1804) are centuries old, and they form the basis of some of the most significant advances in Enlightenment political theory. Thomas Jefferson's formulation in the American *Declaration of Independence* about how "Governments are instituted among Men, deriving their just powers from the consent of the governed," for example, derives directly from contractarian thinking about justice.

Martha Nussbaum argues that social contract approaches are the most powerful theories of justice that we have, especially in comparison to alternative theories, such as utilitarianism, which evaluates justice according to whether institutions, laws, and actions maximize the total aggregate of happiness in a society. Utilitarianism was radical in its day, asserting, in the late eighteenth century, that the happiness of every person, whether peasant or king, counted equally. But among its other problems, utilitarianism has always had an antagonistic relationship with disability. Its metric of overall happiness in society gives us no reason to regard the abortion of fetuses with Down syndrome, the institutionalization of disabled people, or the euthanasia of significantly impaired individuals as morally objectionable. If the sum total of happiness in a population is enhanced by such practices, utilitarianism holds that they are reasonable and just.

The contractarian theoretician whose work Nussbaum both closely follows and extends is the political theorist John Rawls (1921–2002). In a series of books that by all accounts reinvigorated and even revolutionized understandings of social justice, Rawls worked out an approach he called "justice as fairness."[26] His goal was to devise a set of relatively abstract principles that could provide "a way of assigning rights and duties in the basic institutions of society and . . . define the appropriate distribution of benefits and burdens of social cooperation."[27]

Rawls's way of addressing this issue was to ask people to imagine establishing principles of justice without knowing which position they would have in society. So sitting at a negotiation table, you and others hammer out principles, such as how political representation should be determined and how wealth should be distributed in society. But you all do this behind what Rawls called a "veil of ignorance"—that is, without knowing whether you will turn out to be a wealthy entrepreneur or a domestic servant. You would not know whether you would be black or white, female or male, an avowed atheist or a fundamentalist Christian, a gifted musician or a talentless klutz. Of course, this thought experiment means that you are not yet "you"; the whole point is that you have no idea what social position you have, and which desires and goals you will turn out to want to pursue, once the veil of ignorance is lifted. So this is not an exercise of symmetrical reciprocity in which one momentarily tries to put oneself in the position of someone else. The point is to imagine society from multiple, different, and even antagonistic vantage points.[28]

Rawls's idea was that from such a level position of equal vulnerability and uncertainty rational people would devise principles of justice that allow each individual to pursue his or her own advantage on terms that would be fair even to the least privileged in society. A just society, for Rawls, is one based on the principles of justice that we would choose for ourselves if we did not know what our position in society was going to be.

Those principles of justice would also recognize that people have different conceptions of what it means to pursue a good life. For some people, a good life might mean the ability to enhance their own personal happiness, as utilitarianism suggests. But others might wish to devote their lives to helping others, or to become as rich as possible by exploiting others. The contractors negotiating behind the veil of ignorance do not know which version of the good they will want to pursue—will I be an industrial magnate or a Buddhist nun? A radical feminist or a conservative patriarch? For Rawls, this diversity and even discord of preferences and goals is a fundamental feature of society. Therefore, a just society is one that does not dictate the meaning of a good life by telling us all how to live. A just society, instead, is one that recognizes differences and a plurality of life projects and that provides principles for regulating them and distributing the good in ways that both respect the inviolability of individuals and guarantee that "one person's exceeding well being is not permitted to compensate for another person's misery."[29]

Rawls's project is generally recognized to be important because it provides a robust set of principles for justice that balances the distribution of liberties and wealth with respect for a plurality of interests and the worth of individuals. As we have noted, Nussbaum agrees with those who view the Rawlsian version of contractarianism as the most comprehensive and supple approach to social justice that we have. But she also observes that, despite its elegance, Rawls's approach fails to deliver principles of justice for several groups, one of which is people with disabilities.[30] Rawls himself recognized this limitation. In several places he noted that the question of disability is a vexing one—one where his theory of justice as fairness "may fail."[31]

Rawls's concession on this point is an acknowledgment that people with disabilities are not, in his model, fully included in society as subjects of justice. He proposed that one defer the question of their status. This seems an odd suggestion, considering that he could have addressed this problem simply by adding "ability" to the list of characteristics that contracting parties operating behind the veil of ignorance do not know whether they would possess. So just as I do not know, when I am negotiating principles of justice, whether I am going to be male or female once the veil of ignorance is lifted, neither do I know whether I am going to have average intelligence or be intellectually impaired, or whether I will be limbless or have full use of my limbs. This seemingly obvious solution was not suggested by Rawls because it would threaten the starting point of his theory, which is the contractarian idea that all citizens in society will be "normal and fully cooperating members of society over a complete life."[32]

Martha Nussbaum's critique of Rawls hinges on her rejection of this conceptualization of the human as a starting point for a theory of justice. She argues that it is possible to retain the significant strengths of Rawls's theory of justice as fairness and extend it to groups that he was uncertain about if we jettison some of his core assumptions. The idea that people enter into a social contract to be able to better further their own interests, Nussbaum says, should be replaced with the Aristotelian and Marxian premise that people are fundamentally social beings who find fulfillment in relations with others. They can be imagined to enter into a social contract for that reason.[33]

The related assumption that the people who make the social contract are all free, equal, and independent can be replaced with the realization that nobody, throughout the course of his or her life, is the completely independent entity that social contract theories imagine the prototypical human being to be. Therefore, the fiction of autonomy can be replaced with an idea of the person that acknowledges dependency.[34] Understandings of justice can thus extend to include both individuals who require care and those who provide care.

Finally, the idea that people enter into a contract in order to secure mutual advantage from others who are roughly equal to them in power and ability can be replaced by an understanding of people as contractors who see justice as part of their good—that is, who perceive that the purpose of arriving at principles of justice is not necessarily to ensure reciprocal advantage. The purpose of justice is justice: to ensure that even people who offer no reciprocity or mutual advantage are equal subjects of justice.[35]

A key feature of Rawls's theory of justice that makes it so appealing is his argument that the purpose of social justice is to ensure that rights, liberties, and wealth are distributed among a population in ways that are of greatest benefit to the least advantaged people in society. How does one determine who is the least advantaged? Rawls says by a single measure: that of income and wealth. But this reliance on a single metric to index advantage is a weak spot in his theory, and it is the point from which the capabilities approach developed. Disability featured in this development from the beginning. In the original formulation of what has become the capabilities approach, economist Amartya Sen criticized Rawls's reliance on income and wealth to determine a person's relative advantage in society by pointing out that a disabled person might have the same income as someone who is not disabled but nonetheless could be much worse off, if, for example, public space was not accessible to him or her.[36] The relevant question in terms of social inequality, therefore, is not how much resources a person can command, but what that person is actually able to do or be—what capabilities she or he is afforded by society.

Martha Nussbaum extended this focus on capabilities to make them principles of justice. Her argument is that a just society is one that provides affirmative measures that help each individual develop his or her capabilities to the fullest extent possible. Exactly what an individual's capabilities are—exactly what a person can do and be—will vary according to genetic and social inheritance, the vicissitudes of birth, and individual physical and mental abilities. Justice requires that we both acknowledge that variation and accord every human being equal dignity and moral entitlement. This means that our concern should be to construct social policies, laws, and redistributive channels that affirm, facilitate, and further individuals' dignity and sense of self-worth.

So justice, in Nussbaum's approach, is about fostering and ensuring the circumstances that allow individuals to realize a life with human dignity. How do we define that? Nussbaum affirms that dignity is a vague concept, an "intuitive idea."[37] But it is an idea that can be filled with content, and she defines it through ten capabilities that she argues are central requirements for a life with dignity. The ten capabilities include the capability to live to the end of a human life of normal length, to have adequate nourishment, to have attachments to others, and to be able to participate effectively in political choices that govern one's life. The complete list is as follows:

1. *Life.* Being able to live to the end of a human life of normal length; not dying prematurely, or before one's life is so reduced as to be not worth living.

2. *Bodily Health.* Being able to have good health, including reproductive health; to be adequately nourished; to have adequate shelter.

3. *Bodily Integrity.* Being able to move freely from place to place; to be secure against violent assault, including sexual assault and domestic violence; having opportunities for sexual satisfaction and for choice in matters of reproduction.

4. *Senses, Imagination, and Thought.* Being able to use the senses, to imagine, think, and reason—and to do these things in a "truly human" way, a way informed and cultivated by an adequate education, including, but by no means limited to, literacy and basic mathematical and scientific training. Being able to use imagination and thought in connection with experiencing and producing works and events of one's own choice, religious, literary, musical, and so forth. Being able to use one's mind in ways protected by guarantees of freedom of expression with respect to both political and artistic speech, and freedom of religious exercise. Being able to have pleasurable experiences and to avoid non-beneficial pain.

5. *Emotions.* Being able to have attachments to things and people outside ourselves; to love those who love and care for us, to grieve at their absence; in general, to love, to grieve, to experience longing,

gratitude, and justified anger. Not having one's emotional development blighted by fear and anxiety. (Supporting this capability means supporting forms of human association that can be shown to be crucial in their development.)

6. *Practical Reason.* Being able to form a conception of the good and to engage in critical reflection about the planning of one's life. (This entails protection for the liberty of conscience and religious observance.)

7. *Affiliation.*

    A. Being able to live with and toward others, to recognize and show concern for other humans, to engage in various forms of social interaction; to be able to imagine the situation of another. (Protecting this capability means protecting institutions that constitute and nourish such forms of affiliation, and also protecting the freedom of assembly and political speech.)

    B. Having the social bases of self-respect and non-humiliation; being able to be treated as a dignified being whose worth is equal to that of others. This entails provisions of non-discrimination on the basis of race, sex, sexual orientation, ethnicity, caste, religion, national origin and species.

8. *Other Species.* Being able to live with concern for and in relation to animals, plants, and the world of nature.

9. *Play.* Being able to laugh, to play, to enjoy recreational activities.

10. *Control over one's Environment.*

    A. *Political.* Being able to participate effectively in political choices that govern one's life; having the right of political participation, protections of free speech and association.

    B. *Material.* Being able to hold property (both land and movable goods) and having property rights on an equal basis with others; having the right to seek employment on an equal basis with others; having the freedom from unwarranted search and seizure. In work, being able to work as a human, exercising practical reason and entering into meaningful relationships of mutual recognition with other workers.[38]

Nussbaum intends these central human capabilities to be taken as a metric for justice. She says that the list is open-ended and subject to modification. But the point in drawing up such a list is to concretize the idea of human dignity and to establish a threshold below which it is possible to say that justice is lacking. The capabilities are meant to be regarded as fundamental entitlements that all individuals have in any society. Just as Rawls's theory asks us to think about justice by imagining principles we would choose for ourselves if we did not know what our position in society was going to be, Nussbaum asks us to think about justice by considering whether a life without the capabilities she enumerates could be considered a life with human dignity.

Three aspects of Nussbaum's capabilities approach are particularly important for our purposes. The first is her focus on the *minimum* level of entitlements. The capabilities approach does not address the upper limits of the threshold; it is concerned with justice in relation to the very basic level of minimum core entitlements.[39] Thus it asserts that all citizens have an entitlement to be educated (capability 4), but it does not say that everyone has the right to go to college. How the basic minimum level of an entitlement is determined is left variable. An example of this is capability 2 on Nussbaum's list concerning bodily health: "*Bodily Health.* Being able to have good health, including reproductive health; to be adequately nourished; to have adequate shelter." This should be read to mean that a just society is one that provides all citizens with an adequate level of health, nourishment, and shelter. It does not define "adequate"—this is left to be worked out through processes of deliberation and contestation in different societies. But it does insist that the meaning of "adequate" be calibrated with the other capabilities in mind. So does the shelter potentially regarded as adequate facilitate the capability of good health? Of "not having one's emotional development blighted by fear and anxiety" (capability 5)? If the answer to questions like these is no, then the shelter in question should not be regarded as adequate.

Assessing capabilities in relation to one another means that all of the capabilities on the list are inextricably intertwined. This is the second core feature of Nussbaum's approach to justice that is critical to this discussion. Nussbaum insists that the different capabilities she identifies as core entitlements are nonfungible—a lack in one area cannot be compensated by an abundance in another. The reason for this insistence arises from deep misgivings about utilitarian understandings of justice. Rawls criticized utilitarianism for encouraging trade-offs between different goods to produce the greatest aggregate of happiness. So political freedom, for example, could be sacrificed for greater economic security if the result was a greater balance of happiness. Rawls regarded this kind of trade-off as both dangerous and unjust, and Nussbaum agrees.

The nonfungibility of capabilities is directly relevant to sexuality and disability because it disallows any suggestion that a society that provides disabled people with a relatively high standard of living does not need to worry about providing them with possibilities to discover and develop sexual satisfaction. The capabilities approach would regard such an argument as illegitimate. "If people are below the threshold on any one of the capabilities, that is a failure of basic justice, no matter how high up they are on all the others," Nussbaum maintains.[40]

The third feature of the capabilities approach that is particularly significant for our discussion is its insistence on treating each individual as a separate person worthy of a life with dignity. That each person must be regarded as an end—that is to say, as a distinct bearer of value—is a core dimension of Nussbaum's model, as it is of Rawls's (and ultimately of Kant's moral philosophy, which both approaches draw on). Both Nussbaum and Rawls argue at length against the utilitarian calculus of aggregate happiness. Nussbaum, in addition, makes the feminist observation that approaches to justice that focus on groups or societies often shortchange women, either because women's "private" needs are often considered peripheral to the "public" realm of justice or, more simply, because women are not regarded as persons worthy of moral entitlement and human dignity. It is ironic, therefore, says Nussbaum, that "the idea that the individual person should be the focus of political thought has sometimes been given dismissive treatment by feminists, on the grounds that it implies a neglect for care and community and involves a male Western bias toward self-sufficiency and competition, as opposed to cooperation and love." Her response is that

> there is a type of focus on the individual person . . . that requires no particular metaphysical tradition, and no bias against love and care. It arises naturally from the recognition that each person has just one life to live, not more than one; that the food on A's plate does not magically nourish the stomach of B; that the pleasure felt in C's body does not make the pain experienced by D less painful . . . in general, that one person's exceeding happiness or liberty does not magically make another person happy or free. . . . If we combine this observation with the thought, which all feminists share in some form, that each person is valuable and worthy of respect as an end, we must conclude that we should look not just to the total of the average, but to the functioning of each and every person.[41]

It goes without saying that if women have been ignored as subjects of justice, people with disabilities have fared even worse. Until very recently, their dignity as individuals has seldom been recognized—recall, for instance, the ghastly case of the multiply lobotomized young man that we cited in chapter 2 or Swedish writer Gunnel Enby's chilling description of her life in the institution she lived in for many years as a young person with polio, where everyone was given sedatives and put to bed by 7 PM and where the only personal item allowed was a single photograph on a bedside table. We have seen that even a progressive theorist like Rawls had few qualms about simply omitting people with disabilities as subjects of justice. For those reasons, an insistence on treating each person as an end, as an individual who has unique value, desires, and needs, must be an urgent and crucial element of any kind of engagement with regard to the lives of people with disabilities.

The Right to Sex?

Three of the capabilities appearing on Nussbaum's list of central human capabilities are directly relevant to disability and sexuality. They are as follows:

(3) *Bodily Integrity.* Being able to move freely from place to place; to be secure against violent assault, including sexual assault and domestic violence; having opportunities for sexual satisfaction and for choice in matters of reproduction.

(5) *Emotions.* Being able to have attachments to things and people outside ourselves; to love those who love and care for us, to grieve at their absence; in general, to love, to grieve, to experience longing, gratitude, and justified anger. Not having one's emotional development blighted by fear and anxiety.

(7A) *Affiliation.* Being able to live with and toward others, to recognize and show concern for other human beings, to engage in various forms of social interaction; to be able to imagine the situation of another.[42]

When considering these capabilities in relation to people with disabilities, it should be clear at this point what Nussbaum is *not* saying. In claiming that individuals have an entitlement to "opportunities for sexual satisfaction" (capability 3), Nussbaum is not saying that people have a right to sex and that a just society is one that provides its citizens with sexual partners. She is saying that human beings have the capability to develop intimate ties to others and to experience and value sexual satisfaction. The minimal threshold for a life with dignity, therefore, is one in which this capability is acknowledged and facilitated rather than denied and prevented.

How it is facilitated is something that is left be worked out, and will vary. So in a society like Sweden, where there is a strong social consensus against prostitution and where the purchase of sexual services is illegal, sex work or "sex surrogacy" will probably not figure very prominently in policies and assistive practices around sex and disability. More emphasis might be placed on developing services like those provided by the Danish business Handisex, which puts adults with disabilities into contact with helpers who will assist them with sex without actually having sex with them. Danish sexual advisors also assist adults with sex without, themselves, having sex with them, so discussion could also consider instituting and developing the kinds of educational programs that train them.

However the issue is ultimately resolved, the point is that a commitment to the dignity of each individual will entail an approach in which people with significant disabilities are not simply left out of discussions about sexuality, and in which affirmative measures are taken to facilitate their erotic fulfillment.

The capabilities approach's insistence on the nonfungibility of capabilities means, furthermore, that there can be no trade-offs between different entitlements. If we agree with Nussbaum that a core human entitlement is both protection from abuse and the possibility of forming romantic and sexual relations with others, then a just society will be one that both protects its citizens from abuse *and* provides possibilities and opportunities for individuals to develop their sexuality together with others. A society that recognizes one of those entitlements (protection from abuse, for example) but simultaneously makes it clear to people with disabilities that any help they request with sex *constitutes* an abuse, and that their sexuality, if they must have one at all, should be limited to discreet masturbation, is not just a society that discriminates. It is a society that is fundamentally unjust.

The capabilities for attachment, affiliation, and sexuality that Nussbaum lists as fundamental human entitlements bear a strong resemblance to similar entitlements recognized by international bodies, such as the United Nations and the World Health Organization. The UN resolution known as the Standard Rules on the Equalization of Opportunities for Persons with Disabilities, for example, states that "persons with disabilities must not be denied the opportunity to experience their sexuality, have sexual relationships and experience parenthood."[43]

Similarly, the World Health Organization's "working definition" of sexuality asserts that "sexual health requires a positive and respectful approach to sexuality and sexual relationships, as well as the possibility of having pleasurable and safe sexual experiences, free of coercion, discrimination and violence. For sexual health to be attained and maintained, the sexual rights of all persons must be respected, protected and fulfilled."[44]

We have seen how, in Denmark, formulations like these are cited in nationally distributed documents, such as the *Guidelines about Sexuality—Regardless of Handicap*. In chapter 3, we noted how the *Guidelines* document in fact went even further than the UN resolution it cited by changing the resolution's negative liberty ("persons with disabilities *must not be denied* the opportunity . . .") to positive entitlement ("people with reduced functional ability *shall have* the possibility . . ."). Even though this phrase has been removed from the most recent edition of the *Guidelines*, the new version still begins with the following quote from a publication from the WHO's regional office: "Sexuality is an integrated part of every individual's personality. Sexuality is a core need and a part of what it means to be a human being, that cannot be separated from other aspects of life. . . . Sexuality influences our thoughts, feelings, actions and relationships and, thus, our mental and physical health. And just as health is a fundamental right, so is sexual health a basic human right."[45]

This kind of authoritative assertion in a document published by a government ministry provides a crucial justification for both general engagement with the sexual lives of disabled people and for the specific work carried out by sexual advisors and other concerned caregivers.

In Sweden, in sharp contrast, the idea that sexuality might be a right is roundly dismissed. A typical example of how this happens occurred in 2004, when the blind journalist and disability rights activist Finn Hellman wrote an op-ed column in the leftist newspaper *The Worker* (*Arbetaren*). Hellman's column was a response to a televised debate that aired a week after (and as a result of) the CP *Show*'s episode on sex and disability in Denmark discussed in the previous chapter.[46] During that debate, one of the discussants, a politician in her fifties from the Social Democratic Party, explained that she was deeply opposed to the idea of having anyone employed by the state help a disabled person with sex. A young personal assistant who wasn't opposed asked her, "But if a handicapped person can't do it themself? If they can't do it?"

The politician's answer was, "Too bad" (*Tyvärr*).

Finn Hellman's column pointed out the callousness of that answer, and he asked readers to meditate on the question "What would happen if everyone in Sweden woke up one morning and could no longer touch themselves between their legs—if citizens couldn't caress themselves and wank on their own? Probably desperate sex riots would result."

"But today," he continued, "when people who are that seriously disabled are just a minority, peace reigns in the dictatorship of the liberated majority." In language reminiscent of Cheryl Marie Wade's, Hellman asked readers to consider "how it happens that severely disabled people are provided with help with cleaning, dressing, and having their butts wiped, but not with sex?" "What does it mean," he wondered, "to deny others that which one has access to oneself?"[47]

Responses to Hellman's column were quick in coming. Typically for Sweden, rather than focusing on disability, the responses were primarily about prostitution. Although Hellman's four-hundred-word column mentioned prostitution in only two sentences ("The discussion about whether severely disabled people should get help from assistants or sex workers is important. But concrete changes can hardly be expected as long as it is illegal to buy sex in Sweden"), he was dismissed as being a "spokesperson for the prostitution industry" (*prostitutionsförespråkare*) and accused of committing "a serious affront that shows no respect at all for true human value" (*en grov skymf bortom all respekt för sant människovärde*).[48]

In a letter that seemed to channel the spirit of Inger Nordqvist, one response informed Hellman that if people with disabilities wanted to have sex and could not, they should turn to "mechanical sex aids" (*mekaniska sexhjälpmedel*), not to other people.[49] How exactly anyone with limited or no mobility would actually be able to use such sex aids without help was not considered, and that issue was steadfastly ignored when Hellman, in his reply to the ensuing debate, pointed this out.[50]

Another response to Hellman's column was from Mattias Kvick, a man who identified himself in his letter as a "rehabilitation facilitator" (*habiliteringspersonal*), that is, as someone whose profession it is to work with people with disabilities. Kvick had this to say about sexual facilitation:

In my view it is completely impossible [*helt omöjligt*] to attempt to find guidelines for how this kind of help [with sex] might occur in ways that prevent every conceivable risk for abuse and/or feelings of humiliation in relation to any of the people involved.[51]

This remark is a concentrated version of the kind of commentary that saturates Swedish public debate on this topic. Particularly striking is the language: the proclamation, not that it is difficult or challenging—no, it is "completely impossible" to even *attempt* to try to find guidelines for assisting people with disabilities to have a sexual life. An assertion like that does its best to preempt discussion and shut it down before it can even begin. It is another example of the overheated denials described by Bettan in chapter 3, when she recounted the "moral panic" that ensued when she brought up the topic of sex in a group of personal assistants.

Also striking in Kvick's response is the standard of morality to which persons with disabilities who need help are held: they can't have help with sex, he declares, because he doesn't believe it is possible "to prevent every conceivable risk for abuse and/or feelings of humiliation in relation to any of the people involved." A question one might well ask upon reading that concern is how much sex *anyone* would have if we were permitted to engage in sexual relations only after every imaginable precaution had been taken to prevent "every *conceivable* risk for abuse and/or feelings of humiliation in relation to any of the people involved"? Saturday nights after the clubs close would be lonely times indeed.

The heading under which Kvick's letter appeared was "Sex Is Not a Right" (*Sex är ingen rättighet*). A main point of his letter was to argue that Finn Hellman confuses the right to sexuality with the right to sex. This is an erudite distinction; in international human rights discourse, "sexual rights" refers to both individual integrity and the freedom to explore one's sexuality together with others. The right to be gay, after all, does not mean very much if the right to have gay sex is withheld. But the distinction that Kvick articulates is common in Swedish debate when the subject is people with disabilities. It reiterates the Swedish view that sexuality is a private characteristic more than a social relation, but it also serves a specific rhetorical purpose: as a buck-stops-here argument meant to put an end to any suggestion that some people with disabilities might need special accommodations or help in order to experience sex. This need for help *with* sex is framed as demanding a right *to* sex. And to propose that sex is a right, this argument goes, is to sanction abuse. Because how should such a right be facilitated? By a "government or regional sex help hotline where sexual assistants work according to a roster and with overtime compensation after 7 PM?"[52]

The facility and vigor with which Swedish commentators like Mattias Kvick reject the idea that sex is a human right suggests that one of the profound political challenges that sexuality and disability presents is the problem of how we might argue for the sexual rights of people with disabilities without using the language of rights.[53] Even for other reasons, rights language can be awkward in relation to people with significant disabilities, because the notion of "rights" in much political theory and popular understanding is bound up with duties—to work, for example, or to be available for military service. The idea that citizens who have rights also have duties is a difficult link to maintain when it comes to people with severe disabilities, who may be unable to perform many or even any of the duties we incur as citizens.

But rights language in relation to sexuality becomes even more problematic when we realize that for many people with significant disabilities, what is at issue is not so much an extension of rights, but their *facilitation*. An analogy to accessibility is appropriate: nobody could argue that it is enough to just proclaim that people with mobility and other impairments have the right to access public space and then leave the matter at that. For that right to have any meaning, affirmative measures, such as curb cuts, elevators, braille signage, and so on, need to be provided to facilitate disabled individuals' capability to access public space.

What the Danes whose work we have documented in this book have appreciated, and what Swedes like Mattias Kvick seem intent on denying, is that the same kind of logic should apply to the private realm as well. It is meaningless—indeed, it is cynical and even cruel—to proclaim that significantly impaired individuals have the right to their sexuality but that if they cannot manage on their own to experience that sexuality, well, "too bad."

"Excessibility" Guidelines

The stalemate that can ensue when talk about the sexual lives of people with disabilities gets phrased in terms of rights is an important reason why we believe the capabilities approach to social justice has the potential to reframe engagement in positive and far-reaching ways. The capabilities approach is a variety of a human rights approach to justice—Nussbaum characterizes it repeatedly as "a species" of a human rights approach. But the language of capabilities and entitlements, rather than rights, may be able to move perspectives beyond a view that insists that a disabled person who requests help with sex is expressing a demand that society provide him or her with a sex partner.

The capabilities approach weaves together the strands of vulnerability, obligation, responsibility, difference, and justice that we have been discussing throughout this chapter. Its starting point in relation to people with disabilities is that they are "fellow citizens, and fellow participants in human dignity," as Nussbaum puts it.[54] We therefore have a collective obligation and a responsibility to treat people with disabilities not as recipients of charity and goodwill, not as objects of compassion, but as primary subjects of justice. Unlike classical liberal approaches to ethics, the capabilities approach does not ask us to try to imagine ourselves as someone with a disability and to then decide, on the basis of that fantasized substitution, whether or not people with disabilities are entitled to certain kinds of treatment or certain kinds of help. Instead, in a way similar to what Levinas and Derrida propose, the capabilities approach only requires that we acknowledge that people with disabilities exist in our world. We do not have to understand them or gain anything from engaging with them; they share the world with us and are *therefore* deserving of respect and dignity. And that dignity is not just an airy idea; it means something specific, namely, the entitlement to develop and flourish according to each individual's own abilities.

A decent society cannot ensure that people have happy, fulfilling lives. But it can provide them with a threshold level of capability in each of the key areas that Nussbaum enumerates. In the area of sexuality, the capabilities approach argues that fundamental human capabilities include the capability to form attachments to others, to be protected from violence and abuse, and to have opportunities for sexual satisfaction. Those who would dispute any part of that formulation are asked to consider whether a life without those capabilities could truly be considered a life worthy of human dignity—would it be a fully human life, or would it be a subhuman life? The question is not whether one can, oneself, imagine living without sex. The question is whether or not each human life should have the opportunity to develop and explore her or his erotic awareness and capacities and to be given the possibility of extending herself or himself in ways that engage sensations, activities, and relationships that can provide pleasure, comfort, self-respect, and satisfaction.

The capabilities approach to social justice insists that a life with dignity is a life in which those capabilities of extension and pleasure are facilitated at some minimum threshold level. In the case of adults with significant impairments, this means a number of relatively modest things.

It means, first of all, appreciating the fact that physical or intellectual impairment does not necessarily exclude a person from experiencing erotic feelings, curiosity, and pleasure.

It means a willingness to engage with individuals to help them understand and express those feelings and desires.

It means understanding that individuals with disabilities, just like everyone else, need help and support in acquiring ways to comprehend and express their sexuality. This means cultivating an awareness of signs that might indicate an interest in or a curiosity about sexuality.

It means developing an ability to raise the topic of sex and talk about it in ways that highlight sexual expression and sexual pleasure (of saying "yes" to sex) instead of always framing sex exclusively in terms of protection and abuse (of only saying "no").

It means inviting and choreographing those discussions in ways that allow the person with the disability to either pursue the issue or decline to pursue it. Conversations may take time and patience, because the person with the disability may communicate only through a few sounds or with subtle movements of his or her eyes. Or the person may require help to understand the difference between things like the public and private, or affection and erotics. The conversations also may end up involving more than two people, for example, if the desires of the person with the disability are not clear to the helper and he or she needs to get a colleague's opinion before moving forward. This means developing explicit policies around sexuality that make it clear that it is a legitimate and welcome topic of discussion and concern.

Facilitating a disabled person's capability to understand and experience sexuality means many other things besides. Basically, it means doing many of the things that Danish sexual advisors and others have been doing for the past thirty years.

And it means stopping the kinds of things that this book has documented that many Swedes continue to do whenever the topic of sexuality and disability is raised.

During the course of this research, we discovered that the biggest single stumbling block to a constructive engagement with the lives of people with disabilities is a pair of completely erroneous beliefs. The first is that the only way to help a disabled person have sex is to actually *have sex* with him or her. Of course, that is one way, and we have seen how contact with sex workers is a valued dimension of the lives of some women and men with disabilities. But having sex with someone is not the only way of facilitating sex. Danish sexual advisors, for example, are prohibited by their ethical code from engaging in sex with the people they help. But they still help.

The second belief is the related concern that sexual assistance, if offered at all, must somehow be instituted as an obligatory part of every helper's job, like the duty to bathe a person with a disability or help her or him go to the toilet. In this anxious scenario, articulated so clearly in the Swedish CP *Show*'s selectively edited interviews with Jørgen Buttenschøn and sexual advisor Kirsten Klitte Sørensen, sexual services are imagined to be something that every helper will be obligated to perform whether she or he wants to or not. So individuals who work with people with disabilities are not just their helpers; they are, in effect, their sex slaves. And the state, which pays their salary, is a colossal pimp machine.

Once again, a glance at the way that sexual assistance is organized in Denmark demonstrates just how mistaken a panicked idea like this is. Far from being state-sanctioned sex slaves, helpers in Denmark are under no obligation whatsoever to have anything to do with the erotic lives of the people they help. They *are* obliged to respect that the person they help may have pinups of Galina taped to his wall or a matryoshka doll that doubles as a vibrator standing on her nightstand. But they do not even have to talk about sex—much less assist with it—if they don't want to. If they are asked for any kind of assistance in relation to sex, they were, until very recently, obligated to see to it that the person who asked is put in contact with someone who can advise them or assist them—a colleague, for example, who is more knowledgeable or more willing, or a sexual advisor from another group home. But that is the extent of their duty.

Once we get past the misguided and unnecessary beliefs that sexual facilitation necessarily involves sex with the person providing the assistance and that policies about sexual assistance must necessarily demand that all helpers provide it, we are free to explore the landscape that was mapped out long ago by Danish sexual advisors and the people with disabilities they assist. That landscape consists of three kinds of practices that were spelled out clearly in the 2001 version of the *Guidelines about Sexuality—Regardless of Handicap*: those that a helper *may* perform (such as assistance that allows individuals to masturbate or to have sexual relations with partners who have limited mobility and cannot manage on their own); those a helper is *prohibited from* performing (such as having sex with a person you are helping or providing sexual assistance to an underage person or to an adult who has indicated that she or he does not want it); and, crucially, those that a helper *must* perform (such as being responsible for seeing to it that a person who asks for help with sex gets it, even if the helper will not or cannot provide such assistance herself or himself).

The point of this book is that guidelines like these do for the private sphere what guidelines about accessible space do for the public sphere: they open up a world that otherwise would be closed to people with a variety of disabilities, especially people with significant disabilities.

Like accessibility guidelines, what we might as well call *excessibility* guidelines that offer guidance and advice about sexuality affirm that people with disabilities are fellow citizens, fellow human beings, and fellow participants in human dignity. After long, hard-fought, and still very much ongoing struggles by disabled people and their allies, access to the public realm is now generally regarded as a self-evident right for people with disabilities. This book has argued that the private realm of erotic activities and relationships is just as central and just as crucial for a life with dignity. And we have demonstrated that for people with significant impairments, it is just as possible, if we only allow ourselves to think, discuss, extend our perspectives, and engage.

APPENDIX :: breakdown of interviews

We conducted interviews among the groups of people listed in table A.1. Interviews lasted between 20 minutes and 4.5 hours, with an average of 1.5 hours. Several people were interviewed on two or even three occasions, but they are only counted once in the table.

The categorization in the table is oversimplified, because people we have listed in the different categories were not always interviewed exclusively in the capacity listed. For example, several women and men with disabilities were interviewed just as much for their roles as experts or activists in this field as for their personal stories about and experiences of sex. We have listed Danish sexual advisors separately from "Authorities on sexuality and disability," even though sexual advisors are among the foremost authorities on sexuality and disability. Listing them separately is simply a way to make their presence in this study clear.

Table A.1. Breakdown of Interviews Conducted for This Book

Category of person	Female	Male	Danish	Swedish	Total
Person with a disability	20	20	34	6	40
Parents	6	1	2	5	7
Authorities on sexuality and disability (including academics, sexologists, occupational therapists, etc.)	10	8	1	17	18
Sexual advisors (seksualvejledere)	5	3	8	—	8
Sex workers	5	2	6	1	7
People who work in group homes or as personal assistants	7	3	8	2	10
Other (e.g., government spokespeople; people working with sexuality in firms that employ personal assistants)	5	3	7	1	8
Total	58	40	66	32	98

Chapter 1. The Subject of Sex

1 Organisation for Economic Co-operation and Development, "Government Social Spending."
2 Shakespeare, Gillespie-Sells, and Davies, *Sexual Politics of Disability*, 207.
3 Lapper, *My Life in My Hands*, 129.
4 Finger, "Forbidden Fruit."
5 Shakespeare, "Disabled Sexuality."
6 O'Brien, *Man in the Iron Lung*, 80.
7 Kevin McCallum, "Organizers Run Out of Condoms as Active Olympians Score off the Field," *Sunday Independent*, 2 September 2012, 7.
8 Baer, *Is Fred Dead?*; Anderson, *Doing What Comes Naturally?*; Kaufman, Silverberg, and Odette, *Ultimate Guide to Sex and Disability*.
9 Shakespeare, Gillespie-Sells, and Davies, *Sexual Politics of Disability*, 208.
10 Shuttleworh and Sanders, *Sex and Disability*; McRuer and Mollow, *Sex and Disability*.
11 Kulick, *Queersverige*.
12 "Queer spränger alla sexgränser," *Expressen*, 23 September 2001, 10; "Dum flört med homosexuella," *Resumé*, 8 May 2003, 36; "Åsiktsmaskinen," DN-*På Stan*, 8

November 2002. In 2003 the Green Party presented a proposal to parliament demanding that all legislation be revised from a queer perspective (Swedish Riksdag [RD] Motion 2002/2003:L273).

13 Rubin, "Thinking Sex."
14 The development of queer theory in Sweden is summarized by Dahl, "Queer in the Nordic Region."
15 Hellman, "Queer- och handikappkonferens i San Francisco," 21–22.
16 Grönvik and Söder, *Bara funktionshindrad?*; Rydström, "Cripteori."
17 Rich, "Compulsory heterosexuality."
18 McRuer, *Crip Theory*, 149.
19 McRuer, *Crip Theory*, 31.
20 McRuer, *Crip Theory*, 31.
21 Shildrick, *Dangerous Discourses of Disability, Subjectivity and Sexuality*, 2; Shildrick, "Critical Disability Studies," 32; Siebers, *Disability Theory*.
22 Shildrick, *Dangerous Discourses of Disability, Subjectivity and Sexuality*, 79; Siebers, *Disability Theory*, 72; Garland-Thomson, *Staring*.
23 An example in the scholarly literature is Shildrick, *Dangerous Discourses of Disability, Subjectivity and Sexuality*, 73, which claims that, in Denmark, "the use of trained sex workers and sexual surrogates is sometimes subsidised by the state."
24 Shuttleworth, "Bridging Theory and Experience," 55.
25 Sen, *Idea of Justice*, 231; Nussbaum, *Frontiers of Justice*, 193.
26 Shuttleworth, "Disabled Masculinity," 169; Shuttleworth, "Bridging Theory and Experience."
27 Desjardins, "The Sexualized Body of the Child."
28 Earle, "Facilitated Sex and the Concept of Sexual Need"; Sanders, "The Politics of Sexual Citizenship."
29 Bahner, "Legal Rights or Simply Wishes?"
30 Mallander, *De hjälper oss till rätta.*
31 Sundet, *Jeg vet jeg er annerledes—men ikke bestandig*, 69–70.
32 Brown, *Boy in the Moon*; Kittay, *Love's Labor*; Kittay, "The Personal Is the Philosophical Is the Political."
33 Berubé, *Life as We Know It*; Nussbaum, *Frontiers of Justice*; Nussbaum, "The Capabilities of People with Cognitive Disabilities."
34 An example is Hvinden, "Nordic Disability Politics in a Changing Europe."
35 An exception is Apelmo, *Som vem som helst.*
36 Linton, *Claiming Disability*, 8–33; Mackelprang and Salsgiver, *Disability*, 17–23; Wendell, *Rejected Body*, 77–81.
37 Kailes, *Language Is More Than a Trivial Concern!*
38 This subject is discussed in more detail in Kulick, "Danes Call People with Down Syndrome 'Mongol.'"

Chapter 2. The Roots of Engagement

1 "Vårt behov av kärlek," *FUB-Kontakt*, no. 1 (1967): 11.

2 *LEV–Evnesvages Vel*, no. 3 (1967): 20, 22.

3 "Vårt behov av kärlek," *FUB-Kontakt*, no. 1 (1967): 11.

4 Buttenschøn, "Seksualiteten bliver tilladelig—Men hvordan med det private," 122.

5 Denmark's area diminished from 58,000 square kilometers to 39,000 square kilometers, and it lost about 800,000 of its inhabitants. Hvidt, *Det folkelige gennembrud og dets mænd*, 142; Buk-Swienty, *Slagtebænk Dybbøl*, 349.

6 Christiansen et al., *Nordic Model of Welfare*; Johansson, *Fast i det förflutna*.

7 This was in line with the recommendations of the Swedish social engineers Alva and Gunnar Myrdal, whose 1934 book *Crisis in the Population Question* (*Kris i befolkningsfrågan*) warned of a "definitive reduction of the quality of the human material" (*en definitiv kvalitetsnedsättning i människomaterialet*). As a remedy to this, they said, governments needed to simultaneously implement sterilization campaigns and improve the living conditions of the poor. Myrdal and Myrdal, *Kris i befolkningsfrågan*, 213.

8 In Sweden, a law that granted schooling to intellectually impaired individuals who were considered educable was enacted in 1954, and this was replaced fourteen years later by the Swedish Care Law of 1967 that guaranteed education, housing, and "activities for daily life" (ADL; i.e., the training of skills like eating, communicating, or managing a household, depending on the type of impairment) for all intellectually disabled people. Danish Law on Public Care (Lov no. 181 af 20. maj 1933, om offentlig forsorg); Swedish Decree on Invalid Support (Kungl, Maj:ts förordning om invalidunderstöd den 28 juni 1935). The 1954 law granting educational access is Lag (1954:483) om undervisning och vård av vissa psykiskt efterblivna.

9 Lag (1954:483). Lag (1967:940), angående omsorger om vissa psykiskt utvecklingsstörda (Omsorgslagen 1967), entered into force 1 July 1968.

10 Lag (1967:940).

11 Socialtjänstlag (1980:620), in force 1982; Lag (1985:568) om särskilda omsorger om psykiskt utvecklingsstörda m. fl. (Omsorgslagen 1985), in force 1986.

12 Lenger, "Mennesker med et handicap erobrede selv deres frihed."

13 Lov no. 454 af 10. juni 1997, om social service, article 77.

14 Lov om social service as amended in 2009, articles 95 and 96. In April 2012, the number of persons who received personal assistance through the BPA arrangement (section 95 of the Social Services Law) was 1,469. *Statistiske Efterretninger*, no. 3 (Copenhagen: Danmarks Statistik, 2013).

15 This amount includes the obligatory fees to various forms of social insurance, which are paid directly to the state. *Analyse af Borgerstyret Personlig Assistance (BPA) samt Kontakt- og ledsagerordning for døvblinde: Vurdering af de økonomiske styringsmuligheder på områderne* (Århus: Borgmesterens afdeling, 2012), www.kbh-nord.dk/pdf/201210-%20Aarhus_Kommune_Analyse-af-Bruger styret-Personlig-Assistance.pdf (accessed 28 June 2014). Salary information is available from Jobindex.dk/tjek-din-loen (accessed 28 June 2014).

16 In both cases the amount reimbursed, as per January 2013, was 275 Swedish kronor or about US$40 per hour.

17 In 2012, the total number of people in Sweden who received personal assistance under the LSS law was 3,900. *Personer med funktionsnedsättning: Insatser enligt LSS 2012*, Sveriges Officiella Statistik, Socialtjänst (Stockholm: Socialstyrelsen, 2013).

18 Disability pensions are regulated in Denmark by the Law on Social Pensions in its wording from 2013 (Lov om social pension) and in Sweden by the comprehensive Social Insurance Act (Socialförsäkringsbalken), which replaced the old pension laws in 2010. Both of these laws are equally applicable to all people with a disability, regardless of the type of impairment. Sådan beregnes førtidspension, www.borger.dk/Sider/Saadan-beregnes-foertidspension (Denmark); Försäkringskassan, Sjukersättning, Faktablad 2013-02-01, www.forsakring skassan.se/wps/wcm/connect/e863bcd8-8acd-49cc-9edd-7b3c6bb58990/4083 -sjukersattning1302.pdf?MOD=AJPERES (Sweden).

19 Hvinden, "Nordic Disability Politics in a Changing Europe."

20 Forslag til Lov om forsorgen for åndssvage, fremsat den 4. november 1958 af socialministeren, *Folketingstidende* 1958–1959, tillæg A (71), Bemærkninger til lovforslaget, col. 1136, Lov no. 192 af 5. juni 1959 om forsorgen for åndssvage og andre særligt svagt begavede.

21 Kirkebæk, "Er normaliseringens periode forbi?"

22 Quotes from Kirkebæk, *Normaliseringens periode*, 324, and from Hanamura, *Niels Erik Bank-Mikkelsen*, 43.

23 Hanamura, *Niels Erik Bank-Mikkelsen*.

24 Hanamura, *Niels Erik Bank-Mikkelsen*.

25 De-institutionalization was more far-reaching in Sweden than in Denmark. In 2012, 14,907 persons with disability lived in 988 group homes in Denmark, an average of 15.09 residents per home, whereas in Sweden, 24,369 persons lived in about 3,500 group homes, an average of 6.96 persons in each home. *NYT fra Danmarks Statistik*, no. 92, 25 February 2013 (Copenhagen: Danmarks Statistik); *Öppna jämförelser av stöd till personer med funktionsnedsättning 2013—Resultat och metod; Personer med funktionsnedsättning—Insatser enligt LSS år 2012; Personer med funktionsnedsättning—Vård och omsorg 1 oktober*

2012: *Kommunala insatser enligt socialtjänstlagen samt hälso- och sjukvårdsla-gen* (Stockholm: Socialstyrelsen).

26 Nirje, *Normaliseringsprincipen*, 91.

27 Nirje, *Normaliseringsprincipen*, 114.

28 A brief debate erupted in the journal *Svensk Vanföre-Tidskrift* in 1961 in re-sponse to an article by a psychologist who argued that people with a disabil-ity could have a "normal emotional life." Three disabled people responded and offered their own opinions on the matter, but they suggested no concrete proposals. Ulf Kragh, "Får den vanföre ha normalt känsloliv," *Svensk Vanföre-Tidskrift*, no. 8 (1961): 5; Georg Larsson, "Den vanföres känsloliv," *Svensk Vanföre-Tidskrift*, no. 9 (1961): 9; Karin Holmberg, "Vårt behov av kärlek," *Svensk Vanföre-Tidskrift*, no. 10 (1961): 19.

29 Ullerstam, *Erotic Minorities*, 152.

30 Ullerstam, *Erotic Minorities*, 151.

31 Lennerhed, *Frihet att njuta*, 159.

32 Translated into English as Katz, *Sexuality and Subnormality*.

33 Katz, *Samlevnads- och sexualfrågor hos psykiskt utvecklingsstörda*, 12.

34 Katz, *Samlevnads- och sexualfrågor hos psykiskt utvecklingsstörda*, 7.

35 Childs, *Sweden*.

36 Katz, *Samlevnads- och sexualfrågor hos psykiskt utvecklingsstörda*, 17, 21, 26–30.

37 Katz, *Samlevnads- och sexualfrågor hos psykiskt utvecklingsstörda*, 7.

38 Vol. Ö2:B2 1969–1970, Handlingar rörande samlevnadsfrågor och handi-kapp. HS-gruppen. Ser. Ö2, Hjälpmedelsinstitutet Archives, Riksarkivet (RA).

39 Minutes, arbetsgruppen för fortsatt utveckling av handikappades samlevnads-frågor, 5 November 1970, P. O. Lundberg's private archives (POL).

40 Greengross, *Rätt att älska*; Nordqvist, *Utredning om hjälpmedel i sexuallivet för män och kvinnor med funktionshinder*.

41 Minutes, HS-gruppen, 12 August 1974, POL.

42 Inger Nordqvist's extreme isolation and perhaps even ostracization from oth-ers working on disability issues is indicated, among other things, by the strik-ing fact that in the thirty-eight-page appendix to the 1989 Assistive Devices Commission's report that is specifically about Nordqvist's workplace—the Central Committee for Rehabilitation—not only is she *not* one of the thirty-four people interviewed by the commissioner who wrote the report, but not a single colleague who *was* interviewed seems to have mentioned her work on sexuality, which is completely absent from the report. Leif Lundberg 1988-09-26, "Utredning om Handikappinstitutets roll och verksamhet," bilaga [supp.] 8 to SOU 1989:39, 217–254. In a 139-page book about the history of the SVCR,

written by its administrative director, Nordqvist and her group are mentioned only in passing, on a single page. Montan, *SVCK/SVCR:s historia åren 1950–92*, 96.

43 "Jobb med sex- och samlevnad får inte kosta pengar—en trekvartstjänst gör allt," *Svensk Handikapptidskrift*, no. 5 (1978): 11–13. In her inquiry on sexual aids, Nordqvist repeated that, for disability organizations, questions about sex and disability were "taboo." Nordqvist, *Utredning om hjälpmedel i sexuallivet för män och kvinnor med funktionshinder*, 76.

44 This correspondence and minutes were originally destined to be kept as an independent collection in the National Archives (Riksarkivet, RA). However, they ended up being filed under the heading "Miscellaneous" in the archives of the now defunct Swedish Institute for Assistive Devices. This means that anyone who looks for the HS-gruppen in the National Archival Database (NAD) will not find it. Ser. Ö2. Handlingar rörande samlevnadsfrågor och handikapp. Hjälpmedelsinstitutet. RA.

45 The administrative leader of Mose Allé training school at this time was Birgit Kirkebæk, who would become famous in the 1990s for presenting Denmark's first PhD dissertation focused on disability. She has since become one of the foremost representatives of critical disability studies in Denmark.

46 "Seksualvejledning i træningsskolen," *S.Å.-Pædagogen*, no. 18 (1968): 414.

47 Gunnar Wad, "Seksualvejledning i træningsskolen," *S.Å.-Pædagogen*, nos. 19–20 (1968): 450.

48 Niels Erik Bank-Mikkelsen, "Nogle bemærkninger om politimestre, narre og andet godt folk," *S.Å.-Pædagogen*, no. 1 (1969): 10.

49 Niels Erik Bank-Mikkelsen, "Udviklingshæmmede og deres seksualproblemer," *Mental Hygiejne*, nos. 5–6 (1969): 120–125.

50 Bank-Mikkelsen, "Udviklingshæmmede," 123.

51 Bank-Mikkelsen, "Udviklingshæmmede," 124–125.

52 Bank-Mikkelsen, "Udviklingshæmmede," 123–124.

53 In 2007 the Swedish National Board of Health and Welfare decided on a new terminology. From then on, *funktionshinder* designates social or physical obstacles, and a new word, *funktionsnedsättning* (functional reduction), is used for physical, psychological, or intellectual impairment; see http://socialstyrelsen.iterm.se (accessed 26 May 2014).

54 *A.H.-Bulletinen*, no. 4 (1972): 10.

55 Enby's book was translated into English in 1975 with the title *Let There Be Love: Sex and the Handicapped*.

56 Enby, *Vi måste få älska*, 72, 73.

57 Karin Olsson, review of Gunnel Enby, *Vi måste få älska*, *A.H.-Bulletinen*, nos. 1–2 (1973): 22.

58 *Handi-Kamp*, no. 5 (1976): 5.

59 The special issues on sexuality that *Handi-Kamp* published were: no. 22 (1979), no. 32 (1980), no. 38 (1981), no. 46 (1982), no. 51 (1983), no. 54 (1983), no. 55 (1983), no. 61 (1984), no. 74 (1987, on prostitution), no. 84 (1989). The last special issue on sexuality was dedicated to the recently published *Guidelines about Sexuality—Regardless of Handicap* (*Vejledning om seksualitet—uanset handicap*). It was also the last issue of *Handi-Kamp*.

60 *Handi-Kamp*, no. 22 (1979): 2.

61 *Handi-Kamp*, no. 32 (1980): 2.

62 *Handi-Kamp*, no. 33 (1980): 5. Note that this is a kind of counter-example to Tom Shakespeare's observation that "slogans such as 'glad to be gay,' 'black is beautiful' do not tend to have an equivalent in the disability movement"; Shakespeare, *Disability Rights and Wrongs*, 76.

63 *Handi-Kamp*, no. 39 (1981).

64 *Handi-Kamp*, no. 51 (1983): 2.

65 *Handi-Kamp*, no. 33 (1989): 5.

66 *Handi-Kamp*, no. 55 (1983): 17.

67 Elisabeth Levy, Jytte Thorbek, and Lisse Holtegaard Christensen, "Det ældste erhverv: Alfonsens," *Politiken*, 27 November 1983.

68 *Handi-Kamp*, no. 56 (1983): 21–22.

69 "Handicapvisen," "Du er min Venus," "Reklamer." Clippings about the ensemble and song texts are from Lone Barsøe's private archives (LB).

70 Rosa Krotoschinsky, "Hørt i radio: Hvem er det synd for?," *Politiken*, 26 August 1984; "Verbale kølleslag med krykkestokke," *Bornholmeren*, 11 December 1984. Compare Beth Junker, "Børne-TV: Gammel og ny dannelse," *Politiken*, 21 April 1985.

71 *A.H.-Bulletinen*, no. 13 (1974): 26.

72 Buttenschøn, "Seksualiteten bliver tilladelig—Men hvordan med det private," 138.

73 Together—and with their students—Buttenschøn and Løt developed easy-to-read booklets, films, and games, such as "Feelings and senses—at stake: Parlor game about feelings, sexuality, prevention, sexually transmitted diseases, and much more, to be used in sexual education" (*Følelser og fornemmelser—på spil: Brætspillet om følelser, seksualitet, prævention, kønssygdomme og meget mere til brug i seksualundervisningen*), developed as part of the sexual advisor course by Annette Crillesen, Jytte Hjort, and Lars Bjarne Pedersen; "What are you doing? Dialogue game about sexuality—regardless of handicap" (*Hvad gør du? Dialogspil om seksualitet—Uanset handicap*), developed by Vibe-Pedersen, Charlotte Voetmann, Helle Kjærgaard, and Conni Hald. Karsten Løt, with a former student, Anette Løwert, also published widely used educational

materials. Løwert and Løt, *På vej til voksen*. Jørgen Buttenschøn is also the author of a popular book on sexology, *Sexologi, en bog for professionelle og forældre om udviklingshæmmede menneskers sexualitet*.

74 Birthe Søderhamn, "Debataften om åndssvages seksualproblemer," LEV–*Evnesvages Vel*, no. 11 (1974): 33.

75 "Forslag til folketingsbeslutning om handicappede og seksualitet," *Folketings-tidende* 1985–1986, vol. A12, cols. 4565–4566.

76 Mette Aarup, KF, quoted in *Folketingstidende* 1985–1986, col. 9485.

77 "Socialstyrelsens undersøgelse af behovet for forbedringer af handicappedes muligheder for seksualliv," Socialstyrelsen, October 1986, Karsten Løt's private archives (KL). Quotes are from pages 1 and 2 of the appendix and page 6 of the main report.

78 "Socialstyrelsens undersøgelse af behovet for forbedringer af handicappedes muligheder for seksualliv," Socialstyrelsen, October 1986, supp. 1. "Notat med cases der illustrerer problemer i relation til straffeloven for personale der ønsker at forbedre de handicappedes muligheder for et seksuallliv," 2, KL. It has been cited also in Tinning, *Sjovere handicapsex i sigte . . .*

79 Socialstyrelsen, *Vejledning*, 5.

80 Socialstyrelsen, *Vejledning*, 6.

81 Socialstyrelsen, *Vejledning*, 15.

82 *Handi-Kamp*, no. 31 (1980): 4.

83 *Fråga Olle dokumentären*, 2 March 2003, Channel 5, Jarowskij Productions. Some of Spinalis's rehabilitation philosophy and methods are also described in the foundation's book *Ny kraft för skadad ryggmärg*.

84 RD Mot. 1984/85:800; Mot. 1984/85:801.

85 RD Socialutskottet 1984/85:21.

86 The National Association of the Handicapped (De Handikappades Riksförbund, DHR) and the Cooperation Committee of Disability Organizations (Handikapporganisationernas Centralkommitté, HCK).

87 "Sexhjälpmedel utreds," *Svensk Handikapptidskrift*, no. 1 (1986): 6; RD Socialförsäkringsutskottet 1985/86:3; DHR to Riksdagens Socialförsäkringsutskott, 29 June 1985, Socialförsäkringsutskottets Arkiv, Riksdagens Arkiv (RdA).

88 Handikappinstitutet to Riksdagens Socialförsäkringsutskott, 3 June 1985, Socialförsäkringsutskottets Arkiv, RdA.

89 Nordqvist, *Utredning om hjälpmedel i sexualivet för män och kvinnor med funktionshinder*, 4–8.

90 SOU 1989:39, 29, 183.

91 Invalid Care Commission (Vanförevårdutredningen) of 1951: SOU 1954:28; Handicap Commission (Handikapputredningen) of 1965: SOU 1967:53; SOU 1967:60; SOU 1969:35; SOU 1970:64; SOU 1972:30; SOU 1976:20; Handicap

Commission of 1989: SOU 1989:54; SOU 1990:2; SOU 1990:19; SOU 1991:46; SOU 1991:97; SOU 1992:52; Söder, Barron, and Nilsson, *Handikapp och välfärd?*; Söder, *Brukarinflytande, livsinflytande, delaktighet*; *Framtiden och människor med omfattande funktionshinder*; Modig, *Samverkan mellan handikapporganisationer och samhälle*; Modig, *Habilitering för barn och ungdomar med funktionshinder*; Heins, *Gjort och ogjort med utgångspunkt från Handikapputredningens lägesrapport Handikapp och välfärd*; Hydén, *Om rättslig reglering*; *Socioekonomisk situation för personer med funktionshinder.*

92 Nordqvist, *Utredning om hjälpmedel i sexualivet för män och kvinnor med funktionshinder*, 65.

93 Nordqvist, *Utredning om hjälpmedel i sexualivet för män och kvinnor med funktionshinder*, supplement, appendix, 6, 5, 11, 13.

94 Nordqvist, *Utredning om hjälpmedel i sexualivet för män och kvinnor med funktionshinder*, 56.

Chapter 3. How to Impede and How to Facilitate

1 Sundet, *Jeg vet jeg er annerledes—Men ikke bestandig*, 189–190.

2 Sundet, *Jeg vet jeg er annerledes—Men ikke bestandig*, 201–202.

3 Sundet, *Jeg vet jeg er annerledes—Men ikke bestandig*, 192.

4 Sundet, *Jeg vet jeg er annerledes—Men ikke bestandig*, 191.

5 Sundet, *Jeg vet jeg er annerledes—Men ikke bestandig*, 196–197.

6 This is confirmed by a 2003 undergraduate thesis essay titled "Eight occupational therapists' attitudes toward the sexual and people with intellectual impairments." The eight occupational therapists interviewed said that they personally thought sex was an important topic that ought to be discussed but they had no training to do so—to the extent that if the topic had been discussed at all during their education, it was during either a single half-day or full-day seminar. Because they felt uncertain of how to deal with sexuality in a professional manner, they expected someone else to handle it. Backlund, Jerkovics, and Erikson, "Åtta arbetsterapeuters förhållningssätt kring sex- och samlevnad och personer med utvecklingsstörning," 6.

7 Buttenschøn, "Seksualiteten bliver tilladelig—Men hvordan med det private," 129.

8 S. Jørgensen, "Hvad er voldtægt—Og hvad er undervisning," *Funktionærbladet*, no. 1 (1969): 25.

9 Löfgren-Mårtenson, *"Får jag lov?,"* 98, 109–110.

10 Socialstyrelsen, *Sällan sedda.*

11 Sundin, "Personliga assistenter ofredades sexuellt."

12 Löfgren-Mårtenson, *"Får jag lov?,"* 98.

13 Bahner, *Funktionshindrad sexualitet?*, 52.

14 Bahner, *Funktionshindrad sexualitet?*, 58.

15 Linder, "Perspektiv på sexuella uttryckssätt i gruppboende," 27.

16 *I en annan del av Köping* (2008), DVD box, TV4 AB.

17 This manner of establishing a relationship is an example of what Lotta Löfgren-Mårtenson has described in her study of young people with an intellectual impairment. She noticed that the young people she observed at dances did not tend to flirt. Their decisions about relationships were expressed concretely and decisively in words or actions, not by flirting or seduction. Löfgren-Mårtenson, *"Får jag lov?,"* 144–148.

18 In a study conducted by journalism students after the first season had been aired, a focus group consisting of five people with disabilities were asked what they thought of the way romantic relationships were portrayed. The response was negative. Members of the focus group thought that the sequences about relationships and attraction were "namby-pamby" (*daltiga*) and "cutesy-cute" (*gulligulliga*). The focus group thought that the depiction of love in the program was "childish and insipid" (*barnslig och simpel*). Storm and Särnholm, "Gränslös glädje—Vägen till rättvisa?," 51.

19 Socialministeriet, *Vejledning om seksualitet—uanset handicap*, 5.

20 Standard Rules on the Equalization of Opportunities for Persons with Disabilities.

21 Socialministeriet, *Vejledning om seksualitet—uanset handicap*, 33.

22 Socialministeriet, *Vejledning om seksualitet—uanset handicap*, 13.

23 Enby, *Vi måste få älska*, 37.

24 Enby, *Vi måste få älska*, 38.

25 Enby, *Vi måste få älska*, 66–67.

26 Grunewald and Hallerfors, "Kan inte utvecklingsstörda onanera?" See also Margareta Nordeman's reply, "Visst behöver utvecklingsstörda hjälp med onani," and the final, unsigned last word from the editors, which follows Nordeman's reply, and which repeats, in many cases verbatim, the same accusations and criticisms that appear in the original review of the films.

Chapter 4. Shifting Boundaries

Epigraphs: (1) quote from "Birgitta Hulter, vårdlärare"; (2) quoted in Löfgren-Mårtenson, *"Får jag lov?,"* 21.

1 De Lauretis, *Practice of Love*, 235.

2 Wade, "It Ain't Exactly Sexy," 88–89.

3 Shakespeare, Gillespie-Sells, and Davies, *Sexual Politics of Disability*, 37.

4 Löfgren-Mårtenson, *"Får jag lov?,"* 94.

5 Löfgren-Mårtenson, *"Får jag lov?,"* 95.

6 Löfgren-Mårtenson, *"Får jag lov?,"* 97.

7 Löfgren-Mårtenson, *"Får jag lov?,"* 98.

8 Löfgren-Mårtenson, *"Får jag lov?,"* 110.

9 Nordeman mentions the films in her book *När känslan tar över* (When the feeling carries you away), 124.

10 Nordqvist, Supplement to *Utredning om hjälpmedel i sexualivet för män och kvinnor med funktionshinder*, 9–10.

11 Nordeman said that she and the others involved in making the film chose this machine because it did not look like a dildo. "We decided on the massage apparatus because we thought it would look innocent [*ofarlig*] in the eyes of the female staff members. They always have opinions about what looks pornographic."

12 Lennerhed, *Sex i folkhemmet*; Lennerhed, *Frihet att njuta*.

13 This man is Bengt Lindqvist, who went on to become deputy minister for social welfare in the years 1985–1991. It is interesting to note that in his 2012 memoir, *Blindstyre*, his participation in *More from the Language of Love* is passed over in stony silence.

14 Sjölander-Holland, "Komma nära den man vårdar," 16–17.

15 Lunds kommun, "Personalens roll när det gäller vuxna brukares sexualitet."

16 Christina Larsson, "Hotellstädare: stoppa porren; Cecilia sade upp sig: torka sperma är inte ett normalt arbete," *Aftonbladet*, 27 July 2004, www.aftonbladet .se/nyheter/article10474274.ab (accessed 19 April 2014).

17 Andreasson, "Det är en myt att hotellgästerna vill se porr."

18 Hoffman, "Svar på Katarina Engströms inlägg."

19 An undated article in the Swedish web-based journal *FunkaPortalen* details some of the complexities of this relationship. It discusses plans by the Work Environment Authority to inspect the homes of people with disabilities in the event of complaints from assistants, and it describes a concern that the outcome of such inspections could be that people with disabilities may be "forced to change things in their homes and their lives that they see as very personal."

20 In January 2010 a regional Administrative Court of Appeal (Kammarrätten) ruled that restrictions on smoking in public spaces did not apply to the rooms of people with psychiatric impairments who live in a group home. Arguing a case on behalf of the employees of a group home in the city of Eskilstuna, the Work Environment Authority (Arbetsmiljöverket) wanted the law prohibiting smoking in public places to apply to the rooms of the eleven residents of the group home, all of whom needed assistance, and most of whom smoked. In handing down its decision, the court noted that the law

prohibiting smoking in public places did not apply to people's homes. However, it mandated that the group home forbid smoking in the common rooms of the home and also that it provide workers with special masks, and offer any worker who is disturbed by the smoke employment elsewhere. It encouraged residents not to smoke when workers are in their rooms and to open the windows and air out the rooms after every cigarette. Kammarrätten i Jönköping, avdelning 1, 2010-01-14, Mål no. 360-09.

While this court decision would appear to resolve the issue of the legal status of a disabled person's service apartment or room in a group home, in practice the issue remains contentious, and the situation is anything but clear. Everyone we questioned in Sweden who worked as an assistant or in a company that hired personal assistants for disabled people maintained that rooms were both private and public. A typical response to our query about the legal status of a disabled person's living quarters is the following one, from a person who works with educational programs for personal assistants. The issue of what a disabled person has in his or her room, this respondent wrote to us in an e-mail, "only becomes an issue of workplace environment when the person with the disability consciously offends the assistants. This applies to political images, pornographic images and religious symbols." An understanding like this brings us back to square one, and illustrates the background against which conflicts can arise around a disabled person's right to privacy versus a worker's right to a "good work environment."

21 Shakespeare, Gillespie-Sells, and Davies, *Sexual Politics of Disability*, 38.
22 Shakespeare, Gillespie-Sells, and Davies, *Sexual Politics of Disability*, 44–48.
23 Socialstyrelsen, *Sällan sedda*, 41.
24 Löfgren-Mårtenson, *"Får jag lov?,"* 108.
25 Overaa, *Faktisk mangler man ord for det.*
26 Hertz, *Sisyfosbreve*, 304–306.
27 Nordeman, *När känslan tar över*, 68–69; Johansen, Thyness, and Holm, *När seksualitet tages alvorligt*, 136; Elisabeth Vallberg, *"'Vi måste träna deras sexuella förmåga—Handgripligen.' Intervju med Hans Wrenne," Ottar*, no. 4 (1982): 89–93.
28 Buttenschøn, *"Seksualiteten bliver tilladelig—Men hvordan med det private,"* 135.
29 Nordeman, *När känslan tar över*, 144.
30 Nordeman, *När känslan tar över*, 143, 144.
31 Enby, *Vi måste få älska*, 37.
32 Löfgren-Mårtenson, *"Får jag lov?,"* 92.
33 Socialstyrelsen, *Sällan sedda*; Flyckt, *Våld mot kvinnor med psykiska funktionshinder*; Nationellt råd för kvinnofrid, *När man slår mot det som gör ont*; Nils-

son and Westlund, *Våld mot personer med funktionshinder*; Risberg, *"Vem vill vara ihop med mig då?"*

34 Granvik and Wernlid, *Säga ja, säga nej.*

35 The clinic's website is www.offclinic.se (accessed 18 February 2013).

36 This research is reported in Kousmanen and Starke, "Identifying the Invisible."

37 Jørgensen, *Seksuelle overgreb—Nej tak!*; Grünberger, *Seksuelle overgreb mod mennesker med handicap*; Muff, *Seksuelle overgreb på mennesker med handicap.*

38 "Forslag til beredskabsplan ved mistankte eller viden om seksuelt overgreb," Seksualpolitik på specialskoler, www.projektseksualpolitik.dk/default.asp?side =18&uside=38 (accessed 2 May 2014).

39 Forebyg seksuelle overgreb mod mennesker med handicap [Prevent sexual abuse of people with handicap], www.forebygovergreb.dk (accessed 2 May 2014).

40 Lov no. 176 af 11. maj 1935, om Adgang til Sterilisation og Kastration; Lov no. 171 af 16. maj 1934, om Foranstaltninger vedrørende Aandssvage; Lag (1934:171) om sterilisering av vissa sinnessjuka, sinnesslöa eller andra som lida av rubbad själsverksamhet; Lag (1941:282) om sterilisering; Koch, *Tvangssterilisation i Danmark 1929–67*, 381; Tydén, *Från politik till praktik*, 56, 60.

41 Löfgren-Mårtenson, *"Får jag lov?,"* 170.

42 Desjardins, "The Sexualized Body of the Child," 79.

43 This was also the concern that seemed to be raised most often by Swedish parents and staff who discussed the issue with Lotta Löfgren-Mårtenson. Löfgren-Mårtenson, *"Får jag lov?,"* 171.

44 Mollow, "Is Sex Disability?," 286.

45 Mollow, "Is Sex Disability?," 301.

46 Mollow, "Is Sex Disability?," 308.

Chapter 5. Paying for Sexual Services

1 Hertz and her son were also featured in a ninety-minute, verité-style documentary from 1980, directed by Bille August, titled *Tomas—A Child You Can't Reach* (*Tomas—Et barn du ikke kan nå*).

2 The Danish words used were *usentimental, hjerteskærende, rystende, bevægende, hudløse,* and *ærlighed.* Only one review explicitly mentions that Hertz paid a sex worker to visit her son. Marianne Uttrup, "Lone Hertz købte luder til sin søn," *bt* (a popular tabloid), 10 September 1992. The other reviewer who alluded to the incident wrote only that Hertz discusses her son's "attempt at a sex life." Holger Ruppert, "Her skånes ingen," *bt,* September 1992. Other reviews of the book are Annelise Bistrup, "Jeg er i ingenmandsland," *Berlingske Tidende,* 20 September 1992; Bettina Heltberg, "Alle mennesker er af ånd,"

Politiken, 12 September 1992; Ole Schierbeck, "Samtale med en sprogløs," *Politiken*, 11 September 1992; Pia Skogeman, "Kampen om et sprog," *Berlingske Tidende*, 11 September 1992; Henning Thøgersen, "Lad tavsheden tale," *Ekstra Bladet*, 12 September 1992.

3 Johnny Meyer, "Ok, at Lone købte sex til sin søn," *Ekstra Bladet*, 15 January 2009.

4 Hertz, *Sisyfosbreve*, 301.

5 Meyer, "Ok, at Lone købte sex til sin søn"; Kim Kastrup, "Hertz skaffede en luder til sin søn," *Ekstra Bladet*, 15 January 2009.

6 Meyer, "Ok, at Lone købte sex til sin søn."

7 Olsson, "Min son sa att han vill ha en tjej som på film."

8 Thomas Gustavsson, "Min son vill vara med en naken tjej," *Aftonbladet*, 15 February 2007, www.aftonbladet.se/nyheter/article10878680.ab (accessed 19 April 2014). Note the syntax of this headline: it isn't "My son wants to be naked with a girl"—a formulation that would suggest mutuality and reciprocity, and would surely be more in keeping with Olsson's remarks that his son wanted to be "naked together" with a girl. Instead the newspaper reports that "My son wants to be with a naked girl," a formulation that invites readers to imagine voyeurism, nonreciprocity, and even abuse.

9 Anna Krook, "Är det okej att köpa sex till sin son?," *Expressen*, 15 February 2007.

10 Linna Johansson, "Ett behov bland andra," *Expressen*, 17 February 2007.

11 Hillevi Wahl, "Kvinnor är inga sexhjälpmedel," *Metro Riks*, 18 February 2007.

12 Kristina Persson, *Helsingborgs Dagblad*, 5 March 2007.

13 "Diskussionen har spårat ur," *Corren.se*, 25 May 2007, www.corren.se/oster gotland/?articleId=4208883 (accessed 19 April 2014).

14 Interview with Sören Olsson, 10 October 2011.

15 European Court of Human Rights, *Enhorn v. Sweden*, 2005-I, application no. 56529/00, 25 January 2005, http://sim.law.uu.nl/sim/caselaw/Hof.nsf/1d4d odd24obfee7ec12568490035df05/50986ab40fbd3da7c1256f90004d3e2a?Open Document (accessed 3 May 2014).

16 Justitsministeriet, "Straffelovrådet foreslår skærpelser over for seksual-forbrydelser," 21 November 2012, www.justitsministeriet.dk/print/nyt-og -presse/pressemeddelelser/2012/straffelovrådet-foreslår-skærpelser-over -seksualforbrydelser (accessed 3 May 2014); Jesper Vangkilde and Jesper Hvass, "Thorning: Jeg har ændret holdning til købesex," *Politiken*, 21 November 2012.

17 The woman O'Brien writes about, Cheryl Cohen-Greene, wrote a book of her own in 2012 in which she describes the sessions she had with O'Brien and her life more generally. Cohen-Greene (with Garano), *Intimate Life*.

18 Campredon and Chayé, dirs., *L'Amour sans limites*.

19 Steimer and Stommel, "Sexualbegleiterin."

20 Shakespeare, Gillespie-Sells, and Davies, *Sexual Politics of Disability*, 132.

21 Silverberg, "Sexual Surrogacy Revisited." Cheryl Cohen-Greene, citing the International Professional Surrogates Association, writes that the number of trained surrogates in the United States today is fifty. Cohen-Greene, *Intimate Life*, 30.

22 See, for example, the discussion of sex surrogacy in Shakespeare, Gillespie-Sells, and Davies, *Sexual Politics of Disability*, 131–134.

23 Some writers imply that sexual surrogates might be willing to do the deed out of charity instead of cash. Wendy Greengross has a section on "sexual Samaritans" in her book *Entitled to Love*. Like most other descriptions of sexual Samaritans, who they are and what they do, Greengross's is vague and repeats the platitude that a sexual Samaritan would give a disabled person "more than sex: she would give peace of mind and a kind of love, that is to say, that warmth that human contact brings with it" (121). Greengross also strongly implies that anyone providing sexual services to disabled people would do so out of a sense of compassion, not pecuniary gain.

24 *Scarlet Road* was directed by Catherine Scott and produced by Pat Fiske.

25 Wotton, "Conversations with Richard Fidler." Wotton also describes Touching Base in Wotton and Isbister, "A Sex Worker Perspective on Working with Clients with a Disability and the Development of Touching Base Inc."

26 Nordansjö, *Mitt nakna jag*, 172–174.

27 The Swedish words Max used in his e-mail to the woman were that he *har en cp-skada* (literally, "has a cerebral palsy injury"); Nordansjö, *Mitt nakna jag*, 173. This is the politically correct way of saying "I have cerebral palsy," but it is not a common expression, and it is entirely possible that a sex worker like the one described in the book would not know it. The more common way of saying that one has cerebral palsy in Swedish is *Jag är cp-skadad* (literally, "I am cerebral palsy injured/damaged"). The use of the possessive "have" in Max's e-mail mitigates the severity of the "injury," making it seem slight or localized. To the extent that the story Nordansjö recounts is based on an actual event, the sex worker's hasty exit might be explained, at least in part, by her surprise upon actually seeing Max, who is described in the book as quite severely impaired. (We can also note here that the Swedish expression "cerebral palsy injured/damaged" is an exception to the otherwise ardently politically correct language used in most other instances to talk about disability. This expression, along with one other exception to that rule, is discussed in Kulick, "Danes Call People with Down Syndrome 'Mongol.'")

28 Like many other people in his situation, Rasmus is not interested in mediated communication, such as a Bliss board. Different people have different reasons for rejecting this kind of communication. Some—especially those who

were not exposed to the Bliss system as children or young adults—are either uninterested in, or feel like they don't have the energy to learn, the symbols. In Rasmus's case, the social workers at the group home where he has lived for many years say they have talked to him about getting a Bliss board but that he rejects the idea. He is proud of the fact that he is able to communicate without such mediation, and staff members say he has made it clear that he would regard a Bliss board as a sign of defeat.

29 Wingaard, *Migrantprostitution i Danmark*.

30 Nordansjö, *Mitt nakna jag*, 16.

31 Nordansjö, *Mitt nakna jag*, 217.

32 O'Brien, "The Sex Surrogate," 213.

33 O'Brien, "The Sex Surrogate," 214.

34 O'Brien, "The Sex Surrogate," 220.

35 O'Brien, "The Sex Surrogate," 219.

36 Compare Anders's description of the pleasure he feels during sex to the following portrayal, by Edward Hooper, a man who broke his neck ten years previously: "My brain hasn't figured out I'm supposed to be asexual. It keeps sending erotic messages. But the focus of where I receive those messages has changed from my penis to other areas of my body where I do have feeling: my shoulders, neck, lips, ears. With intimate contact in these areas, coupled with the knowledge that I'm giving pleasure too—by kissing, touching and embracing—my heart begins to race, my head gets warm, my mind surges, aggressively pursuing its feelings. The excitement builds to a level of intense pleasure—then subsides toward contentment." Hooper, "New Insights," 80.

37 Löfgren-Mårtenson, *"Får jag lov?,"* 135.

38 Löfgren-Mårtenson, *"Får jag lov?,"* 178.

39 Research among people with disabilities that confirms this hierarchy of desirability is summarized in Deal, "Disabled People's Attitudes towards Other Groups."

40 Kajsa Sigvardsson, "Han vill gå på statlig bordell," *Aftonbladet*, 16 December 2005, www.aftonbladet.se/wendela/relationer/article10728322.ab?service=print (accessed 19 April 2014).

Chapter 6. Why the Difference?

Epigraphs: (1) Bech, "Report from a Rotten State," 47, n. 3; (2) Berggren and Trägårdh, "Social Trust and Radical Individualism," 22.

1 Grunewald, *Från idiot till medborgare*; Grunewald and Bakk, *Omsorgsboken*; Grunewald and Bakk, *Nya omsorgsboken*; Grunewald and Eeg-Olofsson,

Medicinska omsorgsboken; Bakk and Grunewald, *Omsorgsboken*; Söderman and Antonsson, *Nya omsorgsboken.*

2 Falkheimer and Örsten, "Öresundsregionen i medieskugga."

3 The Danish response to Swedish views on alcohol are widely shared by others who have commented on Swedish alcohol politics. "The fact is that a good part of the puritanism, hypocrisy, and tabu that in many countries is concentrated in the sexual area has in Sweden firmly attached to alcohol" is how journalist David Jenkins put it in 1968, succinctly summarizing the majority, non-Swedish view. Jenkins, *Sweden and the Price of Progress*, 243. Susan Sontag described the Swedish attitude toward alcohol as "nutty" and devoted a good part of her essay on Sweden published in *Ramparts* to the issue. Sontag, "Letter from Sweden," 27.

4 Sontag, "Letter from Sweden," 27.

5 Systembolaget, "Bokslutskommuniké 2012."

6 *Health Statistics for the Nordic Countries*, tables 2.1.3 and 3.1.4; "Danskerne har rekord i lav levealder," *Politiken*, 23 January 2011.

7 Hartelius, *Narkotikapolitik i Sverige*, 36; RD Prot. 2001/02:90.

8 Tham, "Swedish Drug Policy," 396–397. For more recent summaries that agree with Tham's evaluation of Swedish drug policy see Svensson, *Narkotikapolitik och narkotikadebatt*, 167–172, and Goldberg, *Hur blir man narkoman?*

9 The mobile injection room has a website, www.fixerum.dk (accessed 20 August 2013).

10 SOU 1976:9; Ahlberg, "Homo-Sverige utanför RFSL"; Thomsson, "Rätten till våra kroppar."

11 Dahlerup, *Rødstrømperne*, 1:529.

12 *Straffelovrådets betænkning om seksualforbrydelser*, 611.

13 Österberg, "Compromise instead of Conflict?"; Österberg, *Folk förr*. Compare Aronsson, *Bönder gör politik*.

14 Österberg, *Folk förr*, 196.

15 Feldbæk, *Den lange fred, 1700–1800*; Bjørn, *Fra reaktion til grundlov, 1800–1850*.

16 Meyer, "*Dansken, svensken og nordmannen*"; Meyer, "A Comparative Look at Scandinavian Cultures"; Bondeson, *Nordic Moral Climates.*

17 Bech, "Report from a Rotten State," 147n13.

18 For instance, journalist Otto Gelstedt, who was a member of the Danish Communist Party, sharply criticized Stalinist orthodoxy and characterized it as "Bolshevik idiocy" already in 1928, ten years before the Moscow trials, when intellectuals in other parts of Europe lost faith in the Soviet Union. Thing, "Kulturradikalismen"; Vind, "Grundtvig og det danske," 25.

19 Møller, *Grundtvigianisme i det 20. århundrede*; Møller, "Grundtvig og Marx"; Thomsen and Mikkelsen, *Hvor blev det grundtvigske af?*

20 Østergaard, "Findes der en dansk politisk kulture?"; Lunde, "De kommune-farvede danskere"; Vind, "Grundtvig og det danske."

21 Huntford, *The New Totalitarians*, 8.

22 Foucault, *Remarks on Marx*, 75.

23 Enzensberger, *Svensk höst*, 17.

24 Bjørn Bredal, "Er svenskeren et menneske?," *Politiken*, 9 September 2006.

25 Sontag, "Letter from Sweden," 28.

26 Berggren and Trägårdh, *Är svensken människa?*, 14.

27 In their work published in English, Berggren and Trägårdh equivocate about whether the model of welfare they describe is specifically Swedish or more generally Nordic. A primary reason for the equivocation appears to be that like social welfare researcher Gøsta Esping-Andersen, who discusses what he calls the "Scandinavian model" as one of his three models of welfare states, Berggren and Trägårdh recognize that some aspects of the welfare state they describe are shared among Scandinavian countries. A problem that their writing (like Esping-Andersen's) never addresses is differences among those countries—in other words, whether and how what they sometimes call the "Nordic model" looks different, or the same, in Sweden, Denmark, Norway, Finland, and Iceland. Instead, *everything* the authors have to say about the "Nordic model" is illustrated with examples from Sweden. Furthermore, in their book in Swedish in which they develop the arguments we present here, other Nordic countries are not discussed—the authors are very specific that they are discussing the cultural proclivities and national history of Sweden. Because we think that Berggren and Trägårdh's analysis of Sweden is so insightful, we ignore the issue that they obliquely raise, but nowhere address, regarding similarities and differences in the development and operation of the welfare state in other Nordic countries. Berggren and Trägårdh, "Pippi Longstocking and the Autonomous Child and the Moral Logic of the Swedish Welfare State"; Berggren and Trägårdh, "Social Trust and Radical Individualism." Compare Esping-Andersen, *The Three Worlds of Welfare Capitalism*.

28 Berggren and Trägårdh, *Är svensken människa?*, 231.

29 Borchorst, Christensen, and Siim, "Diskurser om køn, magt og politik i Skandinavien."

30 This argument basically restates the conclusions of an important and widely cited 1999 study commissioned by the Nordic Council of Ministers that compared gender politics across the Nordic countries. Bergqvist, *Equal Democracies?*, 287.

31 Hirdman, "Könsmagt under behandling."

32 Stetson and Mazur, *Comparative State Feminism*; Halley, *Split Decisions*.

33 Hernes, *Welfare and Woman Power*, 11.

34 SOU 1990:44; "Hon gjorde Bengt Westerberg till feminist," *Expressen*, 11 November 1993.

35 SOU 1998:6, 1.

36 SOU 1994:56; SOU 1995:60.

37 In fact, it was a majority of younger female party members who urged the Socialist Party to abolish gender quotas. Christensen and Damkjær, *Kvinder og politisk repræsentation i Danmark*, 17.

38 Borchorst, Christensen, and Siim, "Diskurser om køn, magt og politik i Skandinavien."

39 Bernstein, "Militarized Humanism Meets Carceral Feminism."

40 Quote is from the European arrest warrant issued by the Swedish prosecution authority on 26 November 2010, which is repeated in the British High Court's 2 November 2011 dismissal of Assange's appeal against his extradition to Sweden, www.judiciary.gov.uk/Resources/JCO/Documents/Judgments/assange-summary.pdf (accessed 4 May 2014).

41 Examples are Ditte Giese, "Fri mig for Big-Mother omklamringen," *Politiken*, 30 May 2011; and Marta Sørensen, "Hold mig ude af jeres kønskamp, medsøstrene," *Politiken*, 22 June 2013.

42 Knausgård, *Min kamp*, 333.

43 Jalving, *Absolut Sverige*, 10, 12.

44 Quote from Hans Hauge, in Danish: "Danskerne tror, at de kan tale problemerne væk, mens svenskerne tror, de kan tie dem væk"; used as an epigraph in Jalving, *Absolut Sverige*.

45 The Public Order Act (Ordningslagen [1993:1617]), Article 14, forbids any public event that constitutes a "pornographic performance" (*pornografisk föreställning*). This phrase has been interpreted by courts to mean that while women working in strip clubs may bare their breasts, they may not expose their genitals. Nor may anyone working in such clubs attempt to "influence the viewer in a sexual manner through enacting sexual events and situations in blatant and provocative ways" (*påverka åskådaren i sexuellt avseende genom att sexuella händelseförlopp och situationer framställts på ett ohöljt och utmanande sätt*). Niklas Silow, "De styr den nya porrvågen," *Aftonbladet*, 19 June 2000, wwwc.aftonbladet.se/nyheter/0006/19/porr.html (accessed 19 April 2014).

46 Ida Gustafsson, "Moderatpolitiker: Sexköp är OK," *Aftonbladet*, 4 February 2013, www.aftonbladet.se/nyheter/article16179640.ab (accessed 19 April); "M-politiker: Sexköp är helt OK," *Dagens Nyheter*, 4 February 2013, www.dn.se/nyheter/sverige/mpolitiker-sexkop-ar-helt-okej (accessed 19 April 2014); Josefine Elfström, "M-politiker i Åre är för prostitution," *Expressen*, 4 February 2013, www.expressen.se/nyheter/m-politiker-i-are-ar-for-prostitution (accessed 19 April 2014).

47 Jeanette Fundin, "Åremoderaterna tar avstånd från prostitutionsuttalande," *Öresunds-Posten*, 4 February 2013, http://op.se/lanet/are/1.5550350-aremo deraterna-tar-avstand-fran-prostitutionsuttalande (accessed 19 April 2014).

48 Per Hansson, "Ofrånkomlig avgång," *Östersunds-Posten*, 6 February 2013, http://op.se/opinion/ledare/1.5557150-per-hansson-ofrankomlig-avgang (accessed 19 April 2014); "Moderatpolitiker backar om sexköp," *Dagens Nyheter*, 4 February 2013, www.dn.se/nyheter/sverige/moderatpolitiker-backar-om-sex kop (accessed 19 April 2014).

49 Åre Kommun socialnämnden, Sammanträdesprotokoll 2013-02-26, no. A2, sida 12, Dnr 071/12 001.

50 Kingdon, *Agendas, Alternatives, and Public Policies*, 165–195.

51 "Så nær det normale som muligt," Forslag til Lov om forsorgen for åndssvage, fremsat den 4. november 1958 af socialministeren, *Folketingstidende* 1958–1959, tillæg A (71); Bemærkninger til lovforslaget, col. 1136, Lov no. 192 af 5. juni 1959 om forsorgen for åndssvage og andre særligt svagt begavede.

52 Interview with Karl Grunewald, 19 December 2012.

53 Grunewald and Bakk, *Omsorgsboken*, 4.

54 For readers who wonder why we do not discuss this feature of Danish political and social life in this book, we can answer that there are three reasons for this.

The first and most important reason is that Danish rhetoric about immigrants never emerged as an especially relevant topic for our areas of interest. The comments by Danish sexual advisors who refuse to contact non-Danish sex workers that we quote in chapter 5 could be interpreted as an expression of anti-immigrant sentiment, but we think a far more accurate analysis would be one that views them as expressing an anxiety generated by anti-prostitution rhetoric—the kind that flourishes in the mass media in the form that anthropologist Carole Vance has termed "melomentaries" and that relentlessly personifies abject victims of sexual trafficking with images of non-Western and Eastern European women. Vance, "Innocence and Experience."

The second reason we do not discuss immigration rhetoric and policies is that the political situation in Denmark has changed since the 2011 elections, when the Social Democrats returned to power in a center-left coalition. This meant that the Danish People's Party (Dansk Folkeparti, DF), which was the driving force behind the anti-immigrant rhetoric and policies, lost its influence on government politics. DF party members held no ministerial posts in the center-right coalition that governed Denmark between 2001 and 2011, but they had a decisive influence over governmental policies because the coalition needed DF's votes to push forward its economic agenda. As an opposition party after 2011, DF continued its populist campaigns, and like other populist anti-EU political parties throughout Europe, it enjoyed great success in the

2014 EU parliamentary elections. But in Denmark, DF's power was curtailed in 2011, and its views on immigration no longer enjoyed official sanction.

The third reason is that the issue of immigrant-Dane relations is a contentious one, and there is an enormous amount of debate about how to approach it and think about it clearly. To try to engage intelligently in those debates is outside the scope of the topics we want to foreground in this book, and it would have necessitated an entirely different study. An example of the complexity of the debates is that while events such as the publication of the Mohammed cartoons in the newspaper *Jyllands-Posten* drew international attention, and while it is true that because of the influence of the Danish People's Party Danish immigration policies have become increasingly restrictive, it is far from clear that these phenomena are indicative of or reflect widespread racism among the Danish population. Sociologist Henning Bech and Middle Eastern Studies scholar Mehmet Ümit Necef recently sifted through all the reports, academic investigations, and surveys taken between 1990 and 2010 that supposedly documented claims like the ones that regularly appear in the Swedish mass media, and also in internal Danish political debates, that Danes have become racists. Their conclusion, presented in a detailed, 350-page book, is that the evidence for those claims, in fact, is lacking. Bech and Necef, *Er danskerne racister?*

55 Falkheimer and Örsten, "Öresundsregionen i medieskugga."

56 Ole Rothenborg, "Sexköp med bidrag," *Dagens Nyheter*, 25 September 2005.

57 *Fråga Olle dokumentären* [Ask Olle documentary], 2 March 2003, Channel 5, Jarowskij Productions.

58 Ljuslinder, "Handikappdiskurser i Svt"; *CP-magasinet*, Svt, ep. 3, 13 May 2004.

59 In an e-mail correspondence with us in August 2012, Sørensen expressed shock that she was portrayed as actually masturbating men. She had never seen the program (she had been promised a copy, she said, but never received one). She wrote: "I NEVER said that we masturbate men to orgasm. I said that some of us [sexual advisors] have given intellectually disabled men instruction about how to masturbate. I'm sure I described the method, and that became twisted to be that we masturbate them to orgasm." (*Jeg har ALDRIG udtalt mig om at vi onanerer på mænd så de får udløsning, men derimod at vi er nogle der har været med til at oplære udviklingshæmmede mænd i at onanere. Så har jeg sikkert beskrevet metoden, som så er blevet lavet om til at vi onanerer dem til udløsning.*)

60 Grönvik, "Kåta Krymplingar."

61 "Tema Funkis," *Ottar*, no. 4 (2005).

62 Svensk, *Hemligheter kända av många.*

63 Sjölander, "Sex i vården."

64 Sjölander, "Lär av Danmark!"

65 Lunds kommun, "Personalens roll när det gäller vuxna brukares sexualitet."

66 Quoted in *Jyllands-Posten*, 25 August 2005.

67 *Socialpædagogen*, no. 18 (2005): 9.

68 *Socialpædagogen*, no. 3 (2007): 4; BR 154/06, Medlemsforslag om københavner-kodeks på prostitutionsområdet [Member's proposal for Copenhagen code on prostitution], Copenhagen Borgerrepresentation [city council], 9 March 2006.

69 In Danish: *At mennesker med handicap ikke må nægtes mulighed for at opleve deres egen seksualitet, have seksuelle forhold og blive forældre.* Socialstyrelsen, *Seksualitet på dagsordenen*, 5.

70 Socialstyrelsen, *Seksualitet på dagsordenen*, 36.

71 Socialstyrelsen, *Seksualitet på dagsordenen*, 12.

72 Nola Grace Gaarmand, "Københavnsk forbud har ikke betydet mindre købe-sex til handicappede," *Information*, 1 February 2012; Jon Bøge Gehlert and Lars Henriksen, "Forbud mod købesex vil diskriminere handicappede," *Kristeligt Dagblad*, 3 February 2012.

Chapter 7. Disability and Sexuality—Who Cares?

Epigraphs: (1) Kittay, *Love's Labor*, 5; (2) Shakespeare, *Disability Rights and Wrongs*, 56.

1 Aliva och livet, "Är sex en rättighet?," blog post, 4 July 2012, http://aliva.word press.com/2012/07/04/vecka-27-ar-sex-en-rattighet (accessed 19 April 2014).

2 Young, "Asymmetrical Reciprocity," 349.

3 Young, "Asymmetrical Reciprocity," 350.

4 Young, "Asymmetrical Reciprocity," 352.

5 Young, "Asymmetrical Reciprocity," 360.

6 Siebers, *Disability Theory*, 148.

7 McRuer, *Crip Theory*, 181–194.

8 Linton, *Claiming Disability*, 12, 138; Siebers, *Disability Theory*, 4, 64–69.

9 Shakespeare, *Disability Rights and Wrongs*, 63.

10 Shakespeare, *Disability Rights and Wrongs*, 63.

11 Wade, "It Ain't Exactly Sexy," 90.

12 Turner, *Vulnerability and Human Rights*; Jain, "Living in Prognosis"; Puar, "Prognosis Time."

13 Derrida, "The Animal That Therefore I Am (More to Follow)," 396.

14 Derrida, "The Animal That Therefore I Am (More to Follow)," 397.

15 Turner, *Vulnerability and Human Rights*, 9.

16 Hudson, *Justice in the Risk Society*, 194.

17 Rorty, "Human Rights, Rationality and Sentimentality," 126.

18 Levinas, *Otherwise Than Being, or Beyond Essence.*

19 Attridge, "Following Derrida."

20 Kittay, *Love's Labor*, 16.

21 Tronto, *Moral Boundaries*, 169.

22 Williams, "In and Beyond New Labour."

23 Sevenhuijsen, *Citizenship and the Ethics of Care*, 147.

24 Nussbaum, "Capabilities as Fundamental Entitlements," 47.

25 Nussbaum, *Women and Human Development.*

26 Rawls, *A Theory of Justice*; Rawls, *Political Liberalism.*

27 Rawls, *A Theory of Justice*, 4.

28 Rawls's actual description of this procedure is more complex, partly in that he distinguishes between the contractors who agree on principles of justice in what he calls the "original position" (an abstract, hypothetical "device of representation" unaffected by contingencies of the social world) and the citizens who subsequently are the subject of those principles. The contractors are said to be the "representatives" of citizens. Rawls, *Political Liberalism*, 26. But Rawls also says that citizens can assume the role of contracting parties: "We can, as it were, enter into this [original] position at any time simply by reasoning for principles of justice in accordance with the enumerated restrictions on information." Rawls, *Political Liberalism*, 27. This invitation to imagine ourselves as contractors in the original position operating under the veil of ignorance is one of the most compelling features of Rawls's model. It underscores the central point that the contracting parties choose principles for a society in which they themselves are going to live. Nussbaum, *Frontiers of Justice*, 16–17.

29 Nussbaum, *Frontiers of Justice*, 80.

30 The other two groups comprise citizens of poor countries in relation to those of wealthy countries, and nonhuman animals. Nussbaum discusses these problematic cases at length in *Frontiers of Justice.*

31 Rawls, *Political Liberalism*, 21.

32 Rawls, *Political Liberalism*, 20.

33 Nussbaum, *Frontiers of Justice*, 85.

34 Nussbaum explains that we are free to "imagine the parties to the social contract as all needy and dependent beings with strong and ineliminable ties to others. But all the major social contract thinkers choose to imagine their parties as rationally competent adults who, as Locke says, are, in the state of nature, 'free, equal, and independent.'" Nussbaum, *Frontiers of Justice*, 104.

35 Although Nussbaum does not mention Levinas or Derrida, this idea reminds one of their insistence that vulnerability always already entails a relationship of responsibility and obligation.

36 Sen, "Equality of What?"

37 Nussbaum, *Frontiers of Justice*, 70.

38 Nussbaum, *Frontiers of Justice*, 76–78.

39 This is why Nussbaum insists that the capabilities approach is a partial account of justice. Nussbaum, *Frontiers of Justice*, 75.

40 Nussbaum, *Frontiers of Justice*, 167.

41 Nussbaum, *Women and Human Development*, 55–56.

42 Nussbaum, *Frontiers of Justice*, 76–77.

43 These Standard Rules (Resolution 48/96, passed by the General Assembly on 20 December 1993) have been superseded by the 2006 Convention on the Rights of Persons with Disabilities in those countries that have ratified it, which include both Sweden and Denmark. We cite the Standard Rules here, though, because they are still regularly appealed to in contexts advocating progressive policies regarding sexuality and disability. A main reason for this is that the Convention on the Rights of Persons with Disabilities is a more conservative document. It importantly calls for governments to respect the right of persons with disabilities to "marry and found a family," to be allowed to "retain their fertility," and to be provided "with the same range, quality, and standard of free or affordable health care and programmes as provided to other persons, including in the area of sexual and reproductive health" (Article 23, "Respect for Home and Family," and Article 25, "Health"). However, unlike the Standard Rules document, nowhere does the Convention mention the right to express sexuality outside the context of marriage and reproduction. In a way similar to the 2012 version of the Danish *Guidelines* document, this later version of the Standard Rules is less progressive than the document it superseded.

44 World Health Organization, *Defining Sexual Health*, 5; see also http://www.who.int/reproductivehealth/topics/sexual_health/sh_definitions/en/ (accessed 26 May 2014).

45 Socialstyrelsen, *Seksualitet på dagsordenen*, 3; the quote is from Langfeldt and Porter, *Sexuality and Family Planning*.

46 *SVT Debatt*, hosted by Lennart Persson, aired on SVT1 on 18 May 2004 from 10 to 11 PM; prod. no. 31-04/0375-019.

47 Finn Hellman, "Inget hindrar att du rannsakar dig," *Tidningen Arbetaren*, no. 22 (2004).

48 Annika Dalén, "Sexhjälp i stället för prostituterade," *Tidningen Arbetaren*, no. 33 (2004); Mattias Kvick, "Sex är ingen rättighet," *Tidningen Arbetaren*, no. 33 (2004).

49 Annika Dalén, "Bekämpa inte ett förtryck med ett annat," *Tidningen Arbetaren*, no. 38 (2004).

50 Finn Hellman, "Män har velat köpa sex av mig," *Tidningen Arbetaren*, no. 34 (2004).

51 In Swedish: *För mig framstår det som helt omöjligt att söka hitta riktlinjer för hur den här hjälpen ska ske för att förhindra varje tänkbar risk för övergrepp och/eller känslor av förnedring hos någon av parterna.* Kvick, "Sex är ingen rättighet."

52 Kvick, "Sex är ingen rättighet."

53 This claim disputes sociologist Bryan Turner's assertion that "the language of human rights is ultimately the only plausible language for expressing the needs of people with impairment and disability." Turner, *Vulnerability and Human Rights*, 90.

54 Nussbaum, "The Capabilities of People with Cognitive Disabilities, 331.

Unpublished Sources

Archives in Denmark
Lone Barsøe's private archives (LB)
Karsten Løt's private archives (KL)

Archives in Sweden
Arbetarrörelsens Bibliotek och Arkiv [Workers' Movement's Library and Archives] (ARAB)
    Archives of the Riksförbundet för Sexuell Upplysning [Swedish Association for Sexuality Education] (RFSU)
P. O. Lundberg's private archives (POL)
Riksarkivet [National Archives] (RA)
    Archives of the De Handikappades Riksförbund [National Association of the Handicapped] (DHR)
    Archives of the Handikapporganisationernas Centralkommitté [Cooperation Committee of Disability Organizations] (HCK)
    Archives of the Hjälpmedelsinstitutet [Swedish Institute for Assistive Technology, SIAT]

Archives of the Socialdepartementet [Social Ministry]
Riksdagens Arkiv [Archives of the Swedish Parliament] (RdA)
    Archives of the Socialförsäkringsutskottet [Standing Committee on Social Insurances]

Laws

Denmark

Lov no. 181 af 20. maj 1933, om Offentlig Forsorg.

Lov no. 171 af 16. maj 1934, om Foranstaltninger vedrørende Aandssvage.

Lov no. 176 af 11. maj 1935, om Adgang til Sterilisation og Kastration.

Lov no. 192 af 5. juni 1959, om forsorgen for åndssvage og andre særligt svagt begavede.

Lov no. 333 af 19. juni 1974, om social bistand.

Lov no. 454 af 10. juni 1997, om social service.

Sweden

Kungl. Maj:ts förordning om invalidunderstöd den 28 juni 1935.

Lag (1934:171) om sterilisering av vissa sinnessjuka, sinnesslöa eller andra som lida av rubbad själsverksamhet.

Lag (1941:282) om sterilisering.

Lag (1954:483) om undervisning och vård av vissa psykiskt efterblivna.

Lag (1967:940), angående omsorger om vissa psykiskt utvecklingsstörda (Omsorgslagen 1967).

Socialtjänstlag (1980:620).

Lag (1985:568) om särskilda omsorger om psykiskt utvecklingsstörda m. fl. (Omsorgslagen 1985).

Periodicals

This list comprises the total number of periodicals covered by our investigation. Some of these titles may not be cited in the endnotes.

Denmark

Funktionærbladet 1969

Handi-Kamp 1976–1969

Handicap-Nyt 1989–2007

LEV–Evnesvages Vel 1961–2007

Mental Hygiejne 1969

S.-Å. *Pædagogen* 1964–1980
Socialpædagogik 2002–2007
Specialpædagogik 1981–2002
Ungdomskredsløbet 1992–2007
Vanførebladet 1926–1988

Sweden
A.H.-Bulletinen 1970–1979
FUB-Kontakt 1966–1984
Handikappsamverkan 1979–1993
HCK-Information 1969–1977
HCK-Rapport 1978–1993
Hillebard 1988–2000
Intra 1994–2000
Kick 1982–2002
Ottar 1981–1998
Psykisk Utvecklingshämning 1971–1987
RBU-Nytt 1976–2009
Steget 1984–1986
Stiletten 1987–2006
Svensk Handikapptidskrift 1965–2009
Svensk Vanföre-Tidskrift 1923–1965
Unik 2004

Books and Articles

Ahlberg, Eva. "Homo-Sverige utanför RFSL: En historisk exposé." In *Homo i folkhemmet: Homo-och bisexuella i Sverige, 1950–2000*, edited by Martin Andreasson, 76–91. Gothenburg: Anamma, 2000.

Anderson, Orieda Horn. *Doing What Comes Naturally? Dispelling Myths and Fallacies about Sexuality and People with Developmental Disabilities.* New Lenox, IL: High Tide Press, 2000.

Andreasson, Johannes. "Det är en myt att hotellgästerna vill se porr." *Hotellrevyn*, 5 March 2003.

Apelmo, Elisabeth. *Som vem som helst: Kön, funktionalitet och idrottande kroppar.* Lund University Dissertations in Sociology. Vol. 104. Lund: Lunds universitet, 2012.

Aronsson, Peter. *Bönder gör politik: Det lokala självstyret som social arena i tre Smålandssocknar, 1680–1850.* Lund: Lund University Press, 1992.

Attridge, Derek. "Following Derrida." www.usc.edu/dept/comp-lit/tympanum/4/attridge.html (accessed 19 April 2014).

Backlund, Christine, Anna Jerkovics, and Anette Erikson. "Åtta arbetsterapeuters förhållningssätt kring sex- och samlevnad och personer med utvecklingsstörning." C-uppsats från Arbetsterapeutprogrammet. Stockholm: Karolinska Institutet, 2003.

Baer, Robert W. *Is Fred Dead? A Manual on Sexuality for Men with Spinal Cord Injuries.* Pittsburg, PA: Domance, 2003.

Bahner, Julia. *Funktionshindrad sexualitet? En kvalitativ studie om personer med funktionsnedsättning och sexualitetsfrågor i vardagen med personlig assistans.* Gothenburg: Göteborgs universitet, 2010.

———. "Legal Rights or Simply Wishes? The Struggle for Sexual Recognition of People with Physical Disabilities Using Personal Assistance in Sweden." *Sexuality and Disability*, published online 10 May 2012.

Bakk, Ann, and Karl Grunewald. *Omsorgsboken: En bok om människor med begåvningsmässiga funktionshinder.* 4th ed. Stockholm: Esselte Studium, 2004.

Bech, Henning. "Report from a Rotten State: 'Marriage' and 'Homosexuality' in 'Denmark.'" In *Modern Homosexualities: Fragments of Gay and Lesbian Experience*, edited by Ken Plummer, 134–147. London: Routledge, 1992.

Bech, Henning, and Mehmet Ümit Necef. *Er danskerne racister? Indvandrerforskningens problemer.* Copenhagen: Frydenlund, 2012.

Berggren, Henrik, and Lars Trägårdh. *Är svensken människa? Gemenskap och oberoende i det moderna Sverige.* Stockholm: Norstedt, 2006.

———. "Pippi Longstocking and the Autonomous Child and the Moral Logic of the Swedish Welfare State." In *Swedish Modernism: Architecture, Consumption and the Welfare State*, edited by Helena Mattson and Sven-Olov Wallerstein, 50–65. London: Artifice Books on Architecture, 2010.

———. "Social Trust and Radical Individualism: The Paradox at the Heart of Nordic Capitalism." In *The Nordic Way: Equality, Individuality and Social Trust*, 13–29. Stockholm: Swedish Institute, 2012.

Bergqvist, Christina, ed. *Equal Democracies? Gender and Politics in the Nordic Countries.* Oslo: Scandinavian University Press, 1999.

Bernstein, Elizabeth. "Militarized Humanism Meets Carceral Feminism: The Politics of Sex, Rights, and Freedom in Contemporary Antitrafficking Campaigns." *Signs* 36, no. 1 (2010): 45–71.

Berubé, Michael. *Life as We Know It: A Father, a Family, and an Exceptional Child.* New York: Pantheon, 1996.

"Birgitta Hulter, vårdlärare: 'Uppmuntra sexualiteten men provocera inte!'" *Upptinget* 8 (1984): 8. www.sexterapi.se/Upptinget_argang8_1984.pdf (accessed 19 April 2014).

Bjørn, Claus. *Fra reaktion til grundlov, 1800–1850*. Gyldendal og Politikens Danmarkshistorie, vol. 10. Copenhagen: Gyldendal, 1990.

Bondeson, Ulla V. *Nordic Moral Climates: Value Continuities and Discontinuities in Denmark, Finland, Norway, and Sweden*. London: Transaction, 2003.

Borchorst, Anette, Ann-Dorte Christensen, and Birte Siim. "Diskurser om køn, magt og politik i Skandinavien." In *Kønsmagt under forandring*, edited by Anette Borchorst, 247–266. Copenhagen: Hans Reitzels forlag, 2002.

Brown, Ian. *The Boy in the Moon: A Father's Search for His Disabled Son*. New York: St. Martin's, 2011.

Buk-Swienty, Tom. *Slagtebænk Dybbøl: 18. april 1864*. Copenhagen: Gyldendal, 2008.

Buttenschøn, Jørgen. *Sexologi, en bog for professionelle og forældre om udviklingshæmmede menneskers sexualitet*. Glumsø: EIBA Press, 2001.

———. "Seksualiteten bliver tilladelig—Men hvordan med det private: Da de udviklingshæmmedes seksualitet blev anerkendt." *Handicaphistorisk Tidsskrift* 11 (2003): 121–159.

Childs, Marquis. *Sweden: The Middle Way*. New Haven, CT: Yale University Press, 1936.

Christensen, Ann-Dorte, and Poul Knopp Damkjær. *Kvinder og politisk repræsentation i Danmark*. Copenhagen: GEP—Forskningsprogram om køn, magt og politik, 1998.

Christiansen, Niels Finn, Klaus Petersen, Nils Edling, and Per Haave, eds. *The Nordic Model of Welfare: A Historical Reappraisal*. Copenhagen: Museum Tusculanum Press, 2006.

Clare, Eli. *Exile and Pride: Disability, Queerness, and Liberation*. Cambridge, MA: South End Press, 1999.

Cohen-Greene, Cheryl T., with Lorna Garano. *An Intimate Life: Sex, Love, and My Journey as a Surrogate Partner*. Berkeley, CA: Soft Skull Press, 2012.

Dahl, Ulrika. "Queer in the Nordic Region: Telling Queer (Feminist) Stories." In *Queer in Europe*, edited by Lisa Downing and Robert Gillett, 143–158. Surrey: Ashgate, 2011.

Dahlerup, Drude. *Rødstrømperne: Den danske Rødstrømpebevægelses udvikling, nytænkning og gennemslag 1970–1985*. Vols. 1–2. Copenhagen: Gyldendal, 1998.

———. "Er ligestillingen opnået? Ligestillingsdebattens forskellighed i Danmark og Sverige." In *Kønsmagt under forandring*, edited by Annette Borchorst, 226–247. Copenhagen: Hans Reitzels Forlag, 2002.

Davis, Lennard J. *Bending over Backwards: Disability, Dismodernism, and Other Difficult Positions*. New York: NYU Press, 2002.

Deal, Mark. "Disabled People's Attitudes towards Other Groups: A Hierarchy of Impairment." *Disability and Society* 18, no. 7 (2003): 897–910.

de Lauretis, Teresa. *The Practice of Love: Sexuality and Perverse Desire.* Bloomington: Indiana University Press, 1994.

Derrida, Jacques. "The Animal That Therefore I Am (More to Follow)." *Critical Inquiry* 28, no. 2 (2002): 369–418.

Desjardins, Michel. "The Sexualized Body of the Child: Parents and the Politics of 'Voluntary' Sterilization of People Labeled Intellectually Disabled." In *Sex and Disability*, edited by Robert McRuer and Anna Mollow, 69–88. Durham, NC: Duke University Press, 2012.

Earle, Sarah. "Facilitated Sex and the Concept of Sexual Need: Disabled Students and Their Personal Assistants." *Disability and Society* 14, no. 3 (1999): 309–323.

Enby, Gunnel. *Vi måste få älska: En bok om handikappade.* Stockholm: Prisma, 1972.

———. *Let There Be Love: Sex and the Handicapped.* Translated from the Swedish by Irène D. Morris. New York: Taplinger, 1975.

Enzensberger, Hans Magnus. *Svensk höst.* Stockholm: Dagens Nyheter, 1982.

Esping-Andersen, Gøsta. *The Three Worlds of Welfare Capitalism.* Cambridge: Polity, 1990.

Falkheimer, Jesper, and Mark Örsten. "Öresundsregionen i medieskugga." *Sydsvenskan*, 13 June 2013.

Feldbæk, Ole. *Den lange fred, 1700–1800.* Gyldendal og Politikens Danmarkshistorie. Vol. 9. Copenhagen: Gyldendal, 1990.

Finger, Anne. "Forbidden Fruit." *New Internationalist*, July 1992. http://newint .org/features/1992/07/05/fruit.

Flyckt, Karin, ed. *Våld mot kvinnor med psykiska funktionshinder: Förekomst, bemötande och tillgång till stöd.* Stockholm: Socialstyrelsen, 2005.

Foucault, Michel. *Remarks on Marx.* New York: Semiotext(e), 1991.

Framtiden och människor med omfattande funktionshinder: Seminarium 1 september 1989. 1989 års handikapputredning. Linköping: Linköpings universitet, institutionen för temaforskning 1989.

Frank, Gelya. *Venus on Wheels: Two Decades of Dialogue on Disability, Biography, and Being Female in America.* Berkeley: University of California Press, 1999.

FunkaPortalen. "Här är hemmet en arbetsmiljöfråga." *Funka Reportage.* www .funkaportalen.se/Reportage/Stod-Service/Assistans/Har-ar-hemmet-en -arbetsmiljofraga (accessed 19 April 2014).

Garland-Thomson, Rosemarie. *Staring: How We Look.* Oxford: Oxford University Press, 2009.

Goldberg, Ted. *Hur blir man narkoman? Och hur hindrar vi det?* Solna: Academic Publishing of Sweden, 2010.

Grealy, Lucy. *Autobiography of a Face.* New York: Houghton Mifflin, 1994.

Greengross, Wendy. *Entitled to Love: The Sexual and Emotional Needs of the Handicapped.* London: National Fund for Research into Crippling Diseases, 1976.

————. *Rätten att älska: Om känslomässiga och sexuella behov hos människor med handikapp*. Translated by Gunnel Enby and Marianne Rutberg; Swedish editing by Inger Nordqvist. Stockholm: Natur och Kultur, 1979.

Grönvik, Lars. "Kåta krymplingar." *Arena*, no. 6 (2005): 31–33.

Grönvik, Lars, and Mårten Söder, eds. *Bara funktionshindrad? Funktionshinder och intersektionalitet*. Malmö: Gleerups, 2008.

Grünberger, Pernille. *Seksuelle overgreb mod mennesker med handicap: Gode råd om at se og forebygge overgreb*. Copenhagen: Socialt Udviklingscenter SUS, 2010.

Grundtvig, N. F. S. *Nordens Mythologi eller Sindbilled-Sprog, historisk-poetisk udviklet og oplyst*. Copenhagen: Schubothe, 1832.

Grunewald, Karl. *Från idiot till medborgare: De utvecklingsstördas historia*. Stockholm: Gothia, 2009.

Grunewald, Karl, and Ann Bakk. *Omsorgsboken: En bok om psykisk utvecklingsstörning*. Stockholm: Esselte Studium, 1973.

————. *Nya omsorgsboken: En bok om människor med begåvningshandikapp*. Stockholm: Esselte Studium, 1986.

Grunewald, Karl, and Orvar Eeg-Olofsson. *Medicinska omsorgsboken: Om psykisk utvecklingsstörning med tillkommande handikapp*. Stockholm: Natur och Kultur, 1989.

Grunewald, Karl, and Hans Hallerfors. "Kan inte utvecklingsstörda onanera?" *Intra* 1 (1997): 12–13.

Gustavsson, Thomas. "–Min son vill vara med en naken tjej." *Aftonbladet*, 15 February 2007. www.aftonbladet.se/nyheter/article10878680.ab (accessed 19 April 2014).

Guter, Bob, and John R. Killacky, eds. *Queer Crips: Disabled Gay Men and Their Stories*. New York: Harrington Park, 2004.

Halley, Janet. *Split Decisions: How and Why to Take a Break from Feminism*. Princeton, NJ: Princeton University Press, 2006.

Hanamura, Haruki. *Niels Erik Bank-Mikkelsen: Father of the Normalization Principle*. Bogense: Niels Erik Bank-Mikkelsen Foundation, 1998.

Hartelius, Jonas. *Narkotikapolitik i Sverige*. Carnegie Dokumentationsserie (CDS) no. 18. Stockholm: Svenska Carnegieinstitutet, 2008.

Health Statistics for the Nordic Countries. Copenhagen: Nordisk Medicinalstatistisk Kommitté, 2011. http://nowbase.org/Publikationer/~/media/Projekt%20sites/Nowbase/Publikationer/Helse/Helse%202011.ashx (accessed 28 May 2011).

Heins, Agneta Berghamre, ed. *Gjort och ogjort med utgångspunkt från Handikapputredningens lägesrapport: Handikapp och välfärd? En översikt av remissynpunkter*. Rapport från 1989 års handikapputredning. Stockholm: 1989 års handikapputredning, 1991.

Hellman, Finn. "Queer- och handikappkonferens i San Francisco: Klarsyn och nytänkande genomsyrade konferensen." *lambda nordica* 17, nos. 1–2 ([2002] 2012): 21–26.

Hernes, Helga Maria. *Welfare and Woman Power: Essays in State Feminism*. Oslo: Norwegian University Press, 1987.

Hertz, Lone. *Sisyfosbreve*. Copenhagen: Gyldendals, 1992.

Hirdman, Yvonne. "Kønsmagt under behandling." KVINFO, 4 September 2002. www.kvinfo.dk/side/559/article/177 (accessed 19 April 2014).

Hoffman, Ulla. "Svar på Katarina Engströms inlägg." *Hotellrevyn*, 24 June 2003.

Hooper, Edward. "New Insights." In *The Ragged Edge: The Disability Experience from the Pages of the First Fifteen Years of The Disability Rag*, edited by Barrett Shaw, 78–81. Louisville, KY: Advocado, 1994.

Hudson, Barbara. *Justice in the Risk Society: Reaffirming "Justice" in Late Modernity*. London: Sage, 2004.

Huntford, Roland. *The New Totalitarians*. London: Allen Lane, 1971.

Hvidt, Kristian. *Det folkelige gennembrud og dets mænd*. Gyldendal og Politikens Danmarkshistorie. Vol. 11. Copenhagen: Gyldendal, 1990.

Hvinden, Bjørn. "Nordic Disability Politics in a Changing Europe: Is There Still a Distinct Nordic Model?" *Social Policy and Administration* 38, no. 2 (2004): 170–189.

Hydén, Håkan. *Om rättslig reglering*. Rapport från 1989 års handikapputredning. Lund: Lunds Universitet, Rättssociologiska avdelningen, 1991.

Jain, Sarah Lochlann. "Living in Prognosis: Toward an Elegiac Politics." *Representations* 98, no. 1 (2007): 77–92.

Jalving, Mikael. *Absolut Sverige: En rejse i tavshedens rige*. Copenhagen: Jyllands-Postens Forlag, 2011.

Jenkins, David. *Sweden and the Price of Progress*. New York: Coward-McCann, 1968.

Johansen, Mona, Else Merete Thyness, and Jan Holm. *Når seksualitet tages alvorligt*. Translated and adapted by Karin Møgelmose. Copenhagen: Gads Forlag, 2001.

Johansson, Peter. *Fast i det förflutna: Institutioner och intressen i svensk sjukförsäkringspolitik 1891–1931*. Lund: Arkiv, 2003.

Jonasen, Viggo. *Dansk socialpolitik 1708–2002*. 7th ed. Aarhus: Den sociale Højskole, 2003.

Jørgensen, Frank Ulmer. *Seksuelle overgreb—Nej tak!* Copenhagen: Socialt Udviklingscenter SUS, 2005.

Kailes, June Isaacson. *Language Is More Than a Trivial Concern!* 10th ed. Pomona, CA: Harris Family Center for Disability and Health Policy, 2010. www.jik.com /language%20FINAL-L-12.27.10.pdf (accessed 19 April 2014).

Katz, Gregor, ed. *Samlevnads- och sexualfrågor hos psykiskt utvecklingsstörda*. Stockholm: Svenska föreningen för psykisk hälsovård, 1970.

————. *Sexuality and Subnormality*. London: National Society for Mentally Handicapped Children, 1972.

Kaufman, Miriam, Cory Silverberg, and Fran Odette. *The Ultimate Guide to Sex and Disability*. San Francisco: Cleis, 2004.

Kingdon, John W. *Agendas, Alternatives, and Public Policies*. Updated 2nd ed. Boston: Longman, 2011.

Kirkebæk, Birgit. *Normaliseringens periode: Dansk åndssvageforsorg 1940–1970 med særlig fokus på forsorgschef N.E. Bank-Mikkelsen og udviklingen af Statens Åndssvageforsorg 1959–1970*. Holte: Forlaget SOCPOL, 2001.

————. "Er normaliseringens periode forbi? Om flyttetvang for udviklingshæmmede." *Centrum for Handicapforskning*, no. 21, article 1, July 2003. www .handicaphistorie.dk/chf/nyhedsbreve/200307/artikel01.php (accessed 9 August 2013).

Kittay, Eva Feder. *Love's Labor: Essays on Women, Equality, and Dependency*. New York: Routledge, 1999.

————. "The Personal Is the Philosophical Is the Political: A Philosopher and Mother of a Cognitively Disabled Person Sends Notes from a Battlefield." In *Cognitive Disability and Its Challenge to Moral Philosophy*, edited by Eva Feder Kittay and Licia Carlson, 393–413. Chichester: Wiley-Blackwell, 2010.

Knausgård, Karl Ove. *Min kamp: Andre bok*. Oslo: Forlaget Oktober, 2009.

Koch, Lene. *Tvangssterilisation i Danmark 1929–67*. Copenhagen: Gyldendal, 2000.

Kousmanen, Jari, and Mikaela Starke. "Identifying the Invisible: The Experiences of Prostitution among Persons with Intellectual Disabilities: Implications for Social Work." *Journal of Social Work* 13, no. 2 (2013): 123–140.

Kulick, Don, ed. *Queersverige*. Stockholm: Natur och Kultur, 2005.

————. "Danes Call People with Down Syndrome 'Mongol': Politically Incorrect Language and Ethical Engagement." In *Byen og blikkets lyst: Festskrift til Henning Bech*, edited by Marie Bruvik and Morten Emmerik Wøldike, 85–105. Seksualiteter (særudgivelse). Copenhagen: Skriftrække fra Center for Seksualitetsforskning, 2014.

Kuppers, Petra, and Neil Marcus. *Cripple Poetics: A Love Story*. Ypsilanti, MI: Homofactus, 2008.

Langfeldt, Thore, and Mary Porter. *Sexuality and Family Planning: Report of a Consultation and Research Findings*. Copenhagen: World Health Organization, Regional Office for Europe, 1986.

Lapper, Alison. *My Life in My Hands*. London: Simon and Schuster, 2006.

Lenger, Jørgen. "Mennesker med et handicap erobrede selv deres frihed." *Modkraft*, February 2013. http://modkraft.dk/blogindlæg/mennesker-med-et -handicap-erobrede-selv-deres-frihed (accessed 8 August 2013).

Lennerhed, Lena. *Frihet att njuta: Sexualdebatten i Sverige på 1960-talet.* Stockholm: Norstedts, 1994.

———. *Sex i folkhemmet:* RFSUs *tidiga historia.* Stockholm: Gidlunds förlag, 2002.

Levinas, Emmanuel. *Otherwise Than Being, or Beyond Essence.* Translated by Alphonso Lingis. Pittsburgh, PA: Duquesne University Press, 1998.

Linder, Åse. "Perspektiv på sexuella uttryckssätt i gruppboende: Hur personal bemöter och förhåller sig till sexuella uttryckssätt i ett gruppboende för personer med utvecklingsstörning." Flemingsberg: D-uppsats i etnologi, Södertörns högskola, 2006.

Lindqvist, Bengt. *Blindstyre.* Stockholm: Hjalmarson och Högberg Bokförlag, 2012.

Linton, Simi. *Claiming Disability: Knowledge and Identity.* New York: NYU Press, 1998.

Ljuslinder, Karin. "Handikappdiskurser i Svt: Exemplet Cp-Magasinet." In *Funktionshinder, kultur och samhälle,* edited by Rafael Lindqvist and Lennart Sauer, 215–238. Lund: Studentlitteratur, 2007.

Löfgren-Mårtenson, Lotta. *"Får jag lov?": Om sexualitet och kärlek i den nya generationen unga med utvecklingsstörning.* Lund: Studentlitteratur, 2005.

Løwert, Anette, and Karsten Løt. *På vej til voksen: Et undervisningsmateriale til seksualvejledning af unge.* Vejle: Forlaget Løwert, 2004.

Lunde, Helle. "De kommunefarvede danskere—En nation af mindretal." *Grus* 9, no. 26 (1988): 23–42.

Lunds kommun. "Personalens roll när det gäller vuxna brukares sexualitet." Lund: Vård- och Omsorgsförvaltningen, Omsorg och habilitering, 2006.

Mackelprang, Romel W., and Richard O. Salsgiver. *Disability: A Diversity Model Approach in Human Service Practices.* 2nd ed. Chicago: Lyceum, 2009.

MacKinnon, Catharine. "Trafficking, Prostitution, and Inequality." *Harvard Civil Rights–Civil Liberties Law Review* 46 (2011): 271–309.

Mairs, Nancy. *Waist-High in the World: A Life among the Nondisabled.* Boston: Beacon, 1996.

Mallander, Ove. *De hjälper oss till rätta: Normaliseringsarbete, självbestämmande och människor med psykisk utvecklingsstörning.* Lund: Socialhögskolan vid Lunds Universitet, 1999.

McCarthy, Michelle. *Sexuality and Women with Learning Disabilities.* London: Jessica Kingsley, 1999.

McRuer, Robert. *Crip Theory: Cultural Signs of Queerness and Disability.* New York: NYU Press, 2006.

McRuer, Robert, and Anna Mollow, eds. *Sex and Disability.* Durham, NC: Duke University Press, 2012.

Meyer, Frank. *"Dansken, svensken og nordmannen"—Skandinaviske habitusfor-skjeller sett i lys av kulturmøtet med tyske flyktninger: En komparativ studie.* 2nd ed. Oslo: Unipub, 2001.

———. "A Comparative Look at Scandinavian Cultures: Denmark, Norway and Sweden and Their Encounters with German Refugees, 1933–1940." *Journal of Intercultural Communication*, no. 12 (2006). www.immi.se/intercultural.

Modig, Arne. *Habilitering för barn och ungdomar med funktionshinder.* Rapport från 1989 års handikapputredning. Sollentuna: IMU-testologen, 1990.

———. *Samverkan mellan handikapporganisationer och samhälle: En enkätunder-sökning.* Rapport från 1989 års handikapputredning. Sollentuna: IMU-testologen, 1990.

Møller, Jes Fabricius. *Grundtvigianisme i det 20. århundrede.* Copenhagen: Vartov, 2005.

———. "Grundtvig og Marx." *Weekendavisen*, 16 May 2008.

Mollow, Anna. "Is Sex Disability? Queer Theory and the Disability Drive." In *Sex and Disability*, edited by Robert McRuer and Anna Mollow, 285–312. Durham, NC: Duke University Press, 2012.

Montan, Karl. *SVCK/SVCR:s historia åren 1950–92.* Vällingby: Stift. Svenska kommittén för rehabilitering (SVCR), 1995.

Moss, Kate, and Robbie Blaha. *Introduction to Sexuality Education for Individuals Who Are Deaf-Blind and Significantly Developmentally Delayed.* Monmouth, OR: National Information Clearing House on Children Who Are Deaf-Blind, 2001. nationaldb.org/documents/products/sex-ed.pdf (accessed 19 April 2014).

Muff, Elsebeth Kirk. *Seksuelle overgreb på mennesker med handicap: Et littera-turstudie.* Copenhagen: Socialt Udviklingscenter SUS, 2001.

Myrdal, Alva, and Gunnar Myrdal. *Kris i befolkningsfrågan.* Stockholm: Bonnier, 1934.

Nationellt råd för kvinnofrid. *När man slår mot det som gör ont: Våld mot kvinnor med funktionshinder.* Stockholm: Nationellt råd för kvinnofrid, 2001.

Nilsson, Lotta, and Olle Westlund. *Våld mot personer med funktionshinder.* Stockholm: Brottsförebyggande rådet, 2007.

Nirje, Bengt. "How I Came to Formulate the Normalization Principle." In *A Quarter-Century of Normalization and Social Role Valorization: Evolution and Impact*, edited by Robert J. Flynn and Raymond A. Lemay, 17–47. Ottawa: University of Ottawa Press, 1999.

———. *Normaliseringsprincipen.* Lund: Studentlitteratur, 2003.

Nordansjö, Johan. *Mitt nakna jag.* Stockholm: Debutantförlaget, 2005.

Nordeman, Margareta. "Visst behöver utvecklingsstörda hjälp med onani." *Intra* 3 (1997): 32.

———. *När känslan tar över: Sexualitet, utvecklingsstörning, autism.* Stockholm: Carlssons Förlag, 2005.

Nordqvist, Inger. *Utredning om hjälpmedel i sexualivet för män och kvinnor med funktionshinder.* Bromma: Handikappinstitutet, 1988.

———. Supplement to *Utredning om hjälpmedel i sexualivet för män och kvinnor med funktionshinder.* Bromma: Handikappinstitutet, 1988.

Nussbaum, Martha. *Women and Human Development: The Capabilities Approach.* Cambridge: Cambridge University Press, 2000.

———. "Capabilities as Fundamental Entitlements: Sen and Social Justice." *Feminist Economics* 9, nos. 2–3 (2003): 33–59.

———. *Frontiers of Justice: Disability, Nationality, Species Membership.* Cambridge, MA: Harvard University Press, 2006.

———. "The Capabilities of People with Cognitive Disabilities." *Metaphilosophy* 40, nos. 3–4 (2009): 331–351.

O'Brien, Mark. *The Man in the Iron Lung.* Berkeley, CA: Lemonade Factory, 1997.

———. "The Sex Surrogate." In Mark O'Brien, with Gillian Kendall, *How I Became a Human Being: A Disabled Man's Quest for Independence*, 213–221. Madison: University of Wisconsin Press, 2003.

Olsson, Sören. "Min son sa att han vill ha en tjej som på film." Krönika av Sören Olsson i Föräldrakraft no. 1. *Föräldrakraft*, 12 February 2007.

Öppna jämförelser av stöd till personer med funktionsnedsättning 2013—Resultat och metod. Socialstyrelsens publikationer 2013-5-31. Stockholm: Socialstyrelsen, 2013.

Organisation for Economic Co-operation and Development (OECD). "Government Social Spending: Total Public Social Expenditure as a Percentage of GDP." *Social Issues: Key Tables from OECD*, no. 1 (2012). http://dx.doi.org/10.1787/20743904 (accessed 20 April 2014).

Österberg, Eva. "Compromise instead of Conflict? Patterns of Contact between Local Peasant Communities and the Early Modern State: Sweden in the Sixteenth to Eighteenth Centuries." In *Agrarian Society in History: Essays in Honour of Magnus Mörner*, edited by Mats Lundahl and Thommy Svensson, 263–281. London: Routledge, 1990.

———. *Folk förr: Historiska essäer.* Stockholm: Atlantis, 1995.

Østergaard, Uffe. "Findes der en dansk politisk kultur?" In *Enhedskultur—Helhedskultur*, edited by Anne Holmen and Jens Normann Jorgensen. Copenhagen: Danmarks Lærerhøjskole, 1989.

Personer med funktionsnedsättning—Insatser enligt LSS år 2012. Sveriges Officiella Statistik. Socialtjänst. Socialstyrelsens publikationer 2013-3-30. Stockholm: Socialstyrelsen, 2013.

Personer med funktionsnedsättning—Vård och omsorg 1 oktober 2012: Kommunala insatser enligt socialtjänstlagen samt hälso- och sjukvårdslagen. Sveriges Officiella Statistik. Socialtjänst. Socialstyrelsens publikationer 2013-4-18. Stockholm: Socialstyrelsen, 2013.

Puar, Jasbir K. "Prognosis Time: Towards a Geopolitics of Affect, Debility and Capacity." *Women and Performance: A Journal of Feminist Theory* 19, no. 2 (2009): 161–172.

Rawls, John. *A Theory of Justice.* Cambridge, MA: Harvard University Press, 1971.

———. *Political Liberalism.* Enl. ed. New York: Columbia University Press, 1996.

Redaktionen. "Kommentar till Margareta Nordemans inlägg." *Intra* 3 (1997): 33.

Rich, Adrienne. "Compulsory Heterosexuality and Lesbian Existence." *Signs* 5, no. 4 (1980): 631–660.

Risberg, Olof. *"Vem vill vara ihop med mig då?" Om behandling, sexuella övergrepp och utvecklingsstörning.* Stockholm: Rädda barnen, 2004.

Rorty, Richard. "Human Rights, Rationality and Sentimentality." In *On Human Rights: The Oxford Amnesty Lectures 1993*, edited by Stephen Shute and Susan Hurley. New York: Basic Books, 1993.

Rothenborg, Ole. "Sexköp med bidrag." *Dagens Nyheter*, 25 September 2005.

Rubin, Gayle. "Thinking Sex: Notes for a Radical Theory of the Politics of Sexuality." In *The Lesbian and Gay Studies Reader*, edited by Henry Abelove, Michèle Aina Barale, and David Halperin, 3–44. New York: Routledge, [1984] 1993.

Rydström, Jens, ed. "Cripteori." Special issue, *lambda nordica* 17, nos. 1–2 (2012).

Sanders, Teela. "The Politics of Sexual Citizenship: Commercial Sex and Disability." *Disability and Society* 22, no. 5 (2007): 439–455.

Sen, Amartya. "Equality of What?" In *Choice, Welfare and Measurement*, 353–369. Oxford: Basil Blackwell, 1982.

———. *The Idea of Justice.* Cambridge, MA: Harvard University Press, 2009.

Sevenhuijsen, Selma. *Citizenship and the Ethics of Care: Feminist Considerations on Justice, Morality and Politics.* New York: Routledge, 1998.

Shakespeare, Tom. "Disabled Sexuality: Towards Rights and Recognition." *Sexuality and Disability* 18, no. 3 (2000): 159–166.

———. *Disability Rights and Wrongs.* London: Routledge, 2006.

Shakespeare, Tom, Kath Gillespie-Sells, and Dominic Davies. *The Sexual Politics of Disability: Untold Desires.* London: Cassell, 1996.

Shildrick, Margrit. *Dangerous Discourses of Disability, Subjectivity and Sexuality.* London: Palgrave MacMillan, 2009.

———. "Critical Disability Studies: Rethinking Conventions for the Age of Postmodernity." In *Routledge Handbook of Disability Studies*, edited by Alan Roulstone and Carol Thomas, 30–41. London: Routledge, 2012.

Shuttleworth, Russell. "Disabled Masculinity: Expanding the Masculine Reper-
toire." In *Gendering Disability*, edited by Bonnie Smith and Beth Hutchinson,
166–178. New Brunswick, NJ: Rutgers University Press, 2004.

———. "Disability and Sexuality: Toward a Constructionist Focus on Access and
the Inclusion of Disabled People in the Sexual Rights Movement." In *Sexual
Inequalities and Social Justice*, edited by Niels Teunis and Gilbert Herdt, 174–
207. Berkeley: University of California Press, 2006.

———. "Bridging Theory and Experience: A Critical-Interpretive Ethnography of
Sexuality and Disability." In *Sex and Disability*, edited by Robert McRuer and
Anna Mollow, 54–68. Durham, NC: Duke University Press, 2012.

Shuttleworth, Russell, and Teela Sanders, eds. *Sex and Disability: Politics, Identity
and Access*. Leeds: Disability Press, 2010.

Siebers, Tobin. *Disability Theory*. Ann Arbor: University of Michigan Press,
2008.

Silverberg, Cory. "Sexual Surrogacy Revisited." *Contemporary Sexuality* 47, no. 1
(2013): 1–6.

Sjölander-Holland, Ann-Christin. "Komma nära den man vårdar." *Kommunalarbetaren*, no. 7 (1999).

———, ed. "Sex i vården." Special issue, *Kommunalarbetaren*, no. 7 (1999).

———. "Lär av Danmark!" *Kommunalarbetaren*, no. 15 (2007): 35.

Skogeman, Pia. "Kampen om et sprog." *Berlingske Tidende*, 11 September 1992.

Socialministeriet. *Vejledning om seksualitet—uanset handicap*. Socialministeriets
7. Kontor, 2001.

Socialstyrelsen. *Vejledning om seksualitet—uanset handicap*. Copenhagen: SIKON,
1989.

———. *LSS: Lagen om stöd och service till vissa funktionshindrade*. Allmänna råd
från Socialstyrelsen 1994:1. Stockholm: Socialstyrelsen, 1994.

———. *Sällan sedda: Utbildningsmaterial om våld mot kvinnor med funktionsnedsättning*. Stockholm: Socialstyrelsen, 2011.

———. *Seksualitet på dagsordenen: En håndbog om professionel støtte til voksne
med funktionsnedsættelse*. Odense: Socialstyrelsen, 2012.

Socioekonomisk situation för personer med funktionshinder: En intervjustudie.
Rapport från 1989 års handikapputredning. Stockholm: Socialdepartementet,
1991.

Söder, Mårten, ed. *Brukarinflytande, livsinflytande, delaktighet: Om situationen
för människor med funktionsnedsättningar i det offentliga hjälpsystemet. Rapport från seminarium 18 augusti 1989*. Uppsala: 1989 års handikapputredning,
1989.

Söder, Mårten, Karin Barron, and Ingrid Nilsson. *Handikapp och välfärd? En lägesrapport*. Bilagerapport: Inflytande för människor med omfattande funktions-

hinder. *Redovisning av en intervjuundersökning*. Stockholm: Allmänna förlaget, 1990.

Söderman, Lena, and Sievert Antonsson, eds. *Nya omsorgsboken*. Stockholm: Liber, 2011.

Sontag, Susan. "A Letter from Sweden." *Ramparts Magazine*, July 1969.

SOU. *See* Statens offentliga utredningar.

Spinalis. *Ny kraft för skadad ryggmärg*. Stockholm: Stiftelsen Spinalis, 1995.

Standard Rules on the Equalization of Opportunities for Persons with Disabilities. Resolution 48/96, passed by the United Nations General Assembly, 20 December 1993. www.un.org/esa/socdev/enable/dissre00.htm.

Statens offentliga utredningar (SOU). 1954:28. *Vanföreanstalterna och Eugeniahemmet: Riktlinjer för organisationen m.m. av ortoped- och spastikervården samt viss arbetsvård för partiellt arbetsföra*, 1951 års vanförevårdsutredning. Stockholm: Inrikesdepartementet, 1954.

———. 1967:53. *Kommunerna och den sociala omvårdnaden: Rapport och förslag*, handikapputredningen. Stockholm: Nordiska Bokhandeln, 1967.

———. 1967:60. *Bättre hjälpmedel för handikappade: Förslag av Handikapputredningen*. Stockholm: Socialdepartementet, 1967.

———. 1969:35. *Bättre utbildning för handikappade: Förslag av Handikapputredningen*. Stockholm: Socialdepartementet, 1969.

———. 1970:64. *Bättre socialtjänst för handikappade: Förslag från Handikapputredningen om bättre färdmöjligheter för handikappade och bättre samordning i handikappfrågor*. Stockholm: Socialdepartementet, 1970.

———. 1972:30. *Bostadsanpassningsbidrag: Förslag från Handikapputredningen*. Stockholm: Inrikesdepartementet, 1972.

———. 1976:9. *Sexuella övergrepp: Förslag till ny lydelse av brottsbalkens bestämmelser om sedlighetsbrott*, betänkande av sexualbrottsutredningen. Stockholm: Liber Förlag / Allmänna förlaget, 1976.

———. 1976:20. *Kultur åt alla: Betänkande från Handikapputredningen*. Stockholm: Utbildningsdepartementet, 1976.

———. 1982:61. *Våldtäkt och andra sexuella övergrepp*, betänkande av 1977 års sexualbrottskommitté. Stockholm: Liber Förlag / Allmänna förlaget, 1982.

———. 1989:39a. *Hjälpmedelsverksamhetens utveckling: Kartläggning och bedömning*, betänkande av Hjälpmedelsutredningen. Stockholm: Allmänna förlaget, 1989.

———. 1989:39b. *Hjälpmedelsverksamhetens utveckling: Kartläggning och bedömning*, bilagor [attachments]. Stockholm: Allmänna förlaget, 1989.

———. 1989:54. *Rätt till gymnasieutbildning för svårt rörelsehindrade ungdomar*, delbetänkande av 1989 års handikapputredning. Stockholm: Allmänna förlaget, 1989.

———. 1990:2. *Överklagningsrätt och ekonomisk behovsprövning inom socialtjänsten*, delbetänkande av 1989 års handikapputredning. Stockholm: Allmänna Förlaget, 1990.

———. 1990:19. *Handikapp och välfärd? En lägesrapport*, delbetänkande av 1989 års handikapputredning. Stockholm: Allmänna Förlaget, 1990.

———. 1990:44. *Demokrati och makt i Sverige: Maktutredningens huvudrapport.* Stockholm: Allmänna Förlaget, 1990.

———. 1991:46. *Handikapp, välfärd, rättvisa*, betänkande av 1989 års handikapputredning. Stockholm: Allmänna Förlaget, 1991.

———. 1991:97. *En väg till delaktighet och inflytande: Tolk för döva, dövblinda, vuxendöva, hörselskadade och talskadade*, delbetänkande av 1989 års handikapputredning. Stockholm: Allmänna Förlaget, 1991.

———. 1992:52. *Ett samhälle för alla*, slutbetänkande. Stockholm: Allmänna förlaget, 1992.

———. 1994:56. *Ett centrum för kvinnor som våldtagits och misshandlats*, delbetänkande av Kvinnovåldskommissionen. Stockholm: Allmänna Förlaget, 1994.

———. 1995:60. *Kvinnofrid*, huvudbetänkande av Kvinnovåldskommissionen. Stockholm: Allmänna Förlaget, 1995.

———. 1998:6. *Ty makten är din . . . Myten om det rationella arbetslivet och det jämställda Sverige*, betänkande från Kvinnomaktutredningen. Stockholm: Allmänna förlaget, 1998.

Steimer, Miriam, and Anna Stommel. "Sexualbegleiterin: 90 Euro für eine Stunde Zärtlichkeit" [Sexual companion: 90 Euros for an hour's tenderness]. *Spiegel Online*, 16 August 2012. www.spiegel.de/panorama/gesellschaft/sex-fuer-behinderte-menschen-die-dienste-einer-sexualbegleiterin-a-850166-druck.html (accessed 3 May 2014).

Stenström, Nils. *Sprutbyte vid intravenöst narkotamissbruk: En longitudinell studie av deltagarna i sprutbytesprogrammet i Malmö.* Östersund: Department of Social Work, Mid-Sweden University, 2008.

Stetson, Dorothy McBride, and Amy Mazur, eds. *Comparative State Feminism.* Thousand Oaks, CA: Sage, 1995.

Storm, Jorie, and Jenny Särnholm. "Gränslös glädje—Vägen till rättvisa? En kvalitativ studie om hur människor tolkar skildringen av intellektuellt funktionshindrade i dokumentären 'I en annan del av Köping.'" Gothenburg: Institutionen för journalistik och masskommunikation, Göteborgs universitet, 2007.

Straffelovrådets betænkning om seksualforbrydelser. Betænkning no. 1534. Copenhagen: Justitsministeriet, 2012.

Sundet, Marit. *Jeg vet jeg er annerledes—Men ikke bestandig: en antropologisk studie av hverdagslivet til fem personer med psykisk utviklingshemning.* Uppsala: Institutionen för kulturantropologi och etnologi, 1997.

Sundin, Jörgen. "Personliga assistenter ofredades sexuellt." *Allehanda.se*, 9 January 2010.

Svensk, Veronica. *Hemligheter kända av många: En metod- och handbok för dig som har personlig assistans.* Stockholm: Förbundet Unga Rörelsehindrade, 2011.

Svensson, Bengt. *Narkotikapolitik och narkotikadebatt.* Lund: Studentlitteratur, 2012.

Sveriges Officiella Statistik. *Kommunala insatser enligt socialtjänstlagen samt hälso- och sjukvårdslagen: Personer med funktionsnedsättning—vård och omsorg 1 oktober 2012.* Stockholm: Socialstyrelsen, 2013.

Systembolaget. *Bokslutskommuniké 2012.* www.systembolaget.se/ImageVaultFiles /id_21669/cf_364/bokslutskommunike_2012.PDF.

Tham, Henrik. *Från behandling till straffvärde: Kriminalpolitik i en förändrad välfärdsstat.* Stockholm: Kriminologiska institutionen, Stockholms universitet, 1996.

———. "Swedish Drug Policy: A Successful Model?" *European Journal on Criminal Policy and Research* 6, no. 3 (1998): 395–414.

Thing, Morten. "Kulturradikalismen: Radikalismens anden fase." In *Den kulturradikale udfordring: Kulturradikalismen gennem 130 år*, 113–130. Copenhagen: Tiderne Skifter, 2001.

Thomsen, Niels, and Hans Vium Mikkelsen, eds. *Hvor blev det grundtvigske af?* Frederiksberg: Aros, 2004.

Thomsson, Ulrika. "Rätten till våra kroppar: Kvinnorörelsen och våldtäktsdebatten." *Kvinnovetenskaplig Tidskrift* 21, no. 4 (2000): 51–63.

Tinning, Steen. "Sjovere handicapsex i sigte . . ." *LEV–Evnesvages Vel*, no. 5, 1987.

Tronto, Joan C. *Moral Boundaries: A Political Argument for an Ethic of Care.* New York: Routledge, 1993.

Turner, Bryan S. *Vulnerability and Human Rights.* University Park: Pennsylvania State University Press, 2006.

Tydén, Mattias. *Från politik till praktik: De svenska steriliseringslagarna 1935–1975.* 2nd, enl. ed. Stockholm: Almqvist and Wiksell 2002.

Ullerstam, Lars. *The Erotic Minorities: A Swedish View.* New York: Grove, 1966.

Vallberg, Elisabeth. "'Vi måste träna deras sexuella förmåga—Handgripligen.' Intervju med Hans Wrenne." *Ottar*, no. 4 (1982): 89–93.

Vance, Carole S. "Innocence and Experience: Melodramatic Narratives of Sex Trafficking and Their Consequences for Law and Policy." *History of the Present* 2, no. 2 (2012): 200–218.

Vind, Ole. "Grundtvig og det danske—Med sideblik til Sverige." In *Grundtvig: Nyckeln till det danska?*, edited by Hanne Sanders and Ole Vind. Gothenburg: Makadam, 2003.

Wad, Gunnar. "Seksualvejledning i træningsskolen." *S.Å.-Pædagogen*, nos. 19–20 (1968): 450.

Wade, Cheryl Marie. "It Ain't Exactly Sexy." In *The Ragged Edge: The Disability Experience from the Pages of the First Fifteen Years of The Disability Rag*, edited by Barrett Shaw, 88–90. Louisville, KY: Advocado, 1994.

Weise, Jillian. *The Amputee's Guide to Sex*. Berkeley, CA: Soft Skull Press, 2007.

Wendell, Susan. *The Rejected Body: Feminist Philosophical Reflections on Disability*. London: Routledge, 1996.

Williams, Fiona. "In and Beyond New Labour: Towards a New Political Ethics of Care." *Critical Social Policy* 21, no. 4 (2001): 467–492.

Wingaard, Majken. *Migrantprostitution i Danmark*. Copenhagen: Servicestyrelsen, 2010.

World Health Organization. *Defining Sexual Health: Report of a Technical Consultation on Sexual Health, 28–31 January 2002*. Geneva: World Health Organization, 2006.

———. "Sexual and Reproductive Health." http://www.who.int/reproductivehealth/topics/sexual_health/sh_definitions/en/ (accessed 26 May 2014).

Wotton, Rachel, and Saul Isbister. "A Sex Worker Perspective on Working with Clients with a Disability and the Development of Touching Base Inc." In *Sex and Disability: Politics, Identity and Access*, edited by Russell Shuttleworth and Teela Sanders, 155–178. Leeds: Disability Press, 2010.

Young, Iris Marion. "Asymmetrical Reciprocity: On Moral Respect, Wonder and Enlarged Thought." *Constellations* 3, no. 3 (1997): 340–363.

Multimedia

August, Bille, dir. *Tomas—Et barn du ikke kan nå* [Tomas—A child you can't reach]. 1980.

Campredon, Samantha, and François Chayé, dirs. *L'Amour sans limites* [Love without limits]. System TV (France), 2008.

Granvik, Margot, and Eva Wernlid, dirs., *Säga ja, säga nej: Vem ska få krama mig?* [Say yes, say no: Who gets to hug me?]. Stockholm: Riksförbundet FUB, 1995.

Kabilio, Eli, dir. *F**k the Disabled: The Surprising Adventures of Greg Walloch*. New York, 2001.

Onaniteknik för kvinnor, onaniteknik för män: En instruktionsfilm från RFSU, riktad till människor med utvecklingsstörning [Masturbation techniques for women, masturbation techniques for men: Two instructional videos on masturbation techniques for people with developmental disabilities]. Screenwriter: Margareta Nordeman. Produced with financial support from

Statens Institut för Handikappfrågor i Skolan (SIH). Stockholm: RFSU, [1996] 2007.

Overaa, Kurt, dir. *Faktisk mangler man ord for det—En film om udviklingshæmmede og seksualitet* [One doesn't have words for it—A film about learning disabilities and sexuality]. Kurt Overaa Videoproduktion, 1994.

Scott, Catherine, dir.; Pat Fiske, prod. *Scarlet Road*. Paradigm Pictures, 2011.

Wickman, Torgny, dir. *Mera ur kärlekens språk* [More from the language of love]. Merry Film, Swedish Film Productions (SFP), 1970.

Wotton, Rachel. Conversations with Richard Fidler, 31 January 2012. ABC Local (Australia) podcast. www.abc.net.au/local/stories/2012/01/31/3419557.htm.

Note: Page numbers in *italics* refer to illustrations.

"able-disabled" (Wade), 268–269
absence-excess paradox, 171–172
abuse, sexual: boundary between affection and, 151–164; capabilities approach and, 287, 292; Danish discussions on, 18, 56; Danish publications and attitudes on, 69, 70, 109, 157–163, 260; disabled men accused of, 90–92; emotional blackmail, 141–142; fears of, 2, 8; "If I don't do anything . . ." formulation and, 90–93; male helper vulnerability to charges of, 90, 142; McCarthy on, 10; plans of action as guarding against, 107; sex work as, 177; Swedish discussions on, 2, 13, 17, 90–92, 136, 138, 240, 263, 289–290, 293, 312n8; Swedish publications regarding, 153–157, 240; talking about sex as preventing abuse, 158; talking about sex considered abuse, 8, 85, 88, 93, 115, 130, 180; unreported sexual assault, 113
access, sexual, meanings of, 19–20
activism: disability rights movement, 5–6, 268–269; leftist and Marxist, 58–63, 226; Lenger and, 65–66
affection-abuse boundary, 151–164
"Affiliation" capability, 283, 286
Aftonbladet, 176
agents of change, 240–246
A.H. Bulletin (A.H.-Bulletinen), 58–60, 63
alcohol policies, 219–220, 315n3
Amour sans limites, L' (Love without limits) (film), 185, 213

amputees, 7, 9, 10, 171

Åndssvageforsorgen. *See* State Services for the Feebleminded, Denmark

Åndssvageloven (Feebleminded Act of 1959, Denmark), 40–41, 48–49

animals and relevance to theorizing disability, 272–273

Ankilewitz, Ami, 139

Anti-Handikapp, 58–60, 63

Apollonia conference (Stockholm, 1966), 39–42, 218, 219

Arbetsmiljölagen (Work Environment Act, Sweden), 136–137, 309n20

Arbetsmiljöverket (Work Environment Authority, Sweden), 309n20

arbetsterapeuter (occupational therapists), 82–83, 307n6

Arena, 256

Århus, Denmark, 45–46, 65, 68, 70, 248, 253, 258

Århus arrangement (Århusordningen), 45–46, 66

Asperger's syndrome, 191, 204–205

Assange, Julian, 236

assault, unreported, 113. *See also* abuse, sexual

Assistance Act of 1974, Denmark (Bistandsloven), 45, 46, 66

Assistive Devices Commission, Sweden, 74–75, 303n42

Association of Dwarves (Dværgeforeningen), 35

Association of Mobility Impaired Youth (Förbundet Unga Rörelsehindrade), 256

Association of Spastics (Spastikerforeningen), 35

asymmetrical reciprocity, 267–268

August, Bille, 311n1

autism, 97, 144–148, 191, 204, 231

aversion techniques, 81

Bahner, Julia, 26, 93

Bank-Mikkelsen, Niels Erik: as agent of change, 242; education section and, 64; on Mose Allé school letter, 56–57; National Board of Social Services and, 66, 68; normalization principle and, 48–49; at Nyborg conference, 40–41; Six Commandments of, 57, 64–65

Barnes, Colin, 47–48

Barsøe, Lone, 61, 243

Beauvoir, Simone de, 270

Bech, Henning, 217, 224, 319n54

Bentham, Jeremy, 272–273

Berggren, Henrik, 217, 228–231, 316n27

Bergström-Walan, Maj-Briht, 131–133

Bernstein, Elizabeth, 236

Berubé, Michael, 28

Bistandsloven (Assistance Act of 1974, Denmark), 45, 46, 66

Bjerrehus, Suzanne, 181–182

Bjørkman, Birgitte, 61–62

blackmail, emotional, 141–142

blindness, 12, 28, 45, 53, 54, 97, 131–133, 141, 211–214, 231, 288, 309n13

Bliss, Charles (aka Karl Blitz), 106

Bliss boards, 106, 313n28

"Bodily Health" capability, 282, 284

"Bodily Integrity" capability, 282, 286

body image, 209–210

Borchorst, Annette, 232–233, 235, 236

Borgerstyret Personlig Assistance (BPA; Citizen-Controlled Personal Assistance, Denmark), 46, 301n14

Bøssernes Befrielses Front (Gay Liberation Front, Denmark), 60–61

boundaries: about, 120; affection vs. abuse, 151–164; disability, sexuality, and paradoxes of, 171–173; Marcus on, 117–118; mothers and love vs. sex,

143–150; private vs. public, 120–134; relationship boundaries and emotional blackmail, 138–143; sex vs. reproduction, 164–171; work vs. intimacy, 112, 134–143

Boy in the Moon (Brown), 27

BPA (Borgerstyret Personlig Assistance; Citizen-Controlled Personal Assistance, Denmark), 46, 301n14

Bramming, Jeannette, 119

"broad-mindedness" (*frisind*), 217, 224–227

Brosbøl, Kirsten, 259

Bureau for Handicap Issues, Sweden (Byrån för Handikappfrågor), 39, 217

"But's 4-step plan" (*But's 4 trins plan*), 65, 70

Buttenschøn, Jørgen, 66, 68, 71, 85, 124, 245; as agent of change, 242–243, 258; *Cerebral Palsy Show* interview, 250, 252–254, 258, 294; on food used to repress sexual feelings, 42; "4-step plan" of, 65, 70; Nadja Mac's speech recalled by, 148–149; recruited by Bank-Mikkelsen, 64–65; as sexual education advisor, 70, 101, 305n73

Bylund, Christine, vii

Byrån för Handikappfrågor (Bureau for Handicap Issues, Sweden), 39

capabilities approach, 21–22, 264, 265, 276–287, 291–293, 322n39

capitalism, 58–59

care, feminist ethics of, 273–277

Care Book, The (*Omsorgsboken*) (Grunewald), 217–218

Care Law, Sweden (1967), 45, 301n8

Care Law, Sweden (1985), 46

case examples: Alida (sexual advisor), 161–163; Anders, 210–211; Anna, 214; Anne (sexual advisor), 196–197; Annette (sex worker), 206; Axel Branting, 1–2, 12; Bettan, 88–90, 106, 290; Camille (sex worker), 188–192, 200–201, 207; David and Lisa, 111–112, 117; Dorte and Ragnar, 161, 162–163; Eva, 182–184, 216; Eva (sexual advisor), 168–170; Flemming, 193, 197; Gull-Marie (mother), 146–148; Helle Rasmussen, 106–108, 116, 269; Inger, 209; Ingrid, 110, 116; Jonas, 211–213; Jute (sex worker), 191, 206–207, 210–211; Karin (personal assistant), 93; Krister Andersson (occupational therapist), 82–83; Lars, 106–107; Lena and Carina from *Say "Yes," Say "No"* (film), 155–156; Linda and Mats from *In Another Part of Köping* (reality series), 94–96, 98; man with Asperger's syndrome, 204–205; Marcus's interview statement, 117–118; Maria, 213–214; Max from *My Naked Self*, 192, 207–208, 313n27; Pernille, 152–153, 163–164, 213, 231; Peter (sex worker), 191, 194–195, 198–200, 205, 231; Rasmus, 193–195, 198–200, 205, 214–215, 231, 269, 313n28; Sanne (sex worker), 190–192, 207; side-of-the-highway case, 126–127; Søren (sexual advisor), 202–205; Steen and Marianne, 97–102, 101, 111, 215, 231, 269; Susanne, 166–171; Viktoria (personal assistant), 79, 87, 93, 114; woman who blackmailed her personal assistants, 141–142; woman who experienced orgasm by being lifted, 1–2, 12, 142, 264

cerebral palsy, persons with: assistance and, 117–118, 122–123, 140; body image and, 210; Danish word for, 35; Dorte and Ragnar, 161, 162–163; Hansen and, 258–260; hierarchy of desirability and, 214–215; impairment

cerebral palsy, persons with (*continued*)
vs. disability and, 34; Marcus's interview statement, 117–118; Pernille,
152–153, 163–164; plans of action for,
106; Rasmus, 193–195, 198–200, 205,
214–215, 231, 269, 313n28; relaxation
after sex, 216; Sesha Kittay, 27, 28;
sexual education and, 110; sex workers
and, 182, 191, 200, 207; Shuttleworth
on, 19, 26; Swedish words for, 248,
249, 254, 313n27; sympathy and, 3
Cerebral Palsy Show, The (CP *Show*;
CP-*magasinet*), 248–255, 258, 294,
319n59
certification of sexual advisors, 101–102
change, model of, 240–246
Childs, Marquis, 52
Christensen, Ann-Dorthe, 232–233, 235,
236
Citizen-Controlled Personal Assistance,
Denmark (Borgerstyret
Personlig Assistance, BPA), 46, 301n14
Civil Servant Magazine (*Funktionærbladet*), 84–85
Cohen-Greene, Cheryl, 158, 208–210,
312n17
Coming Home (film), 8
Commission on Power, Sweden (Mak-
tutredningen), 234–235
Commission on Violence against
Women, Sweden (Kvinnovåldskommissionen), 235
Commission on Women's Power,
Sweden (Kvinnomaktutredningen),
235
Communist Party: Danish, 226; Swed-
ish, 241
compulsory able-bodiedness, 14
conformity in Sweden, 237–238
consensus, Swedish culture of, 223, 224,
237–238, 247

contraception, 57, 59, 108, 166, 170–171,
263
contractarian theories of justice,
278–281, 321n28
"Control over one's Environment"
capability, 283
Copenhagen code of conduct (Københavner kodeks), 259–260, 261
couples: David and Lisa, 111–112, 117;
Dorte and Ragnar, 161, 162–163; Linda
and Mats from *In Another Part of
Köping* (reality series), 94–96, 98;
Steen and Marianne, 97–102, 111, 215,
231, 269
CP-*magasinet* (*The Cerebral Palsy Show,
CP Show*), 248–255, 258, 294, 319n59
crip theory, 13–17, 269
Crutch Ensemble (Krykensemblen),
62–63, 243
cultural studies approaches, 10, 11, 13–17,
172
culture, political and public: Danish
"broad-mindedness," 217, 224–227;
political authority and, 223–224;
Swedish statist individualism and
"theory of love," 217, 227–232

Dagens Nyheter, 248, 299n12
Dahlerup, Drude, 222
Danish national parliament, 65–66
Danish People's Party (Dansk
Folkeparti, DF), 226, 318n54
Dansk Folkeparti (DF; Danish People's
Party), 226, 318n54
Davies, Dominic, 9
Davis, Lennard, 27
deafness and the deaf, 15, 29–30, 45, 97,
100, 231
De Handikappades Riksförbund (DHR;
Swedish National Association for the
Handicapped), 58

de-institutionalization, 49, 302n25

Denmark: abuse, publications and attitudes on, 157–163; alcohol policies, 219–220; Bank-Mikkelsen's Six Commandments, 56–57; "But's 4-step plan," 64–65, 70; certified sexual advisors, 101–102; drug policies, 221; engagement and discussion in, 18; *frisind* ("broad-mindedness"), 217; group home, description of, 30–31; group home discussions, role playing, and policy, 108–110; group homes where sexuality is unacknowledged, 112–113; immigration rhetoric and policies, 247, 318n54; leftist disability activism in, 60–63; Left Socialist Party proposal, 65–66; National Board of Services report, 66–68; normalization principle and, 48–50; Nyborg Conference (1967), 40–41, 55; political incorrectness and language issues in, 35–38; profile and history, 43–45; recent trends in, 258–261; rumors about, 18; satisfaction in, 265; "sleeping bear" reasoning in, 84–85; sterilization laws, 165; subsidized sex aids proposal and debate, 73–77; Sweden, 178–179; Sweden compared and contrasted with, 3–4, 43–45; welfare assistance laws and pensions, 45–47. *See also* difference factors between Sweden and Denmark; *Guidelines about Sexuality—Regardless of Handicap*; *specific agencies, organizations, and persons*

Derrida, Jacques, 272–276, 292

desirability, hierarchy of, 214–215

Desjardins, Michel, 26, 27

De Vanföras Riksförbund (National Association of Cripples, Sweden), 50

difference factors between Sweden and Denmark: agents of change and windows of opportunity, 240–246; alcohol, drug, and sexuality policies and laws, 219–223; Danish "broad-mindedness," 217, 224–227; engagement, scope of, 245–246; feminism, types of, 232–240; Grunewald on, 217–219; political authority structures, 223–224; recent trends, 255–261; satisfaction and, 265; Swedish misconceptions of Danish practices, 246–255; Swedish statist individualism and "theory of love," 217, 227–232

dignity, in capabilities approach, 285, 287, 292

disability, as identity, 15, 270

disability, defined, 34. *See also specific impairments and issues*

disability pensions: laws, 45–47; regulations in Denmark, 302n18

disability rights movement, 5–6, 268–269

disability studies, 10, 13–17, 27, 34, 256, 269, 271

disciplining and policing of sexuality, 80–81, 86, 124, 153–154, 166

dissociative behavior, 122

"Don't wake the sleeping bear" (*Väck inte den björn som sover*), 84–86

Down syndrome, persons with: Danish words for, 36, 37; Morten Piilmann, 143–144; in *Say "Yes," Say "No"* (film), 156; sex workers and, 175–176, 201, 207; sympathy and, 3

drug policies, 219–221

Dværgeforeningen (Association of Dwarves), 35

Earle, Sarah, 26

Eek, Louise, 215–216, 266

Ekstra Bladet, 175, 181, 195–196

emotional blackmail, 141–142

"Emotions" capability, 282–283, 286

Enby, Gunnel, 59–60, 71, 74, 113–114, 153, 244, 286, 304n55

engagement, ethics of. *See* ethics of engagement

engagement, scope of, 245–246

entitlement, in capabilities approach, 284, 287

Enzensberger, Hans Magnus, 227

erections: aids to, 72; disciplining, 80; paraplegics and inability to achieve, 206–207, 210; as "problem," 80, 83, 89, 123–124; public domain issue and, 123; sex workers and, 199, 201

erotiska minoriteterna, De (*The Erotic Minorities: A Swedish View*) (Ullerstam), 50–51, 180

Esping-Andersen, Gøsta, 316n27

ethics, space of, 117

ethics of engagement: capabilities approach, 277–287, 291–293, 322n39; contractarian theories, utilitarianism, and, 278–281; erroneous beliefs and, 293–294; "excessibility guidelines" approach, 291–295; inability, predicament, and vulnerability, 270–273; obligation and ethics of care, 273–277; right to sex, question of, 286–291; symmetrical vs. asymmetrical reciprocity, 266–268

eugenics, 4, 40, 45, 165–166

European Court of Human Rights, and Sweden, 178

excess-absence paradox, 171–172

"excessibility guidelines," 291–295

experts and passing the buck, 81–83

Expressen, 176, 238–239

facilitation, sexual: Bank-Mikkelsen's Six Commandments of, 57, 64–65;

hesitance to ask for, 122; Katz booklet and, 52; in practice, in Denmark, 106–112; rights language and, 291; rights vs. social/emotional engagement and, 20; unclear wishes and, 110–111. *See also* case examples; *Guidelines about Sexuality—Regardless of Handicap*; specific issues, such as masturbation

fairness, justice as, 279–280

Faktisk mangler man ord for det (*One Doesn't Have Words for It*) (film), 142–144

fear: Danish, about pregnancy, 169–170; Swedish, about engaging with sex, 87–88

Feebleminded Act of 1934, Denmark, 165

Feebleminded Act of 1959, Denmark (Åndssvageloven), 40–41, 48–49

feeding as a way of repressing sexual desire, 42

feminism: contrast between Denmark and Sweden, 177, 221–222, 232–240, 255, 265; ethics of care and, 276–277; governance feminism, 234, 236, 239; in Norway, 232; Nussbaum and, 285; "the personal is political" and, 245; political parties and, 234–235; porn-free hotels campaign and, 137, 236; pornography and prostitution policies and, 174, 177, 221–223

film: *L'Amour sans limites* (Love without limits), 185, 213; *Coming Home*, 8; *Hyde Park on Hudson*, 9; *The Intouchables*, 9; *The Language of Love* (*Kärlekens språk*), 130–131; *Masturbation Techniques for Men* (*Onaniteknik för män*) and *Masturbation Techniques for Women* (*Onaniteknik för kvinnor*), 86, 114–115, 124–134, 219, 255; *More*

from the Language of Love (*Mera ur kärlekens språk*), 130–133, 309n13; *Murderball*, 8–9; *One Doesn't Have Words for It* (*Faktisk mangler man ord for det*), 142–144; representations in, 8–9; *Rust and Bone*, 9; *Say "Yes," Say "No": Who Gets to Hug Me?* (*Säga ja, säga nej: Vem ska få krama mig?*), 154–157; *Scarlet Road*, 186; *The Sessions*, 9; *Tomas—A Child You Can't Reach*, 311n1. *See also* pornography
Finger, Anne, 5
Flanagan, Bob, 269
Folkehøjskoler ("folk high schools"), 226
forældreevne projekt ("parenting project," Denmark), 168–170
Föräldraföreningen för Utvecklingsstörda Barn. *See* FUB
Föräldrakraft (*Parent Power*), 176
Förbundet Unga Rörelsehindrade (Association of Mobility Impaired Youth), 256
Förening för Barn, Unga och Vuxna med Utvecklingsstörning. *See* FUB
Försäkringskassan (Social Insurance Agency, Sweden), 47
Foucault, Michel, 227, 234
Franksson, Jonas, 249, 254–255
frisind ("broad-mindedness"), 217, 224–227
FUB (Förening för Barn, Unga och Vuxna med Utvecklingsstörning; Swedish National Association for Persons with Intellectual Disability [previously Föräldraföreningen för Utvecklingsstörda Barn; Parents' Association for Mentally Retarded Children]), 39, 49, 154
Funktionærbladet (*Civil Servant Magazine*), 84–85

funktionshinder (functional impediment), 34, 58, 304n53
funktionsnedsättning (functional reduction), 34, 304n53

Garland-Thomson, Rosemarie, 28
Gay Liberation Front, Denmark (Bøssernes Befrielses Front), 60–61
gay men, 193–195, 198–200
gay movement, 61
Gelstedt, Otto, 315n18
"gendered power regime," Sweden (*könsmaktsordning*), 236
Gilbert, Stephen, 186
Gillespie-Sells, Kath, 9
governmentality, 234
Greengross, Wendy, 313n23
group homes: described, 30–31; discussions and role playing in, 108–19; fieldwork in, 30–34; parental influence and, 149–150; pregnancy fears and, 169–170; smoking in, 309n20; varied attitudes among, 112–113; written policies in, 109–110. *See also specific issues*
Grundtvig, Nikolaj Frederik Severin, 225–227, 245
Grunewald, Karl, 39, 40, 41, 51, 71, 115, 127, 130, 217–219, 223, 237, 242, 244, 256–258, 272, 308n26
Gruppen för Handikapp och Samlevnadsfrågor (HS-gruppen; Handicap and Relationships Task Force, Sweden), 53–55, 304n44
Guidelines about Sexuality—Regardless of Handicap (Denmark's Ministry of Social Affairs): acknowledgement of sexuality in, 69; agents of change and, 242–243; Board of Social Services report and, 68; Buttenschøn's memoir on, 148–149; contents of, 103–105,

Guidelines about Sexuality (*continued*)
294; *Handbook* (2012) edition of,
260–261, 288; history of adoption of,
64–70; local overrule of, 259–260;
necessity of intervention as feature
of, 69–70, 294; plans of action and,
107; presentation of, 68–69; responsibility, locus of, 105; revisions of, 102,
260–261; sexual advisor education
program, 70; as source of change, 8;
Swedes' knowledge about, 246

Halley, Janet, 234
Hammar, Linda, 95–96, 98
Hammer Bakker institution, 56
Handicap and Relationships Task Force,
Sweden (Gruppen för Handikapp
och Samlevnadsfrågor, HS-gruppen),
53–55, 304n44
Handicap Commission of 1965,
Sweden, 75
Handicap Institute, Sweden, 73–75
Handi-Kamp, 60–63, 243, 305n59
Handisex, 182–183, 287
Hansen, Torben Vegener, 258–259
Hanzen, Glenn, 256
Hawking, Stephen, 138–139
Hegeler, Inge, 131
Hegeler, Sten, 131
Hellman, Finn, 12–13, 288–290
Helsingborgs Dagblad, 177
Hemligheter kända av många (*Secrets
Known by Many*) (Svensk), 256
Hertz, Lone, 144–146, 173, 174–175, 177,
193, 311n1
hierarchy of desirability, 214–215
Hirdman, Yvonne, 233–235
HIV, laws pertaining to, 178
Hobbes, Thomas, 278
Holländer, Vivi, vii
Hooper, Edward, 314n36

"Horny Cripples" ("Kåta krymplingar")
(*Arena*), 256
Hudson, Barbara, 274
Hulter, Birgitta, 119
Hultling, Claes, 71–72, 244, 255
humiliation, 2, 59, 142, 192, 266, 274,
290. *See also* shame
Huntford, Roland, 227
Huxley, Aldous, 227
Hyde Park on Hudson (film), 9

I en annan del av Köping (*In Another
Part of Köping*) (television reality
series), 94–96, 308n18
"If I don't do anything, at least I haven't
done anything wrong" (*Om jag inte
gör något så har jag i alla fall inte
gjort något fel*), 86–94, 101, 240
immigration rhetoric and policies, Danish, 247, 318n54
impairment: "disability" vs., 34, 58; engagement with, 262; as predicament,
270–271. *See also specific impairments*
Implanon contraceptive rod, 166, 170
"inability," theoretical importance of,
270–273
In Another Part of Köping (*I en annan
del av Köping*) (television reality
series), 94–96, 308n18
independence, 7, 45–46, 269
individualism, statist, 227–232, 269
"Individual vibrator adaptation for
woman who can only move her
head" (Nordqvist), 76, 77
Ingvardsson, Margó, 73
Institute for the Self-Determination of
Disabled People (Institut zur Selbst-
Bestimmung Behinderter), 185
intellectual impairment: abuse concerns
and, 151; agents of change and,
242–244; *In Another Part of Köping*

(reality series), 94–96, 308n18; Apollonia and Nyborg conferences on, 39–42; containing sexuality and, 124; important discussions about sexual facilitation and, 71, 124; *Masturbation Techniques* films and, 86, 114–115, 126–134, 219, 255; Mose Allé school letter, 55–57, 84–85, 304n45; Norwegian group home study by Sundet, 26, 33, 80–81; pregnancy concerns and, 164–171; sex workers and, 200–205. *See also* case examples; Löfgren-Mårtenson, Lotta; Nordeman, Margareta

International Professional Surrogates Association, 185

Intouchables, The (film), 9

Intra, 115, 117, 127, 218

Invalid Care Commission of 1951, Sweden, 75

in vitro fertilization, 72

Issues in Relationships and Sexuality among the Mentally Retarded (Katz), 51–53

Jain, Sarah, 272

Jalving, Mikael, 237–238

Jämting, Göran, 238–239, 247

Jefferson, Thomas, 278

Jenkins, David, 315n3

Johansson, Linna, 176–177

Jørgensen, S., 85, 86

justice. *See* social justice

Kant, Immanuel, 285

Kärlekens språk (*The Language of Love*) (film), 130–131

"Kåta krymplingar" ("Horny Cripples") (*Arena*), 256

Kingdon, John, 240

Kirkebæk, Birgit, 304n45

Kittay, Eva Feder, 27, 262, 276

Knausgård, Karl Ove, 237

Knutte the Cripple (*Knutte Krympling*), 63

Københavner kodeks (Copenhagen code of conduct), 259–260, 261

Kommunalarbetaren (*Municipal Worker*), 136, 256

könsmaktsordning ("gendered power regime," Sweden), 236

Krykensemblen (Crutch Ensemble), 62–63, 243

Kuppers, Petra, 7

Kvick, Mattias, 289–291

Kvinnomaktutredningen (Commission on Women's Power, Sweden), 235

Kvinnovåldskommissionen (Commission on Violence against Women, Sweden), 235

Lag om stöd och service till vissa funktionshindrade (LSS; Swedish Law on Support and Service to Certain Disabled People), 46–47, 230, 258, 302n17

Landsforeningen Evnesvages Vel (LEV; National Association for the Well-Being of the Feebleminded, Denmark), 48, 65, 68

Landsofreningen af Vanføre (National Association of Cripples, Denmark), 58, 60

language: political correctness and translation issues, 34–38; of rights, 291, 323n53; sex workers and, 196; in Sweden vs. Denmark, 43

Language Is More Than Just a Trivial Concern! (Kailes), 36, 37

Language of Love, The (*Kärlekens språk*) (film), 130–131

Lapper, Alison, 5, 32

Law on Social Pensions, Denmark (Lov om social pension), 302n18 leftist activism, 58–63

Left Socialist Party (Ventresocialisterne), 65

Lenger, Jørgen, 65–66

Lennerhed, Lena, 51

LEV (Landsforeningen Evnesvages Vel;
National Association for the Well-
Being of the Feebleminded, Den-
mark), 48, 65, 68

Levi, Richard, 72

Levinas, Emmanuel, 274–276, 292

Liberal Party (Venstre), 227

"Life" capability, 282

Linder, Åse, 93–94, 114

Lindqvist, Bengt, 54, 309n13

Linton, Simi, 27, 34

lobotomy, as way of dealing with sexuality, 42, 67, 286

locked-in syndrome, 79

Löfgren-Mårtenson, Lotta, 26, 27, 52,
255; on dances, 85–86, 126, 308n17;
on desire for nondisabled partners,
214; on infatuation, 142; on policing of activities, 153–154, 166; on
private-public boundary, 124–125; on
uncertainty, 92

Løt, Karsten, 64–65, 66, 68, 70, 101, 242,
243, 305n73

love, Swedish theory of, 217, 230–232,
239–240

Lov om social pension (Law on Social
Pensions, Denmark), 302n18

Løwert, Anette, 305n73

LSS (Lag om stöd och service till vissa
funktionshindrade; Swedish Law on
Support and Service to Certain Disabled People), 46–47, 230, 258, 302n17

Lyttseminariet (Crip seminar), 13

Mac, Nadja, 148–149

Mackelprang, Romel, 34

MacKinnon, Catherine, 177, 236,
258

Maktutredningen (Commission on
Power, Sweden), 234–235

Mallander, Ove, 26

Marcus, Neil, 7

marriage law and intellectual impairment in Denmark, 41

Marxist movements, 59, 226

massage, 79, 90–91, 195, 199–200

mass media: prostitution, messages
about, 188, 318n54; role in social
change, 241; role in Sweden, 247–248

masturbation: CP Show discussion of,
251–252, 319n59; discussing, 140; Katz
on, 52; Mose Allé school letter on,
55–57, 84–85; orgasm and instruction
in, 147–149; plans of action for,
106–107; public, 126–127, 143, 147;
side-of-the-highway case, 126–127

Masturbation Techniques for Men
(Onaniteknik för män) and Masturbation Techniques for Women (Onaniteknik för kvinnor) films, 86, 114–115,
126–134, 219, 255

McCarthy, Michelle, 10, 25, 27

McRuer, Robert, 13–15, 27, 269

medical model of disability, 48, 157, 263

"Mentally Retarded and the Sexual
Question, The" conference (Apollonia Hotel, 1966), 39–42, 218, 219

Mera ur kärlekens språk (More from the
Language of Love) (film),
130–133, 241, 309n13

Metro Riks, 176–177

"middle way" (Sweden), 50–55, 224

Ministry of Social Affairs, 8, 66

Mitt nakna jag (My Naked Self) (Nordansjö), 192, 207–208, 215–216, 313n27

Møller, Tor Martin, 253–254

Mollow, Anna, 171–172

mongol, Danish use of word, 36–37, 200, 300n38, 313n27

moral panic, 88, 106, 290

More from the Language of Love (Mera ur kärlekens språk) (film), 130–133, 241, 309n13

Mormors Bordel (Grandmother's Brothel) (TV), 181–182

Mose Allé school, 55–57, 71, 84–85, 245, 304n45

mothers, 143–150

Müller, Frigg Birt, 181–184, 191, 205, 209, 213, 216

Municipal Worker (Kommunalarbetaren), 136, 256

Murderball (film), 8–9, 10

muscular dystrophy, 61, 71, 139, 182, 214

My Naked Self (Mitt nakna jag) (Nordansjö), 192, 207–208, 215–216, 313n27

Myrdal, Alva, 301n7

Myrdal, Gunnar, 301n7

National Association for the Handicapped, Sweden (DHR), 74

National Association for the Well-Being of the Feebleminded, Denmark (Landsforeningen Evnesvages Vel, LEV), 48, 65, 68

National Association of Cripples, Denmark (Landsofreningen af Vanføre), 58, 60

National Association of Cripples, Sweden (De Vanföras Riksförbund), 50

National Board of Social Services, Denmark (Socialstyrelsen), 66–68, 158, 260

national ethos stereotypes, 218–219

Necef, Mehmet Ümit, 319n54

"negotiation state," Sweden as, 223–224, 237

Nirje, Bengt, 49–50

nonpower (Derrida), 273

Nordansjö, Johan, 192, 207–208, 215–216, 313n27

Nordeman, Margareta, 52, 86, 127, 130, 151, 255, 309n11

Nordic Association of Mental Retardation (NFPU), 148–149

"Nordic model," 316n27

Nordic model of disability protection, 47

Nordic Symposium on Relations and the Mobility Impaired (Rörelsehindrades Samlevnadsfrågor), 53

Nordqvist, Inger, 26, 53–55, 58, 71, 73–77, 129, 133, 244, 245, 255, 258, 289, 303n42, 304n43

normalization principle, 40, 47–51, 241–242

Norwegian group home study (Sundet), 26, 80–81, 85

Nussbaum, Martha, 21–22, 28, 277–287, 291–292, 321nn34–35, 322n39

Nutcakes (Nötkakor), 63

Nyborg conference (1967), 40–41, 55, 57

obligation, ethical, 273–277

O'Brien, Mark, 6, 7, 184–185, 208–209, 210, 312n17

occupational therapists (*arbetsterapeuter*), 82–83, 307n6

Oliver, Michael, 28, 47–48

Olsson, Sören, 175–176, 180, 312n8

Om jag inte gör något så har jag i alla fall inte gjort något fel ("If I don't do anything, at least I haven't done anything wrong"), 86–94, 101, 240

Omsorgsboken (The Care Book) (Grunewald), 217–218

One Doesn't Have Words for It (Faktisk mangler man ord for det) (film), 142–144

oppression: gendered, 232–234, 236; sexuality linked with, 239–240
orgasm instruction, 2, 147–149
Österberg, Eva, 223–224
"ostrich policy" in Sweden, 92–93
"Other Species" capability, 283
Ottar, 256
out-of-body dissociation, 122

Palmlöf, Olle, 249, 254
Paralympic Games, 6
parental involvement, 143–150
parenthood by in vitro fertilization, 72
"parenting project," Denmark (forældreevne projekt), 168–170
Parent Power (*Föräldrakraft*), 176
Parents' Association for Mentally Retarded Children, Sweden. *See* FUB
paying for sexual services and prostitution: attitudes of sex workers toward disabled clients, 205–207; body image and, 209–210; congenital disability and, 179–180; contacting a sex worker, 195–200; Copenhagen code of conduct on, 259–260; *CP Show* discussion of, 249–250, 253–254; Danish leftist discussions on, 61; feminist activism and Swedish vs. Danish policies on, 221–223; financial concerns, 202–203; Hansen lawsuit on, 258–259; intellectual impairments and, 200–205; public discussion and debate on, 174–177; reasons for, 207–216; responses to Hellman column and, 289; sex surrogates, myth of, 184–187; sex workers and disabled clients, 187–192; significant physical impairments and, 192–195; Swedish and Danish laws on, 177–179; Thai prostitutes, 196–198; Ullerstam's "erotic Samaritans," 50–51; women who pay for services, 180–184

Pedersen, Lasse Bjarne, 66–67
penisdödargreppet ("penis-killer grip"), 80, 124, 266
personal assistants: "If I don't do anything . . ." formulation and, 90–93; infatuation with, 138–142; Marcus's interview statement, 117–118; pornographic images, encountering, 134–138
"Personalens roll när det gäller vuxna brukares sexualitet" ("Staff's Role in Relation to the Sexuality of Adults with Disabilities"), 136
"personal is political, the," 245
personligassistent.com, 91, 136
Persson, Kristina, 177
philosophy of engagement. *See* ethics of engagement
physical disabilities. *See specific impairments and issues*
Piilmann, Käthe, 142–144, 173
plans of action (*handleplaner*), 106–107, 111, 116, 148, 210; Swedes' knowledge about, 246–247
"Play" capability, 283
pleasure, tension over, 140
policy documents in group homes, 92–93, 109–110, 136, 257
policy entrepreneurs, 242–244
political authority structures, 223–224
political correctness, 34–38
political culture. *See* culture, political and public
political parties, 61–62, 65–66, 226–227, 234, 235, 259
pornography: feminist activism and Swedish vs. Danish policies on, 221–223; helpers encountering, 134–138, 294; sexual harassment issues and, 91–92, 136; Swedish porn-free hotels campaign, 137, 236;

unmentioned in sexual education films, 133

power relations in modern welfare states, 229

"Practical Reason" capability, 283

predicament, impairment as (Shakespeare), 270–271

pregnancy, risks and fears about, 144, 164–171

prejudice. *See* stereotypes

privacy: Danish conception of, 115–117; defensive, silencing use of, in Sweden, 113–115; dissociative behavior and, 122; lack of, in Sundet Norwegian study, 81; locking doors and, 18, 81, 114, 125, 128, 129, 133, 143–144, 172, 263, 266; strategies for, 121–122

private-public boundary: body ministrations and, 121–123; challenge of, 120–121; home space and, 138; hotels and, 137; *Language of Love* films and, 130–133; *Masturbation Techniques* films and, 126–130, 133–134; public space and, 123–126

private sphere, capabilities approach and, 22

Projekt Seksualpolitik på specialskoler, Denmark (Project on sexuality in schools for people with disabilities), 158

prostitution. *See* paying for sexual services and prostitution

protection and self-determination, tension between, 153–154, 163

psychiatric impairments, 29

Puar, Jasbir, 272

public culture. *See* culture, political and public

public sphere and capabilities approach, 22. *See also* private-public boundary

queer theory, 11–14, 272, 300n14

Rawls, John, 21, 279–281, 284, 285, 286, 321n28

reciprocity, symmetrical and asymmetrical, 266–268, 274

Relax vibrator, 129

reproduction-sex boundary and pregnancy risk, 164–171

RFSU (Riksförbundet för Sexuell Upplysning; Swedish Association for Sexuality Education), 73, 86, 115, 127, 129, 130, 256

Rich, Adrienne, 14

rights: language of, 291, 323n53; to "private life," 115; right to sex as ethical question, 286–291; social justice vs., 18–19

Riksförbundet för Sexuell Upplysning (RFSU; Swedish Association for Sexuality Education), 73, 86, 115, 127, 129, 130, 256

Roks (Riksorganisationen för kvinnojourer och tjejjourer i Sverige; National Organization of Shelters for Young and Adult Women, Sweden), 137

role playing, 108–109

Rörelsehindrades Samlevnadsfrågor (Nordic Symposium on Relations and the Mobility Impaired), 53

Rorty, Richard, 274

Rousseau, Jean-Jacques, 278

Rubin, Gayle, 12

Rust and Bone (film), 9

sadomasochism, 214

Sahlin, Mona, 11

Sällan sedda: Utbildningsmaterial om våld mot kvinnor med funktionsnedsättning (*Seldom Seen: Educational Material on Violence against Women with Disabilities*), 141–142

Salsgiver, Richard, 34

Samaritans, sexual or erotic, 50–51, 191, 313n23

Samlevnadsoch sexualfrågor hos psykiskt utvecklingsstörda (Katz), 51–53

Sanders, Teela, 26

S.Å. Teacher (*S.Å.-Pædagogen*), 55–56

satisfaction in Denmark vs. Sweden, 265

Say "Yes," Say "No": Who Gets to Hug Me? (Säga ja, säga nej: Vem ska få krama mig?) (film), 154–157

"Scandinavian model," 316n27

Scarlet Road (documentary), 186

Secrets Known by Many (Hemligheter kända av många) (Svensk), 256

seksualvejledere. See sexual advisors

Seksualvejlederforeningen (Sexual Advisors' Union), 261

seksualvejlederuddannelse (sexual advisor education), 70, 242, 243, 253

Seksuelle overgreb—Nej tak! (Sexual Abuse—No Thanks!) (SUS), 158, 159–161

Seldom Seen: Educational Material on Violence against Women with Disabilities (Sällan sedda: Utbildningsmaterial om våld mot kvinnor med funktionsnedsättning), 141–142

self-determination and protection, tension between, 153–154

Sen, Amartya, 21, 278, 281

"Senses, Imagination, and Thought" capability, 282

Sessions, The (film), 9

Sevenhuijsen, Selma, 276–277

sex aids subsidy debate in Sweden, 73–77, 241

Sex and Disability (McRuer and Mollow), 10–11

Sex and Disability (Shuttleworth and Sanders), 10–11

"Sex in Health Care" ("Sex ivården") (Sjölander), 256

"Sexköp med bidrag" ("Subventions to buy sex") (*Dagens Nyheter*), 248

sexologists, passing the buck to, 82–83

"Sexpo," 194–195

"Sex Surrogate, The" (O'Brien), 184–185, 208–209

sex surrogates, myth of, 184–187

Sexual Abuse—No Thanks! (Seksuelle overgreb—Nej tak!) (SUS), 158, 159–161

sexual advisor education (*seksualvejlederuddannelse*), 70, 242, 243, 253

sexual advisors (*seksualvejledere*), 18, 27, 31, 32; abuse prevention and, 113, 158–161; certification of, 18, 101–102; contraception and pregnancy, engagement with, 164–171; *Guidelines about Sexuality—Regardless of Handicap* and, 101–105; plans of action and, 106–107, 111, 116; political climate in Denmark, responses to changes in, 261; role of, 107; Swedish beliefs about, 18, 105–106, 248–255, 293–294; on teaching masturbation, 148–149

Sexual Advisors' Union (Seksualvejlederforeningen), 261

sexual education: agents of change and, 242; in Bank-Mikkelsen's Six Commandments, 57; Buttenshøn and Løt's materials for, 305n73; contrast of Swedish vs. Danish attitudes toward, 22; in *Guidelines about Sexuality—Regardless of Handicap*, 69, 70; HS Task Force and, 53; Ingvardsson and, 73; Lenger bill and, 66; on masturbation and orgasm, 147–149; *Masturbation Techniques* films, 86, 114–115, 126–134, 219, 255; National Board of Social Services report (Denmark) on, 68; Nordqvist interviews on, 26; Swedish tradition of, 130; taking the initiative in, 116. *See also* Mose Allé school; Swedish Association for Sexuality Education

sexual harassment, 90–93, 110

sexuality: aggression and abuse associated with, in Sweden, 154–155; in memoirs and poetry on disability, 7–8; neglect of, in disability rights movement, 5–6; as sex, in *Guidelines*, 103; UN Standard Rules on the Equalization of Opportunities for Persons with Disabilities definition of, 287; WHO working definition of, 288. *See also specific issues, such as* masturbation

Sexuality and Women with Learning Disabilities (McCarthy), 10

Sexuality—Possibilities Different Conditions (Sexualitet—möjligheter olika förutsättningar) conference, 157

sexual orientation, 193–195

Sexual Politics of Disability, The (Shakespeare et al.), 4, 9–10, 122, 139, 185, 269

sex workers. *See* paying for sexual services and prostitution

Shakespeare, Tom, 9, 28, 262, 270–271, 273, 305n62

shame, 121, 122, 144. *See also* humiliation

Shildrick, Margrit, 14, 28, 300n23

Shuttleworth, Russell, 19, 26

Siebers, Tobin, 14, 27, 269

Siim, Birte, 232–233, 235, 236

silence in Swedish discourse, 89, 238, 245, 256

Singer, Peter, 273, 275

Sisyphus Letters, The (*Sisyfosbreve*), 144–146, 174–175

Sjölander, Ann-Christin, 256

"sleeping bear" reasoning, 23, 84–86, 265

smoking, court decision on, 309n20

social contract theories, 278–281, 321n34

Social Democratic parties, 11, 44, 54, 73, 178–179, 181, 234, 235, 239, 259, 288

Social Development Center (Socialt Udviklingscenter, SUS), 157–158

Social Insurance Act, Sweden (Socialförsäkringsbalken), 302n18

Social Insurance Agency, Sweden (Försäkringskassan), 47

social insurance schemes, 44–45

Socialist Party, 61–62, 317n37

Socialist People's Party (Socialistisk Folkeparti), 259

social justice, 3, 4, 17, 25, 38; capabilities approach to, 21–22, 264, 265, 276–287, 291–293, 322n39; contractarian theories and utilitarianism, 278–281, 321n28; Rawls's theory of justice as fairness, 279–281, 321n28; "rights" vs., 18–19; vulnerability and, 277. *See also* ethics of engagement

social model of disability, 47–48, 270

Socialstyrelsen (National Board of Social Services, Denmark), 66–68, 158, 260

Socialstyrelsen (Swedish National Board of Health and Welfare), 165, 304n53

Sonoma State Hospital (California), 48

Sontag, Susan, 228, 237, 315n3

Sørensen, Kirsten Klitte, 250–251, 319n59

space, public vs. private, 123–126. *See also* private-public boundary

spastiker, Danish use of word, 35, 37, 196, 198

Spastikerforeningen (Association of Spastics), 35

spinal cord injuries: congenital impairments contrasted with, 29; hierarchy of desirability and, 214; Hultling and, 72; locus of erotic messages and, 314n36; materials available on, 29, 82; Nordqvist on sexual aids for, 77; Swedish focus on rehabilitation and, 71

Spinalis rehabilitation clinic, 29, 72, 82, 244

"Staff's Role in Relation to the Sexuality of Adults with Disabilities" ("Personalens roll när det gäller vuxna brukares sexualitet"), 136

state feminism, 234. *See also* feminism

State Services for the Feebleminded, Denmark (Åndssvageforsorgen): Bank-Mikkelsen's Six Commandments and, 57; education section, 64; normalization principle and, 49; Nyborg conference, 40–41; *S.Å. Teacher (S.Å.-Pædagogen)* journal, 55–56

statist individualism, 227–232, 269

stereotypes: asexual child/innocence, 5, 6, 171–172; of Denmark in Swedish media, 247–248; hypersexual, 6–7, 171–172; of national ethos, 218–219

sterilization, 40–41, 57, 165, 167–169, 263

Sterilization Act (1935), Sweden, 165

Sterilization and Castration Act of 1935, Denmark, 165

Stichting Alternative Relatiebemiddeling, 185

strip clubs, 238–239, 317n45

Sundet, Marit, 26, 27, 33, 80–81, 85

surveillance, 52, 86, 125–126, 266

Svensk, Veronica, 256

Svenska Centralkommittén för Rehabilitering (svcr; Swedish Central Committee for Rehabilitation), 53, 303n42

Svensk Vanföre-Tidskrift (Swedish Cripple Journal), 50, 303n28

Sweden: abuse, publications and attitudes on, 153–157; alcohol policies, 219–220, 315n3; Apollonia conference (1966), 39–42, 218, 219; Denmark compared and contrasted with, 3–4, 43–45; disciplined sexuality in, 80–81; dissatisfaction in, 265; "Don't wake the sleeping bear" formulation, 84–86; drug policies, 220–221; engagement through disavowal in, 17–18; guidelines, lack of, 113; "If I don't do anything . . ." formulation, 86–94; ignored sexuality in, 79; *In Another Part of Köping* (reality series), 94–96, 308n18; leftist disability activism in, 58–60, 63; "the middle way," 50–55, 224; as "negotiation state," 223–224; "ostrich policy" in, 92–93; political correctness in, 34–35; practical questions as obstacle in, 105–106; privacy, defensive and silencing use of, 113–115; "problem" passed along to experts in, 81–83; profile and history, 42–45; prostitution and HIV laws, 177–179; recent trends in, 255–258; statist individualism, 227–232; sterilization laws, 165; types of professionals in, 81–82; welfare assistance laws and pensions in, 45, 46–47, 230; Work Environment Act, 136–137. *See also* difference factors between Sweden and Denmark; *specific agencies, organizations, and persons*

Swedish Association for Sexuality Education (Riksförbundet för Sexuell Upplysning, RFSU), 73, 86, 115, 127, 129, 130, 256

Swedish Central Committee for Rehabilitation (Svenska Centralkommittén för Rehabilitering, svCR), 53, 303n42

Swedish Cripple Journal (*Svensk Vanföre-Tidskrift*), 50, 303n28

Swedish feminism, 232–240, 255, 265. *See also* feminism; state feminism

Swedish Institute for Assistive Devices, 304n44

Swedish Law on Support and Service to Certain Disabled People (Lag om stöd och service till vissa funktionshindrade, LSS), 46–47, 230, 258, 302n17

"Swedish model" of prostitution policy, 179

Swedish National Association for Persons with Intellectual Disability. *See* FUB

Swedish National Association for the Handicapped (De Handikappades Riksförbund, DHR), 58

Swedish National Board of Health and Welfare (Socialstyrelsen), 165, 304n53

Swedish National Organization of Shelters for Young and Adult Women (Riksorganisationen för kvinnojourer och tjejjourer i Sverige; Roks), 137

Swedish national parliament, subsidized sex aids debate, 73–75

"Swedish theory of love," 217, 230–232, 239–240

Sydney, Australia, 43, 186, 187

symmetrical reciprocity (Young), 266–268, 274, 279

telephone sex, 91

television: CP-*magasinet* (*The Cerebral Palsy Show*), 248–255, 258, 294, 319n59; *In Another Part of Köping* (reality series), 94–96, 308n18; *Mormors Bordel* (*Grandmother's Brothel*),

181–182; pornography in hotel rooms, 137

Tham, Henrik, 220–221

theater troupes, 62–63

39 Pounds of Love (documentary), 9, 139

Thisted, Karen, 181–182

Thorning-Schmidt, Helle, 179, 235

Tomas—A Child You Can't Reach (*Tomas—Et barn du ikke kan nå*) (documentary), 311n1

torsk (a person who pays for sex), 249, 253, 254

Touching Base, 186

Trägårdh, Lars, 217, 228–231, 316n27

translation issues, 34–38

Treaty of Roskilde (1658), 43

Tronto, Joan, 276

Turner, Bryan, 272, 274, 323n53

Ullerstam, Lars, 50–51, 180

United Nations Convention on the Rights of Persons with Disabilities, 322n43

United Nations Standard Rules on the Equalization of Opportunities for Persons with Disabilities, 19, 103, 104, 260, 287–288, 322n43

utilitarianism, 278–280

Väck inte den björn som sover ("Don't wake the sleeping bear"), 84–86

Vance, Carole, 318n54

veil of ignorance, 279–280, 321n28

Ventresocialisterne (Left Socialist Party), 65

vibrators, 70, 76–77, 105, 106–107, 129, 133, 136, 183, 245, 294

Vi måste få älska (*We Must Be Allowed to Love*) (Enby), 59–60, 71, 113–114, 153, 244, 286

vulnerability, 268, 271–274, 277, 321n35

Wad, Gunnar, 55–57, 69, 149, 261
Wade, Cheryl Marie, 121–122, 124, 268, 271, 289
Wahl, Hillevi, 176–177
Weise, Jillian, 7
welfare assistance laws, 45–47, 230
welfare state model, 44, 229–230
We Must Be Allowed to Love (*Vi måste få älska*) (Enby), 59–60, 71, 113–114, 153, 244, 286
Wendell, Susan, 28, 34
When the Feeling Carries You Away (Nordeman), 151
Williams, Fiona, 276
women's caucuses, 235
Work Environment Act, Sweden (Arbetsmiljölagen), 136–137, 309n20

Work Environment Authority, Sweden (Arbetsmiljöverket), 309n20
Worker, The (*Arbetaren*), 288–289
work-intimacy boundary, 134–143
World Health Organization (WHO), 288
Wotton, Rachel, 186–187

"You Are My Venus" (Crutch Ensemble), 62
Young, Iris Marion, 266–268, 274
Youth Circle (Undgdomskredsen) of the National Association of Cripples, 60

Zylka, Eva, 185–186